COPING WITH
Chemotherapy

Also by Nancy Bruning

Breast Implants: Everything You Need to Know

Female and Forgetful

Natural Medicine for Menopause and Beyond

Natural Relief for Your Child's Asthma

The Natural Health Guide to Antioxidants

Natural Medicines for Colds and Flu

Ayurveda: The A–Z Guide to Healing Techniques
  from Ancient India

Healing Homeopathic Remedies

Swimming for Total Fitness

Rhythms and Cycles: Sacred Patterns in Everyday Life

COPING WITH
Chemotherapy

Authoritative Information
and Compassionate Advice
from a Chemotherapy Survivor

NANCY BRUNING

Avery
A MEMBER OF
PENGUIN PUTNAM INC.
NEW YORK

Every effort has been made to ensure that the information contained in this book is complete and accurate. However, neither the publisher nor the author is engaged in rendering professional advice or services to the individual reader. The ideas, procedures, and suggestions contained in this book are not intended as a substitute for consulting with your physician. All matters regarding health require medical supervision. Neither the author nor the publisher shall be liable or responsible for any loss, injury, or damage allegedly arising from any information or suggestion in this book. The opinions expressed in this book represent the personal views of the author and not of the publisher.

While the author has made every effort to provide accurate telephone numbers and Internet addresses at the time of publication, neither the publisher nor the author assumes any responsibility for errors or for changes that occur after publication.

Most Avery books are available at special quantity discounts for bulk purchase for sales promotions, premiums, fund-raising, and educational needs. Special books or book excerpts also can be created to fit specific needs. For details, write Putnam Special Markets, 375 Hudson Street, New York, NY 10014.

AVERY

a member of
Penguin Putnam Inc.
375 Hudson Street
New York, NY 10014
www.penguinputnam.com

Library of Congress Cataloging-in-Publication Data

Bruning, Nancy.
Coping with chemotherapy : authoritative information and compassionate advice from a
chemotherapy survivor / Nancy Bruning.
p.   cm.
Includes index.
ISBN 1-58333-131-X
1. Cancer—Chemotherapy—Popular works.   2. Antineoplastic agents—
Side effects—Popular works.   I. Title
RC271.C5B783   2002   2002018538
616.99'4061—dc21

Printed in the United States of America
1   3   5   7   9   10   8   6   4   2

Book design by Jennifer Ann Daddio

Acknowledgments

There are so many people who believed in this book and helped me in so many ways that I scarcely know where to begin to offer my appreciation.

Perhaps at the beginning, I'd like to extend my thanks:

To the editor of the original Doubleday edition, Fran McCullough, and my agent, Susan Protter, whose encouragement and guidance were instrumental in its inception and indispensable to its completion; also to Michael Ross and to my good friend Kathleen O'Reilly, who read the manuscript, understood the magnitude of the task, and offered valuable support and suggestions when I needed them most. My deepest gratitude and appreciation to Dani Grady, long-time friend and breast cancer survivor. I would like to thank the folks at Avery Books, the publisher of this new edition, in particular Rudy Shur, who started the ball rolling and prompted me to rethink the way I organized the material to make it more user-friendly; Laura Shepherd, who continued where Rudy left off; and Dara Stewart, whose gentle editing hand improved the manuscript significantly.

To the cancer patients who shared with me their experiences with chemotherapy in the hope that others might benefit from them.

My thanks—and admiration—to the oncologists and other cancer-care professionals who graciously took time from their busy schedules to answer my questions, in some cases for both the original and revised edi-

tions. (Many of them have moved to other institutions since I first interviewed them, but I have preserved their original affiliations since those
are a reflection of their positions at the time they spoke.)

From Memorial Sloan-Kettering Cancer Center: Grace Christ, former
director of the Department of Social Work; Dr. Thomas Fahey, deputy
physician-in-chief; Dr. Richard Gralla, former associate attending physician; Dr. Thomas Hakes, associate attending physician; Patricia Henry,
former oncology nurse; Jimmie Holland, M.D., chief of psychiatry; Linda
James, former planning analyst of the Department of Strategic Planning;
Matthew Loscalzo, assistant director of social service; Donna Park, former
assistant director of nursing, ambulatory care; and Sister Rosemary
Moynihan, former assistant director of social service and current coordinator of the HIV Mental Health Project at St. Joseph's Hospital and Medical Center in Paterson, New Jersey.

Pam Felling, staff physical therapist; M. L. Frohling, biofeedback
technician; Lisa Logan, clinical dietitian; and Regina Schmidt, oncology
nurse/team coordinator, all formerly at the Denver Presbyterian Medical
Center.

From the University of Texas MD Anderson Cancer Center: Katherine
Crosson, former director of patient education; Dr. Gabriel Hortobagyi,
head of Medical Oncology Breast Service; Mary Hughes, psychiatric clin-
ical nurse specialist; Dr. Irwin Krakoff, head of Division of Medicine; Dr.
Peter McLaughlin, associate professor of the Department of Hematology;
Dr. James A. Neidhart, former chairman of the Department of Medical
Oncology; and Dr. Karen Ritchie, chief of psychiatry.

From St. Vincent's Hospital and Medical Center: Dr. Judith Bukberg,
clinical associate professor and associate attending physician in psychiatry; and Dr. William Grace, chief of oncology.

Special thanks to New York oncologists Dr. Ward F. Cunningham-
Rundles and Dr. Ronald Bash; Los Angeles oncologist Dr. Michael Van
Scoy-Mosher; and Dr. Richard Cohen, clinical professor of medicine, University of California—all extraordinary oncologists and remarkable human
beings.

I would also like to thank the following: Barbara Blumberg, Linda Anderson, and Betty MacVicar from the National Cancer Institute; Diane

Blum, executive director of Cancer Care, Inc.; Dr. Michael Schachter; Dr. Philip Schulman, associate professor of clinical medicine at North Shore University Hospital; Patricia Fobaire, radiation social worker at Stanford University Medical Center; Dr. Maryl Winningham, exercise physiologist; Dr. Charles Vogel, director of the Comprehensive Cancer Center for the State of Florida; Lari Wenzel, medical psychologist of the Memorial Cancer Institute at Long Beach Memorial Medical Center; Sylvia Weissman, former associate director of social services at Cancer Care, Inc.; Shari Lieberman, Ph.D., New York dietitian and nutritionist; Lin Perkin, Denver exercise physiologist; Mr. Nicholas, wig stylist for the Kenneth Beauty Salon of New York; Joseph Rodriguez, general manager of the Vidal Sassoon Salon in New York; Edith Imre, proprietor of Edith Imre Hair Fashions, Inc.; the late Evelyn Ricki Dienst, former professor of psychology at the California School of Professional Psychology; Michael Lerner, president of Commonweal; Susan Liroff, director of the Women's Cancer Center; Barbara Carter, R.N., D.N.Sc.; Mary Wieneke, R.N., M.S.; and Peggy Knight.

Finally, I would like to extend very, very special thanks to the late Victoria Wells, cofounder and director of the Cancer Support Community in San Francisco—I only wish she had been in my life when I was going through chemo in 1980; and to the late Rose Kushner and Elenore Pred, who continue to serve as an inspiration to me and countless other activists who are working to improve the state of cancer care: wish you were here.

To all of us who have gone through chemotherapy or who will be going through chemotherapy, and to those who love and care about us.

Contents

PART THREE
Guide to Complementary Therapies

Foreword

A diagnosis of cancer is unquestionably a life-challenging event. Many times it comes when there have been no outward signs of disease—you feel just fine, except that you've been told you have cancer. Hearing the word "chemotherapy" often comes as a second wave and can douse you in fear and confusion. For some people, the thought of chemotherapy is so frightening that they will not consider it, even if it could be their best option.

I had the good fortune to pick up the first edition of *Coping with Chemotherapy* in 1987. At that time, my first chemotherapy had failed and a new tumor had emerged, rendering my breast cancer "inoperable." I had sought several opinions from top oncology teams in the country and was trying to find the treatment that was right for me. In the midst of this whirlwind effort to save my life, *Coping with Chemotherapy* became my talisman and constant companion. The thorough research of all the relevant issues, the clear and concise writing, and the warm and friendly tone from someone who had been there helped me to navigate one of the most challenging and frightening journeys of my life. I came back to the book many times during the course of my various treatments. It was my lifeline, an unfailingly reliable guide and a source of reassurance, as it has been, and continues to be, for so many.

When *Coping with Chemotherapy* came out in 1985, cancer was still a taboo subject. People seldom discussed their diagnosis with others, there were few support groups, and there was little public acknowledgment of the challenges faced by cancer patients. By frankly and openly presenting a "how to" book about the process of coping with chemotherapy as if it were no more a cause for shame than home improvement, Nancy Bruning laid the groundwork for what has become a national grass-roots movement of cancer patients and survivors. The effects of this movement have already been seen in the greater public awareness of cancer, the increased attention to the urgency of finding better treatments, and in the proliferation of support treatments, programs, and organizations for those going through chemotherapy.

At each decision point—whether to start chemotherapy, change it, or pursue another treatment option—information is your best ally. At such moments, when we need to be at our strongest, things can seem the most daunting and it can be the most difficult to see clearly.

Coping with Chemotherapy is one of the best tools available to help you achieve that clarity in making these decisions and in coming to grips with the process that you will be going through. It is a book that people pick up before starting treatment, and that they come back to repeatedly during the process. Whether it is read for health information, for advice on relieving side effects, for psychosocial issues, or for an explanation of what to expect and how others have weathered the difficulties, Nancy Bruning's book has been an invaluable tool for almost two decades. And in her new edition of this well-loved classic, she has updated the content so that it includes the latest information on cutting-edge and emerging treatment modalities.

Despite the fact that some cancer treatments have become standardized, in most cases there are many choices for the patient to make. These choices can be a challenge in themselves, calling upon you to make decisions about matters that are likely to be totally foreign to you. Nonetheless, the process hinges on two simple, important concepts: *Only you will know the right decision to make—it's your life—and no one can care about this more than you.* The process of becoming informed and making your treatment choice is one of the most positive and empowering projects you can embark upon. Once you do this and truly "own" your decision, you have changed your relationship to the disease and taken control. When you come out the other side, you will be better and stronger emotionally than you ever thought you could be. This essential coping tool is perhaps one of the most important messages of the book and of Bruning's life.

You are on a journey to find your best path to new health and happiness. If you take it one step at a time, you can do it. So many before you have—there are nine million cancer survivors in the United States alone. Whatever choices you make, they will ultimately be the right ones for you—if you own them, take action, and look forward. Through this process, you may well find a new strength that you never thought possible and an ability to live each day to the fullest. *Coping with Chemotherapy* is the guidebook to get you there.

—Dani S. Grady,

Director of Development and Institute Relations,
San Diego Cancer Research Institute;
Board Member, National Coalition for Cancer
Survivorship; Cofounder, Board of Trustees, Cancer
Survivorship: San Diego; Director's Advisory
Committee, University of California, San Diego
Comprehensive Cancer Center; Member, Institute
Review Board, University of California San Diego.

Introduction

Whether you are still in the process of deciding on a therapy, about to begin treatment, or already undergoing it, it is important to remember that many people before you have gone through chemotherapy, that they did manage to cope, and that there are ways that have been developed to help you get through it, too. The same strength that stems from the will to live and enables people to make the tough decision to undergo chemo continues to stand them in good stead during the actual treatment. So do a positive attitude, a good doctor-patient relationship, and a realistic picture of what to expect in the way of results and side effects. —Nancy Bruning

In 1980, at the age of thirty-one, I discovered I had breast cancer. A biopsy had revealed that the lump that had grown alarmingly large over the last few months was not a cyst. It was a malignancy. In order to save my life—so my surgeon said—I had to have the standard surgical procedure, a modified radical mastectomy, the very next day. Although this removed all the visible tumor, unfortunately some lymph nodes were involved, and this meant that the cancer might have spread to other parts of my body. The only way to kill those stray cancer cells was with chemotherapy, which I was advised to have "just in case."

Without a doubt, I found the idea of chemotherapy more frightening than the surgery I had just been through. The fact was that in spite of major, mutilating, and supposedly life-saving surgery, my surgeon might not have "gotten it all." It wasn't over yet: Cancer might still be somewhere in my body, and I was now being offered a treatment about which I knew very little, and what little I did know was all bad. I had allowed my surgeon to lop off my breast without investigating my options, and, by his own admission, it hadn't worked. I felt betrayed and, mistrustful of medical advice, was not about to be rushed into something else I didn't know a lot about.

So I went to a chemotherapist other than the one recommended by my surgeon. Through sheer luck—referral from a friend of a friend who also had cancer—I found a capable, compassionate cancer specialist whom I liked, respected, and trusted immediately. (And during the course of treatment I grew to like, respect, and trust him even more.) He explained the statistics: Without chemotherapy my chances of remaining disease-free for ten years would be about 15 percent. According to the latest scientific study, published in 1979, the best standard chemotherapy increased my chances to about 70 percent—at least for the next eight years. He described the course of therapy—the scheduling of the drugs and their likely side effects—and then assured me he would do everything he knew, nutritionally and otherwise, to help minimize the side effects. Clearly, 70 percent was better than 15 percent. A quick assessment of the unorthodox therapies revealed no comparative figures, which made those therapies more frightening than chemo. Under the circumstances, I agreed to the plan. I wanted to live, and chemo seemed the best chance there was.

If I had to do it all over again, I would. Looking back, chemotherapy was not as bad as I had thought it would be. I continued to work and enjoy most of my usual activities, even though I didn't feel exactly wonderful. I had a relatively hopeful prognosis, I got relatively "low-dose" chemo under the care of a good physician, and I was surrounded by people who cared. Everyone thought I coped amazingly well, and I suppose I did. But I know I would have coped even better if I had done some things a little differently.

It wasn't until about two years after my treatment was over and life had settled down to a semblance of normality that I could begin to look back at my experience with a critical eye.

I realized after the fact what I couldn't see while I was busy grappling with the awful, earth-shattering possibility of my own death: that I should have been better informed about my disease and its treatment, and I should have been better prepared to deal with some of the side effects, especially the complete hair loss. I realized that I would have coped better if I had had more psychological support than my doctor, family, and friends could give me and that I did not have to suffer alone in my feelings of depression, anxiety, doubt, fear, anger, confusion, sadness, ignorance, and isolation.

I realized, too, that a book about chemotherapy—one that really talked about what it's like, what I might expect, and what could be done to make the experience more bearable—would have been a great comfort to me. As a journalist, I naturally thought that maybe I should be the one to fill this information gap.

Although there were by then several informative books on cancer and its treatment, there was still nothing for the general audience—patients and their families—that focused solely on chemotherapy. No books were around that helped answer the questions foremost on people's minds: Should I have chemotherapy? And if I do have chemo, how on earth am I going to get through it? Just as important, no books were around that would help caregivers, friends, and family who want to help those undergoing chemotherapy but don't know how.

And so the idea and the conviction to write a book on coping with chemotherapy came about, a book based in part on the methods that I found successful and in part on the experiences of others.

While doing the research for the first edition of this book, published in 1986, I absorbed (or tried to absorb) the medical literature and spoke with more than fifty cancer specialists, social workers, nurses, and cancer patients all over the country. I learned that chemotherapy is a highly individual matter. There are hundreds of different chemotherapy treatments, and people's diseases, personalities, life circumstances, prognoses, levels of tolerance, and reactions to the drugs can and do vary. So do the will to live and the ability to fight. I learned that if it is given wisely and well to informed patients, chemotherapy can cure some people and extend the comfortable productive life spans of many others.

The cruel facts are that there are patients who might be helped by chemotherapy but who are not getting it, there are those who might be *better* helped by it, and there are some who are harmed rather than helped by chemotherapy and who shouldn't be getting it at all. Chemotherapy is clearly not for everyone. Anyone who is faced with its mixed blessings should be fully informed before making decisions about it. No one should accept, refuse, continue, or stop chemotherapy out of ignorance or fear.

Since the 1980s, and even since 1993 when the second edition of this book was published, cancer has come out of the closet—in particular, breast and prostate cancers—as health consumer activists and celebrities advocate for more awareness and better care. We can talk about cancer now, but the chemotherapy experience can still fall short of what it might be because the nitty-gritty of chemotherapy is still shrouded in mystery. Most people, even after they have been diagnosed and their treatment has begun, suddenly find themselves plunged into a maze without a map. Cancer care for most people is completely foreign territory—full of half-truths, myths, and misconceptions, of personal issues and dilemmas, of complicated new words and procedures, of hot and cold running hope and fear.

To be sure, there have been a number of improvements in chemotherapy, making it more beneficial for some people and more tolerable, too. Although these developments are for the most part small, incremental steps, there have been enough of them to make a difference and to require a third, updated edition of this book.

For one thing, there are new chemotherapy drugs that attack cancer cells in totally new ways. There are new ways of administering anticancer drugs to make them not only more effective but less toxic, too. For another, the cancer profession is finally recognizing the extent of the physical and psychological burdens experienced by patients and their families and acknowledging that these burdens must be considered when treatment choices are made. The realization that in addition to improving the effects of chemo on the cancer they must work harder to reduce the emotional and physical side effects means they are more likely to offer support therapies. There are several new drugs used along with chemo to reduce the distressing side effects, particularly fatigue, nausea and vomiting. Thanks to the incredible increase in acceptance and popularity of natural therapies in general, nutrition, exercise, acupuncture, mind-body therapies, and emotional support are becoming much more accepted as adjuncts to chemotherapy drugs.

This information is gradually trickling into the world of chemotherapy, thanks in large part to patients becoming more active in their own care. When I first wrote *Coping with Chemotherapy,* I had to scramble and dig deeply to find research and practitioners who used complementary therapies along with standard, mainstream medicine. Today there is an emerging new discipline called *integrative medicine,* which formally, responsibly, and creatively seeks to do exactly that.

Chemotherapy has changed dramatically since its inception. Doctors are encouraging people to become more involved in making treatment choices. More and more patients and their loved ones are asking how the coping process can be made easier, swifter, and better. More and more patients are taking it upon themselves to make sure they are getting the best chemotherapy regimen available and asking their doctors and nurses for help in getting through it as easily as possible. More and more are investigating and taking advantage of ways and people to help make their treatment less formidable in order to help patients, their families, and their friends meet new challenges from a position of strength rather than weakness.

Despite these advances, as a chemotherapy patient you are still in dire need of a map to get you through the maze. In *Coping with Chemotherapy,* I provide that map. I give you:

- *Information* so you may weigh your options sensibly.
- *Guidance* so you can help your cancer specialist help you.
- *Practical suggestions* to make living with chemotherapy more comfortable.
- *Reassurance* that others have entered the special world of chemotherapy, have come out the other end, and are managing to adapt to the new life the experience has presented to them.

This new edition presents not only information on new drugs and medical support to blunt the side effects, but also the latest information on combining chemotherapy with other therapies. Does taking vitamin supplements help or interfere with the effectiveness of chemotherapy? Does acupuncture really help mitigate nausea and fatigue? Should I rest or get some exercise? If I should be exercising, what kind should I engage in? Is there any way I can safely keep my hair from falling out? How can I lessen the hot flashes and vaginal dryness from the premature menopause that chemo is causing? What's happening with my sex life—will it ever be normal again? Will I ever get my energy back? I answer these and many other questions you may have.

In Part One, I help you make decisions about your treatment and address the important question of whether or not you should have chemotherapy and if so, what kind, and where. I begin with a few chapters that provide background and practical information about chemotherapy—the different types, the various goals, how it works, and how to make sure you are getting the best treatment currently available. Ideally, I'd like you to read these introductory chapters first, but I also understand that you're probably not too interested in the history of chemotherapy if your hair has just begun to fall out in handfuls.

Whether you've already begun chemo or are deciding whether to undergo it, you'll want to turn to Part Two—a comprehensive guide to coping with the most common physical and emotional side effects. Under each heading, I tell you what's happening, why it's happening, and what to do about it, including using natural therapies such as diet, nutritional supplements, exercise, herbal therapy, and acupuncture.

In Part Three, I provide a fuller discussion of the complementary therapies suggested in the A-to-Z section. I also devote individual chapters to the emotional impact of cancer and chemotherapy and the whys and wherefores of getting emotional support.

Although many patients, family members, nurses, doctors, and other health-care professionals have thanked me for writing this book, a few have also told me that the book is too frightening. The last thing I want to do is frighten people unnecessarily. Getting a diagnosis of cancer is frightening, too; yet few people today would say, "It's best not to tell her." Gone are the days when doctors and families felt they needed to protect the poor passive patient, to keep her in the dark about her disease. Why should it be any different when discussing the treatment for the disease?

There's no getting around the fact that chemotherapy can be a highly toxic therapy; not knowing this will not make it less dangerous—only more. This isn't to say that people don't vary in the amount of information they need and want, and it isn't to say that you need to absorb all this information at one time. Too much information, for certain people or at certain times, does not help them cope better—they cope worse.

So, a few words of advice: Be aware that you may not be ready to learn certain details now but may welcome them later. At times, you may feel overwhelmed by it all and overloaded with information. If you sense this is happening to you, back off for a while. You don't need to know everything at once—it's not likely you'll be able to process it. But for when you do need to know, I have tried my best to provide it. I hope you will be able to take from this book what you need when you need it. Remember that chemotherapy is an evolving field, so this book is by no means the final word on this treatment. Nor can it take the place of a qualified physician or other health-care professional. I encourage you to do your own additional research if that makes you feel more secure and in control. The Internet, in particular, has a growing number of sites for information, support, and encouragement. But be aware that numerous surveys have found that the quality of the information on the Web varies tremendously from site to site. I have listed many—but, of course, not all—of the most reputable sites in the Resources section (Appendix B) of this book.

Coping with Chemotherapy should be used as a supplement to your doctor's care and a resource to learn about the many other aspects of cancer in which you may be interested. This book necessarily concentrates on the aspects that are most directly related to the issue at hand—chemotherapy. But where does cancer end and chemotherapy begin? Chemotherapy does not exist in a vacuum: A chemo patient is, after all, a cancer patient. I have touched briefly upon many areas that concern all cancer patients in the hope that this will pique further interest and self-education in this endlessly fascinating subject that will on some level be of concern for the rest of our lives. Volumes have been written about areas I have kept brief; for example, about other forms of therapy and psychosocial concerns. I have also not included childhood cancer, because that is a whole other world that could not have been treated adequately here. Many sources of information about these and related subjects are listed in the Appendices, to which you may want to refer.

Anyone facing chemotherapy surely has a big job ahead. The physical and psychological changes and challenges in your life begin at the time of diagnosis; they may come to a peak sometime during the treatment; and they can continue for long afterward. It is not an easy road you travel, and in spite of the proliferation of support groups and counseling resources, it may often be a lonely one. *Coping with Chemotherapy* was written for you to turn to again and again, whenever you need information, inspiration, or simply a hand to hold. I hope you will be able to draw strength, comfort, courage, assurance, and wisdom from these pages and the people who have given of themselves in order to help others who are going through a similar difficult time. But no matter how much help you have, it is still up to you and your own strength and determination to make it as you pick your own way along the path to coping with chemotherapy.

PART ONE

Decisions, Decisions

Coping with chemotherapy begins with making the decision whether or not to undergo it. This decision is not an easy one, but then, important decisions rarely are. Though you may rely on others for information and advice, ultimately the choice is up to you. However, whether you are on the threshold of chemotherapy or already well into it, information about cancer and its treatment helps you to make the choice to begin—or to continue—much more wisely and responsibly.

Many patients and cancer-care professionals find that learning something about cancer is the first step in a sound decision-making process. It's also essential that you understand what chemotherapy is, how it works, and its advantages and shortcomings, as well as have a realistic picture of its goals, your prognosis, your alternatives, and how chemotherapy fits in with and compares to other forms of treatment. You also need to find a competent, caring cancer specialist (oncologist) who will be responsive to your needs and who will give you the most effective treatment with the fewest possible side effects. Access to the many methods used to support chemotherapy patients is also paramount.

Admittedly, some of these factors carry more weight than others, depending on the individual. But all contribute to your making informed, intelligent choices throughout your therapy, to a basic conviction that you are doing the right thing, and to your having a feeling of control over your life. These are all fundamental to accepting treatment and learning to live with it . . . and after it.

CHAPTER ONE

Understanding Cancer

When I was diagnosed with cancer, I knew very little about the disease. That probably put me at a disadvantage. Most cancer patients are in the same position.

No one can expect to become a cancer specialist overnight, but acquiring a basic understanding of your disease is worth the effort and is a necessary preliminary to understanding all cancer therapies. As an oncologist at Memorial Sloan-Kettering Cancer Center told me:

> *People try to understand cancer without understanding very much about biology in general. I think people do not understand their disease because they don't understand much of the basic science that goes into it. And yet you hear people complain that when your doctor tells you something, you have no choice; you have to listen to him. What choice do you have if you don't know very much about these things in general?*

Cell Biology

Your body is made up of many different types of tissue—skin, muscle, bone, blood, glands, and other organs. The tissues, in turn, are made up of tiny specialized cells that perform specific functions. Within each cell is a *nucleus* that contains *chromosomes*. Each chromosome can contain up to several thousand genes. The genes, in turn, are made up of *deoxyribonucleic acid* (DNA), which takes the form of two spiraling strands. The DNA can be likened to a foreman who controls the cell's activities; it is the DNA that ultimately makes up the genetic program of each cell.

One of the activities the DNA oversees is reproduction. Cells reproduce themselves in order to replace those that have become damaged or have died or if more cells are needed for some special reason. Some cells, like those making up the blood, are replaced more often than others are. For example, your white blood cells are replaced completely every six hours, a rate of production that steps up during infection, when you need more of them than under normal conditions.

Cells reproduce by division—one cell splits in half to produce a "daughter" cell. There is a time in every cell's life when it reproduces; a time when it is "fertile" and a time when it is not. Cells go through four phases during each of their reproductive cycles in which the DNA makes an exact copy of itself to pass on to the nucleus of the next generation. Some types of cells reproduce within hours; others may take days, weeks, months, or years. After division, the cell begins the next four-phase reproductive cycle, perhaps after first passing through a resting phase.

Normal human cells are obedient and altruistic. They "know" when they should reproduce and when they should not. They stay where they belong. They perform whatever functions they are programmed to perform. Whatever their functions and rates of growth, they exist for the good of the entire body. (Cells also respond to other stimuli, such as the commands given by the hormones produced in our endocrine glands.)

Cancer cells, however, do not obey the commands of the body. Unlike normal cells, whose motto might be "One for all and all for one," cancer cells behave as if it were every man for himself. They reproduce wildly, more often than the normal cells that surround them. They are usually unable to perform any useful function for the good of the entire body. On the contrary, they are malignant, meaning they invade and injure vital organs of the body, thus interfering with those organs' ability to perform needed functions. In advanced stages of cancer, these cells spread and grow in other parts of the body to wreak havoc there, too.

Though they arise from normal cells, cancer cells usually don't look exactly like the other cells in the tissue of origin. They may be oddly misshapen, have a strange membrane or nucleus, or contain the wrong number of chromosomes.

Causes of Cancer

It is believed that cancer cells arise from normal cells that have undergone a change called *carcinogenesis*. Throughout history, there have been various theories as to how the original cancer cell is produced. Recently, researchers have identified and isolated single genes in several types of human cancer called *oncogenes* ("onco" comes from the Greek word *onkos*, meaning "mass" or "tumor"). It is believed that these genes transform normal cells into cancer cells. Many scientists believe that oncogenes are commonly present in our cells in another form, but remain dormant unless damaged or "turned on" by carcinogens.

It is natural to wonder why such troublemakers exist in the first place. Scientists believe that oncogenes were once *proto-oncogenes*, or normal genes involved in normal growth before becoming cancer-causing. They may be needed at some point in human development—before birth, during childhood, or during the healing process—and then are "switched off" when they are no longer needed. Oncogenes, it is believed, are formed and become troublemakers only when they are activated by an inherited defect or exposure to an outside agent called a carcinogen.

Oncogenes are normally suppressed by "suppressor" genes also called *anti-oncogenes*. In some cases, these controlling genes may be missing or themselves damaged. Recently, researchers have identified a gene known as p53, which is normally an anti-oncogene. This gene seems to be defective in about 90 percent of all cancers. Perhaps you have heard of BRCA1 and BRCA2, which have been characterized as the breast cancer and ovarian cancer genes. These are normally anti-oncogenes, but they can mutate. When a woman passes the mutated version down to her daughter, her daughter is at higher risk for developing these cancers. Once we know what turns a healthy proto-oncogene into an unhealthy oncogene, perhaps we will learn what turns it off. This would open up a whole new area of research that could ultimately lead to a cure for cancer. Of course, it would still be preferable to prevent the damage to the healthy proto-oncogene or protective anti-oncogene in the first place.

For this, we must also consider the theory that cancer is a two-step process of *initiation* and *promotion*. According to this theory, the initiators prime the genes of the cell and so set the stage for cancer development. Initiators include viruses, radiation, and chemicals such as those contained in tobacco, toxic waste, or food. But these initiated cells are harmless and behave normally and eventually die—they may even be repaired or normalized by the body—unless promoters are also present. Promoters include anything that enhances the effect of an initiator, such as diet, hormones, chemicals, environmental conditions, and an inherited predisposition.

Current theory holds that cells usually require a number of "hits" to switch on the cancer process. This theory looks promising and would help to explain why everyone who smokes doesn't get lung cancer, why all X-ray technicians don't get leukemia, and why a diet of junk food doesn't guarantee the development of gastrointestinal cancer.

How Cancer Grows and Spreads

Cancer, as we now understand it, consists of well over 100 different diseases. These, however, fall into four main categories: carcinomas, lymphomas, leukemias, and sarcomas. *Carcinomas* are the most common— between 85 and 90 percent of all cancers are of this type. They are solid tumors or "lumps" originating in the lining (epithelium) of the organ. Examples are carcinoma of the breast, lung, uterus, intestines, esophagus, stomach, and kidney. *Lymphomas,* cancers of the lymphatic system, cause the spleen and lymph nodes to produce abnormal cells. Lymphomas can cause solid tumors to grow in various parts of the body. *Leukemias* are disseminated (circulating) tumors that involve bone marrow, which is the blood-forming system, where they cause abnormal white blood cells to be produced. *Sarcomas,* the rarest form of the four, are solid tumors that develop on the connective tissue of the muscles, bones, nerves, and other organs.

The carcinomas share a common pattern of growth and spread. Cancer of this type begins as a single abnormal cell, which reproduces itself over and over again until it becomes a mass, or a tumor, at which point it can begin to cause problems for the host. If the cancer has spread to other, distant parts of the body, more problems can arise.

All abnormal growths, including cancers, are called *lesions* or *neoplasms.* Precancerous conditions are termed *dysplasia.* The earliest cancer is called *in situ* (meaning "in its place") or *preinvasive cancer.* At this point the cancer is still *localized* and highly curable.

If early cancer goes untreated, it begins to invade the surrounding tissue. Though it is still considered localized and the cure rates are high, *invasive cancer* is a serious condition. The tumor may grow so large that it crowds out the healthy cells, destroys them, and reduces their function; forms an obstruction in a vital pathway of the body; or exerts dangerous pressure on nearby vital organs. Surgical removal of the tumor is usually still possible as a cure, though some or all of the cancerous organ being invaded may be removed as well. Radiation therapy may also successfully destroy cells of *locally invasive* cancer. When a tumor has spread to a new but still nearby organ, it is called *regional extension,* and it may also still be curable with surgery and/or radiation.

But cancer is not content to grow in one place. At some point during the growth of a tumor, cancer cells begin to break off. They hitch a ride from the bloodstream or the lymphatic system and circulate freely throughout the body like seeds on the wind. This tendency to spread (metastasize) is perhaps cancer's most frightening and deadliest characteristic. When metastatic or advanced cancer has spread to vital organs such as the brain, bones, liver, or lungs, it cuts off the organ's blood supply or crowds the organ and crushes it. Either way, the organ is no longer able to perform its function. It is not uncommon, for instance, for a woman with metastatic breast cancer to die of liver failure caused by her cancer spreading to that organ. (Even though the cancer is in the liver, its place of origin was the breast, so is still considered to be breast cancer.)

In general, the longer a tumor exists, the greater the likelihood that it has shed cells, and the greater the number of those cells there will be. It is thought that our immune system plays a large role in defending our bodies from cancer, just as it protects us against undesirable creatures, such as bacteria and viruses. It is widely believed that the immune system controls early cancer cells routinely, before they reproduce to the point where the cancer is large enough to be detected. The immune system may also be able to control advanced cancer, which would explain how the rare but documented "spontaneous remissions" can happen.

But sometimes the immune system slips up, even at the early stage. There are many reasons why it may not successfully destroy the abnormal cells our bodies are constantly churning out, but they all boil down either to a system that is too weak or to cancer cells that are too clever. The immune system may be weak because of age, stress, overwhelming systemic infection, factors in the environment, or nutritional deficiencies. Cancer itself may suppress the immune response. There may be a constitutional deficiency. Cancer cells have the unique ability to produce a protective coating that fools the immune system into ignoring them. Unfortunately, surgery, radiation, and chemotherapy—three major conventional treatments now used against cancer—can also suppress our natural immunity. The fourth major form of treatment—immunologic therapy—seeks to do just the opposite.

Although our immune systems may battle valiantly against proliferating cancer cells, there may eventually be too many of them and our natural defenses may become overwhelmed. Our immune system has fumbled the ball, so to speak, and you may now decide to call upon some form of treatment to try to save the game. I'll discuss cancer treatment in the next chapter.

CHAPTER TWO

How Cancer
Is Treated

Since no one cancer treatment has proved to be perfect in its effectiveness or in not producing undesirable side effects, chemotherapy is rarely offered as the only treatment. The trend is moving increasingly toward using combined modality therapy—chemotherapy in combination with one or more other forms of therapy, usually the conventional therapies of surgery and radiation but sometimes with the less common, emerging therapies such as biologic/immunotherapy. In addition, aspects of unconventional cancer therapies have come to be taken seriously and integrated into the overall treatment plan.

Surgery

Surgery is the primary treatment for most of the major forms of cancer. However, it is effective alone as a cure only in early, localized solid-tumor cancer. In such cases, the object of the surgery is to remove all traces of the malignancy. When, as in my case, there is good reason to believe that the cancer has spread to distant parts of the body, the object of surgery is to remove as much of the tumor as possible so that additional treatment—radiation, chemotherapy, or immunotherapy—will be better able to control or destroy the remaining cells that have escaped the scalpel. Some experts believe, however, that a tumor begins to shed cells from the very beginning of its growth, and so even in "early cancer" there is the possibility of spread. Surgery may still be able to cure cancer in these cases because few enough cells were shed for the immune system to handle. Surgery may also be used to remove metastases in some types of cancer and for palliation of symptoms such as pain.

Cancer surgery is often extensive, and recuperation is often painful. A percentage of patients do not even survive cancer surgery. A commonly overlooked effect of surgery is the distressing change in body image that it leaves in its wake. It's not unusual to feel mutilated or somehow "not whole" afterward, especially if the affected area is highly visible, useful, or symbolic. As is the case with chemotherapy, thanks to advances, surgery is a safer and less mutilating option than it was in the past. And researchers continue to refine the technique. For example, in breast cancer, laser surgery to kill the tumor is being tested. This technique is far less disfiguring than surgery with a knife. In Germany, surgeons have successfully "zapped" breast tumors with ultrasound, killing the cancer cells. For both laser and ultrasound, the tumors must be very small (half inch in diameter or smaller) for best results.

Radiation Therapy

Radiation therapy, or radiotherapy, is the recommended primary treatment of choice for some forms of cancer, such as early Hodgkin's disease, some lung cancers, and head and neck cancers. You may undergo radiation therapy alone, but it is often used in conjunction with surgery or chemotherapy to cure or control cancer. Radiation is also effective as a palliative therapy to relieve symptoms of cancer.

Radiotherapy may be administered externally via machines whose radiation penetrates deep inside the body, avoiding healthy tissue as much as possible. Or it may be administered internally with a radioactive isotope encapsulated in a needle, tube, or seed and implanted in the body, either directly into the cancer or nearby. Sometimes radioisotopes are injected into an organ or into the bloodstream, where they enter the tumor directly.

Radiation therapy changes cancer cells' chemistry with rays or charged particles. When the radiation reaches the tumor cells, it either kills the cells directly or damages the DNA and makes it impossible for the present cells or the next generation of cells to reproduce. In effect, the tumor becomes "sterile."

Radiation has its own set of advantages and drawbacks. Radiation therapy kills normal cells along with cancer cells but targets primarily cells that are actively dividing. That means cancer cells are more vulnerable because they generally divide more rapidly than normal cells and will die at a far greater rate than normal cells. Like surgery, this treatment is most effective when it can be used locally. Unlike surgery, radiotherapy can destroy a tumor without grossly disfiguring the patient; it leaves vital structures intact. It does not work on widely spread metastases unless wide-field radiation is used, but this technique does have serious side effects on healthy tissue. Cancers vary greatly in their "radiosensitivity": Radiation is highly effective for certain types of cancers, somewhat effective for some, and not at all effective for others. A big drawback is that the tumor must be in a location where the radiation can reach it.

Even with improved technology, some normal tissue is damaged by radiation. This results in a wide spectrum of side effects, depending on the area being irradiated, the dose, and your individual constitution. You may experience skin reactions such as dryness, itchiness, and burns; loss of hair; lowered energy and appetite; constipation or diarrhea; sore mouth or throat; changes in taste perception; tooth and ear problems; and nausea and vomiting. In addition, radiation has been shown to have the ability to cause leukemia, fertility problems, and birth defects in some cases.

An innovative type of radiation therapy called *stereotactic radiosurgery* has been used for many years to treat some types of brain tumors, for which it has been very effective and has resulted in fewer side effects than if the whole brain was treated. In this technique, radiation beams are aimed at the tumor from many different angles with computers and CT scans assuring that the beams converge on the tumor and deliver a very high dose there and nowhere else. The Karolinska Institute in Sweden and the Staten Island Hospital in New York City have extended the use of this technique to both primary and metastatic tumors. It has been used for patients who are newly diagnosed, as well as those with recurrent diseases including lung and liver cancer, pancreatic cancer, sarcomas, and prostate cancer. Doctors at the Karolinska Institute have published their promising results using their technique, but Staten Island has published only on radiosurgery of the head and neck. For information about Staten Island Hospital's technique, go to http://www.siuh.edu/conindex5.html.

Chemotherapy

You will find a more detailed picture of chemotherapy later in this book, but for now I'm going to supply a quick sketch to help you understand where chemo fits in with the other types of cancer therapies.

Chemotherapy literally means the treatment of disease with chemicals, or drugs. Usually, though, the term is understood to mean treatment with anticancer drugs. The post–World War II era is generally considered the beginning of its development. Now dozens of drugs are in standard use alone or in various combinations. In addition, new drugs and new combinations of drugs are constantly being investigated and evaluated and are available to patients participating in clinical trials and, in some cases, outside of the trials.

Chemotherapy is unique among the major conventional approaches to cancer treatment because it is not just a local treatment. Chemicals have the ability to circulate throughout the body. Only circulating chemicals can reach cancer cells that have broken off solid tumors and spread to distant sites and that may be undetectable and/or untouchable by local treatments; only chemicals are useful in treating disseminated tumors of the blood and lymph. Chemotherapy works because it is *cytotoxic*—it poisons the cells, especially those that reproduce rapidly, as cancer cells do. But as with other therapies, chemo doesn't always work. And because normal cells are also vulnerable to varying degrees, there are many potential side effects, the most common of which are loss of energy, loss of hair, nausea and vomiting, and susceptibility to infection.

Originally, chemotherapy was used only as a last resort after all else had failed. But using chemotherapy as a second line of defense, after a recurrence has already happened, has failed to improve the survival rate of many patients with the most common solid tumors. So, the way chemo is used has changed drastically. Today, doctors are giving chemotherapy much earlier during the course of the disease because, as with the other modalites, that seems to be when it works the best. Today, chemotherapy may be the treatment of choice to actually cure certain cancers. But a newer strategy is to use chemotherapy as *adjuvant therapy* (a therapy used to increase the efficacy of another) as soon as possible right after surgery or radiation has "debulked" a tumor or "reduced the tumor burden." It is hoped that when used this way, chemotherapy will prevent or postpone suspected micrometastases from causing a recurrence. Chemotherapy is also being used after surgery to shrink already evident inoperable metastases. It is sometimes used before surgery to reduce the size of a tumor and make it more operable ("neoadjuvant" chemotherapy) or along with radiation to make a tumor more susceptible. Chemotherapy cures only a few types of cancers; however, even when it does not achieve a cure, chemo may control a person's cancer for many years and allow him to live longer than he would have without it. Though inroads are being made in minimizing side effects, these effects are still a problem for many people, and whether the risk is worth the benefit is always an individual choice. Researchers are busy trying to come up with new, more effective, less toxic cytotoxic drugs. And as you will see, they are also working on drugs that are not directly cytotoxic, but show promise of controlling cancer for a long time, much like we control diabetes.

Hormone (Endocrine) Therapy

Hormones are chemicals produced by our endocrine glands to stimulate other organs. If a cancer begins in tissues that are affected by hormones, usually the tumor will be affected by them, too, as cancers generally arise and thrive in hormone-affected tissues. Such tumors are called hormone-sensitive or hormone-dependent; by changing the hormonal environment, we can affect a tumor's growth.

Originally, hormone therapy consisted of the surgical removal of the glands that produced the hormones (ablative surgery). This method is still used. But in addition, oncologists often give synthetic hormones or hormone suppressants alone or along with other anticancer drugs for certain types of cancer, including cancers of the breast, uterus, prostate, thyroid, and kidney and lymphomas, leukemias, and myelomas. Even though its action is very different from that of the other drugs, hormone therapy is a type of chemotherapy. At this time it is unclear exactly how hormones, and thus hormone-blocking drugs, affect cancers. This field is considered to be somewhat experimental, but these substances are in fact incorporated into many standard treatments.

Cancer specialists are beginning to use hormone therapy much more often than in the past, particularly to treat breast cancer. Now tumor cells are routinely tested for hormone sensitivity (with tests called hormone receptor assays). These assays, for example, help identify women who have tumors that are highly dependent on estrogen or progesterone and so are most likely to benefit from hormone therapy. By the beginning of the twenty-first century, tamoxifen, which blocks estrogen in breast cells, had become the most widely used endocrine drug for treating all stages of breast cancer in women with estrogen-dependent tumors, regardless of their age or menopause status. It was also unrivalled as the standard hormone therapy for postmenopausal women with advanced breast cancer. But tamoxifen may soon be knocked off its throne—there are several new compounds that inhibit the production of estrogen by affecting an enzyme called *aromatase*.

These new drugs work in a different way than tamoxifen does. Aromatase is needed by the body to produce estrogen, and the drugs that block this effect are not surprisingly called *aromatase inhibitors*. They appear to be less toxic and more effective than tamoxifen, and several (as of this writing: anastrozole [Aridimex], letrozole [Femara], formestane, and exemestane) have been FDA-approved for treating breast cancer in postmenopausal women. Their use as "second-line" treatment—that is, to further improve and extend life after other therapy, such as tamoxifen, has failed—is well established in postmenopausal women.

In addition, recent studies show that postmenopausal women with advanced breast cancer who take anastrozole as first-line treatment live twice as long as women who take tamoxifen, and preliminary data show that letrozole is also more effective than tamoxifen in these women. Other studies show that anastrozole or letrozole may be used as "neoadjuvant" therapy *before* surgery to shrink breast tumors. In one study of postmenopausal women with estrogen-rich, or estrogen-sensitive breast tumors, fifteen out of seventeen women who would have had mastectomies were able to have breast-conserving surgery instead—over the course of three months, letrozole shrank the tumors by about 80 percent.

Unlike the other drugs used in chemotherapy, hormone therapy is not cytotoxic —it does not kill cells directly. These drugs don't cure, but they may cause long-term remissions or enhance the effect of cytotoxic drugs. Their side effects are usually mild compared with those of their more toxic cousins. In addition to their antitumor activity, steroidal hormones may reduce certain side effects of chemotherapy, including loss of appetite, and they may increase a sense of well-being.

Though hormone therapy is used for several kinds of cancer because of its relatively few and mild side effects, when I refer to "chemotherapy" I am referring generally to the cytotoxic group of drugs, except when hormones are specifically mentioned. For more information about hormones and their side effects, see Guide to Anticancer Drugs (Appendix A).

The New Wave of Anticancer Drugs

Many researchers and clinicians are encouraged by a new wave of anticancer drugs or agents, some of which have been approved by the Food and Drug Administration (FDA) and some of which are still in the pipeline. These represent a more targeted approach than either cytotoxic or endocrine therapy in that they aim to affect only the cancer cells and leave the healthy cells alone.

Immunotherapy

Many of the new approaches are forms of immunotherapy. Immunotherapy is based on the fact that our immune systems, which can recognize and eliminate foreign substances such as bacteria and viruses, also can destroy cancer cells. Immunotherapy utilizes a number of natural and synthetic substances called biological response modifiers (BRMs) or biologicals, which are known to boost, direct, or restore the body's normal immune system defense mechanisms. Some BRMs themselves have antitumor properties. Biological therapies being used and investigated include the use of interleukins, interferons, tumor necrosis factor, colony-stimulating factors, vaccines, and monoclonal antibodies. Biologicals may be used along with standard therapy, such as chemotherapy, to help the body recover from the damage done by these treatments and perhaps to prolong a remission and increase survival time.

This new approach to cancer treatment is appealing because it appears to be more "natural"—its goal is to harness and enhance the body's own ability to take care of itself. While they do not have the same side effects as surgery, radiation, and chemotherapy, immunologic substances have their own set of possible disturbing side effects, including flulike symptoms like chills, fever, nausea, malaise, and body aches; severe allergic reactions and seizures; kidney problems; ulcers and scarring at the injection site; skin rashes; and even death. In spite of the brouhaha with which immunology was originally greeted, this approach has not yet lived up to the expectations of its being a gentle but powerful cure. Although this type of therapy is accepted as treatment for a few cancers, in most instances, it is still considered experimental.

GENETIC THERAPY

Genetic therapy is a hotly pursued Holy Grail. Some forms of gene therapy seek to supply you with healthy versions of missing or flawed genes. With this approach, the genetic makeup of your cells is corrected, instead of giving you drugs to treat or control the disease. Because gene therapy is a targeted treatment that attacks cancer cells directly, it seems to have minimal side effects.

One form of gene therapy uses the body's natural defense system to fight cancer. Your immune system's white blood cells are often fooled into ignoring cancer cells. To counteract this blind spot, doctors inject the tumor with a foreign gene in order to get the tumor cells to "express" the new gene. If this is successful, the immune system may recognize the cancer cells as foreign invaders and attack them.

Some forms of genetic therapy are designed to disrupt the processes that cause normal cells to grow and turn cancerous. Even if these treatments do not kill cells, they may be able to suppress their cancerous tendencies for as long as the cells survive. If so, the compounds could be used in long-term therapy and cancer might be controlled like other chronic diseases such as diabetes. Researchers have engineered specific tumor cells in mice to suppress the growth of metastases. Since the metastases— not the original tumor—are usually the cause of disability and death, this, too, could be a major means of controlling, but not curing, cancer.

Some approaches target specific proteins. Some of these therapeutic agents shut down proteins that signal cells to grow; others encourage proteins that suppress tumor growth. Since at least one-fifth of all human genes make proteins that signal cells to grow or to stop growing, this approach may prove to be "a more rational form of therapy," according to one researcher. Drugs in this category are called *signal transduction inhibitors* (STIs). Gleevec (STI-571), for example, blocks one such hyperactive protein and was approved by the FDA in 2001. Thus far, this agent works in two rare cancers—a form of leukemia and stomach cancer. But in these two diseases, this approach netted spectacular results early on, at least for the short term: speedy remissions in 60 to 90 percent of patients. In a study presented in December 2001, researchers found that some people do become resistant to Gleevec. After one year of therapy, 8 percent become resistant and 3 percent died. However, this is still superior to the 20 percent annual death rate with traditional treatment. Iressa, still being tested as of this writing, shuts down a growth protein in non-small-cell lung cancer. Another STI called phenoxodiol holds much promise because instead of targeting one signal pathway, it targets an enzyme believed to control all the pathways.

Another avenue for gene therapy is being used for breast cancer in certain women: A drug called herceptin is an antibody that slows tumor growth by counteracting the protein HER-2/neu, which is produced by a gene. Still another type of genetic therapy seeks to activate or repair anti-oncogenes, such as the p53 gene. This gene appears to stop the growth of certain cancers and, not surprisingly, is damaged in 90 percent of cancers. One interesting approach being tested is to use genetically altered viruses that grow only in cells with inactivated suppressor proteins (produced by anti-oncogenes), such as the p53 gene. Onyx-015, for example, used in head and neck cancers as well as in advanced colorectal cancers, is injected directly into the tumor, where it attacks the cancer cells and causes tumors to "melt" away.

ANTI-ANGIOGENETIC DRUGS

A different type of approach seeks to stop tumor growth by cutting off the tumor's blood supply. Tumors stimulate the growth of their own blood supply in a process called *angiogenesis,* and there are drugs being tested that slow or halt new blood vessel growth. Early animal studies are very promising, but the first generation of these drugs, such as endostatin and angiostatin, overall have had more modest results in humans with advanced disease, and they have been shown to be far from harmless. Still, this approach shows promise. The pioneer in the field. Dr. Judah Folkman, professor of cell biology at Children's Hospital in Boston, believes these drugs will best be used in conjunction with conventional therapy and radiation (see Chapter 3, "Low-Dose Chemotherapy"). He says the problem with the early research in this field is that they mistakenly thought all new capillaries were the same. Claude Hariton, of Aeterna Laboratories, a manufacturer of an angiogenesis inhibitor, says that drugs need to be stronger acting because angiogenesis depends on several complex processes, and "shutting one door" won't solve the problem; rather, "you have to shut, if possible, all the doors by which the vessels will grow around the tumor."

Angiogenesis inhibitors seem to work best in early stages of the disease, and they seem to stabilize tumors rather than eradicate them. They may need to be administered daily, instead of on the twice-weekly schedule used in testing thus far. Dozens of anti-angiogenetic drugs are being developed and tested and may be more effective when used in the early stages of cancer. In the meantime, "accidental" anti-angiogenetic drugs are already available and being given to some cancer patients. These drugs, which have been approved for other uses but also inhibit blood vessel growth, include thalidomide, Celebrex, Vioxx, and COX-2 inhibitors. A 2002 study suggests that herceptin, described above, may also inhibit the growth of blood vessels, and this may be contributing to its effectiveness. Interestingly, several nutrients and natural plant chemicals such as green tea, genistein (found in soy isoflavones), curcumin (found in turmeric) and n-acetyl-cysteine, also have anti-angiogenetic properties.

Complementary and Alternative Therapies

Thus far, I have discussed only the "conventional" cancer therapies that are offered by mainstream American medicine. Although some of these therapies are still experimental, their basic approach is accepted by mainstream medicine and they are being investigated under the auspices of major cancer institutions and the National Cancer Institute.

However, now that we are recognizing that conventional therapy has its limitations, particularly in the treatment of cancer, many people are becoming interested in therapies that fall outside the offerings of mainstream, or conventional medicine. Cancer patients are no exception and in fact may be at the forefront of this movement. These therapies are known collectively by many names, including alternative, unconventional, adjunctive, unorthodox, or unproven therapies. Perhaps most accurate and least pejorative is "unconventional." Unconventional therapies can be used two ways: As complementary therapy and as alternative therapy.

Certain unconventional therapies are used as *complementary* therapies, *in addition to* conventional therapy. Complementary unconventional therapies include diet, nutritional therapies, some herbs, exercise, mind-body techniques, and psychosocial support such as support groups. They have become so widespread and accepted that when used as complements to conventional cancer therapy, they are almost conventional! These are the most accepted, most available, and most compatible with conventional treatment. These are the therapies I discuss in Part Three of this book. They can be used *before, during, and after* chemotherapy to build up your strength, minimize side effects, improve your quality of life, enhance the anticancer effects of your chemotherapy regimen, help you to recuperate after therapy, and continue to support your body's own efforts to fight cancer.

As *alternative* therapies, they are generally used *instead of* conventional therapy. Many of them are also used as a last-ditch effort *after* standard or experimental treatment has failed. In addition to the therapies mentioned above, these include Emanuel Revici's method, Stanislaw Burzynski's antineoplastons, Virginia Livingston's therapy, Gerson Therapy, and Lawrence Burton's antineoplaston therapy, herbal therapies, laetrile therapy, chelation therapy, and homeopathic treatments. An explanation of these alternative therapies is beyond the scope of this book, but there are many excellent resources on this topic, and several are listed in the Resources section (Appendix B). Sometimes these anticancer therapies are used to complement conventional treatment, but generally their practitioners reject conventional cancer therapy's "cut, burn, and poison" approach as being too harsh on the body and too harmful to the very healing mechanisms they try to employ.

Combining Conventional
and Unconventional Therapies

In modern cancer care, it is becoming rare to use only one type, or modality, of treatment. Today a combination of two or more types of therapies is increasingly favored, because one enhances the effect of another or supplies a therapeutic strength where the others are weak. Though the conventional therapies—surgery, radiation, chemotherapy, immunotherapy, and the newer drugs such as anti-angiogenesis drugs—are most often combined, more and more cancer-care providers and their patients are also dipping into the pool of unconventional therapies.

And why not? It is becoming clear that all unconventional therapies cannot forever be dismissed as completely worthless in light of continuing revelations about the interrelationship of the immune system, the mind, nutrition, the environment, and cancer. As a result, some practicing oncologists are beginning to suggest—or at least not object to—a more *holistic* approach for their patients undergoing traditional therapies.

Although most oncologists are still skeptical of claims that these therapies have any anticancer effect, many are increasingly comfortable with the idea that certain unconventional therapies can make chemotherapy an easier treatment to take. Not all unconventional therapies are compatible with chemotherapy, but in general this seems to be a reasonable road to take, at least until we have more evidence that any of these alternative therapies alone can help control the disease, especially in its advanced stages.

I'm happy to report that an increasing number of researchers are interested in studying how unconventional therapies can help patients undergoing chemotherapy and in providing us with evidence that they do help. For example, a now classic study by Stanford University's David Spiegel, M.D., and colleagues looked at the effect of psychotherapy on survival time and quality of life. Patients who attended support groups lived twice as long as did those who did not. Another example exists in the growing evidence of links between cancer and nutrition and an appreciation of dietary support during chemotherapy. The National Cancer Institute is conducting major studies of the role that nutrients such as specific vitamins and minerals, fiber, and fat play in preventing, inhibiting, or developing cancer. There are already completed studies that show that certain nutritional supplements such as vitamin E protect against the damaging effects of chemotherapeutic drugs on the heart, improve energy, make chemotherapy more effective, and according to a panel of experts at a National Institutes of Health Consensus Conference in 1997, increase life span. Acupuncture can improve the immune response; reduce side effects such as nausea, vomiting, and fatigue; and increase the effectiveness of chemotherapy.

As a result of these studies, today, the best cancer centers are offering some degree of complementary medicine—they are offering patients nutrition, exercise, psychological support, and education along with chemotherapy. They may suggest acupuncture or a hands-on therapy such as massage—or even have practitioners on staff.

This is a big step in the right direction, but it is still difficult for the average cancer patient to find a holistic program. We usually have to run around and piece it together ourselves. How much better it would be if the care could be coordinated and integrated, and if medical students learned about them along with the conventional approaches they now study and practice. In fact, there is a movement afoot, spearheaded by Dr. Andrew Weil, to reform this country's medical system by integrating alternative and conventional medicine. The name of this new form of health care would be "integrative medicine." This seems to me to be a wonderful direction for medicine to go in, and patients would enjoy the best of both worlds. Sometimes this is referred to as complementary and alternative medicine (CAM).

BEING OPEN-MINDED

The overwhelming problem with unconventional therapies used as alternative therapies is that we are not sure about the possibility of benefit because by and large they have not undergone the kind of scientific support and testing that the standard and experimental mainstream-endorsed therapies have received. Unfortunately, almost all the evidence about their effectiveness is anecdotal or testimonial in nature or remains unpublished by accepted medical journals. The medical mainstream says this lack of concrete proof of efficacy is why it does not recommend these treatments to its cancer patients as primary treatments. Although the direct risk is attractively low, many doctors feel they are indirectly harmful because patients who go for alternative therapy are lured away from effective traditional treatment and possibly a cure.

Until recently, the cancer establishment had lumped all these therapies together, branded them as quackery, and dismissed them as totally worthless. To be sure, there is a lot of quackery and bad medicine out there, just as there is in conventional medicine. You want to be open-minded, but not so open-minded that your brains fall out.

But here, too, times are changing, and the federal government has taken steps to separate the wheat from the chaff. In 1990, the Office of Technology Assessment (OTA), a research arm of Congress, commissioned the evaluation of unconventional cancer treatments, and the results were published as a government report. And in 1992, the National Institutes of Health (NIH) established the Office of Alternative Medicine (OAM) to facilitate the evaluation of alternative medical treatment. In 1994, the OAM issued a report called *Alternative Medicine: Expanding Medical Horizons.* The resulting reports are available to anyone and are listed along with other excellent sources of information about unconventional therapies in the Resources section (Appendix B) of this book. The OAM has been reorganized and is now called the National Center for Complementary and Alternative Medicine (NCCAM). Instead of merely a coordinating body, it is able to initiate research studies on its own. With its new mandate, new leadership, and bigger budget, it is funding exciting research projects including a research project involving 15 cancer centers to study the impact of complementary therapies. It is also sponsoring a small but relatively long-term study of the Gonzalez regimen which uses pancreatic enzymes, coffee enemas, and dietary supplements to treat pancreatic cancer. The new director, Dr. Stephen E. Strauss, told the *Los Angeles Times* that NCCAM decided to study the Gonzalez regimen because the preliminary data suggested that it prolonged life in patients who would otherwise die of pancreatic cancer, a disease for which there is no effective standard treatment and which kills nearly 30,000 Americans each year.

We still don't have universally accepted scientifically conducted studies on which you can base an informed decision, but at least these and other more recent books shed some light and provide more evenhanded discussions. You will find clear descriptions of the most widely used therapies—what they involve, what they claim, where they are offered, whom to call, and how much they cost. You will also get guidelines for evaluating the treatment as best as you can, and you will be able to get a clearer understanding of the history and current state of the field. For the first time, you may actually be able to make an informed choice, but the choice is still a difficult one.

UNCONVENTIONAL CHOICES

If you are lucky, your oncologist will understand your dilemma and help you make the best decision for you: straight conventional treatment, chemotherapy plus complementary therapies, or alternative therapy. You will still find a great deal of resistance to alternative therapy, but many doctors are softening their stance on combining therapies.

Michael Van Scoy-Mosher, M.D., says that when patients come to him to discuss unconventional treatments:

> I don't belittle their beliefs—people who explore these therapies tend to be intelligent. If a person wants to do it instead of conventional treatment, but conventional treatment has a lot to offer, I would try to talk her out of it. If conventional treatment has little to offer, I wouldn't take much of a stand. However, I do feel I owe people my honest opinion about these treatments. If she wants to do it in addition to conventional treatment, I would tend to support that because these treatments are relatively nontoxic and if a person believes in it, it helps increase their sense of empowerment and to that extent they are useful.

Michael Lerner, Ph.D., has studied unconventional cancer treatments since 1981, when his father was diagnosed with a life-threatening cancer. He subsequently served as special consultant for the OTA report *Unconventional Cancer Treatments*. He has also written his own thoroughly researched, evenhanded, well-respected book on the subject, *Choices in Healing*. Here's what this leading authority on the objective evaluation of these therapies has to say:

> People ask me, as someone who has studied unconventional cancer therapies, what to do. First, I never recommend therapies to anyone

because I am not a physician. Second, the question is very difficult to answer even at a general level because there are so few scientific studies available assessing most of these unconventional therapies. Third, as a general rule, I believe that the open and intrinsically health-promoting spiritual, psychological, nutritional, and physical therapies, undertaken in a balanced way with appropriate professional guidance, can be sensible adjuncts to appropriate mainstream therapies in enhancing health and quality of life. On the other hand, my father never used any of the unconventional therapies that I researched, and he has done exceptionally well with mainstream therapies alone.

What my whole experience has taught me is that unconventional therapies are not appropriate for everybody with cancer. In fact, I think they are really appropriate only for a minority. Unconventional cancer therapies can be considered most appropriate for cancer patients who are strongly drawn to them, who are inclined to believe in them, who want to be engaged actively in their own treatment, and who have the good sense to integrate the best of these therapies with the best mainstream medicine. At the same time, I usually suggest that cancer patients who are not drawn to unconventional treatments can comfortably put them aside. Until there is robust scientific evidence of real benefit from any therapy, alternative or mainstream, no patient should be pushed in the direction of therapies that have not proved themselves.

You may find it helpful to discuss the issue with a knowledgeable professional. For example, Michael Lerner is the president of an organization called Commonweal, a health and environmental research institute. Located in California, Commonweal offers weeklong retreats designed especially to help people with cancer think through treatment options and make informed, considered decisions. However, only a few of us live in California, and I hope that you will find guidance closer to home. Even if your oncologist doesn't "believe" in alternative therapies, he or she should at least try to answer any questions you may have and be willing to discuss the issue calmly. Your oncology nurse, the social service department, and the dietary department of your hospital are other potential sources for information.

Although it is a subject that is being brought up increasingly frequently, some patients may still be afraid to bring up unconventional therapies with their conventional health-care practitioners. It is, however, part of their job to be informed and to help you become informed in order to make an intelligent decision—one that is right for you. And it is your right and responsibility to still any doubts you might have about your therapy. Many people find it excruciatingly difficult to decide between following a conventional or unconventional therapy. Using both approaches—simultaneously or sequentially—enables you to enjoy the benefits of both and spares you the agony of making an either/or decision. If you would prefer to use an alternative therapy but your cancer is so far advanced that alternative therapies may not be powerful enough, David Bognar, in his book, *Cancer: Increasing Your Odds for Survival*, suggests that you "consider that one of the benefits of conventional treatment is that it can cause tumor regression and may even put the cancer in remission, buying you valuable time. This time can then be used for following up with other treatment modalities and complementary therapies." This is essentially the approach I took, as I discuss in more detail in Chapter 13. However, people often turn to alternative therapies once they are told that they cannot be helped with conventional treatment.

Perhaps the most persuasive argument for opening up the traditional treatment plan to some elements of the alternative therapies does not rest directly on any claims about their possible anticancer abilities. It lies rather in the fact that some of these practices do foster better overall health, help minimize the side effects of cancer and chemotherapy, and allow patients to participate more actively in their treatment and assume some control over some aspects of their lives. In a medical world where generally we passively wait around for people in white coats to pump us full of toxic chemicals, doing health-building things for ourselves, preferably under the guidance of a qualified but accessible professional, is a welcome change.

In contrast to surgery, radiation, chemotherapy, and current immunologic approaches, which have side effects because they harm normal tissue, alternative therapies are usually nontoxic and noninvasive and do not endanger normal tissue. This, combined with their strong holistic philosophy, makes this approach immensely appealing.

Even Barrie R. Cassileth, Ph.D., of the University of Pennsylvania Cancer Center, who is no advocate of unconventional therapies, understands their value and appeal. In the June 17, 1982, issue of the *New England Journal of Medicine*, she wrote to her colleagues:

> *The anti-medicine, pro–self-help bias of the new alternative treatments arises in the context of increasing mistrust and dissatisfaction with the standard health-care system and with researchers' failure to cure malignant disease. Traditional multimodality care of cancer, often fragmented and associated with a passive role for the patient, contrasts starkly with the active, personalized, nontoxic, home-based alternatives. . . . There is something to be learned from the seductive draw of alternative remedies. We may not wish to recommend wheatgrass therapy or spiritual healing in lieu of chemotherapy, but we might well consider the merits of patients' needs for involvement in their own care, their interest in helping themselves through attention to diet, their requirements for personalized attention to self as opposed to disease.*

Clearly, there is no single "magic bullet" against cancer as yet, and the best approach seems to be an intelligently designed eclectic one.

CHAPTER THREE

Understanding Chemotherapy

Cancer chemotherapy is part of a long medical tradition of using chemical compounds to treat disease. From natural herbs to sophisticated synthetic substances, effective medicines were usually discovered accidentally, and chemotherapy is no exception.

The lucky accident that made modern cancer chemotherapy possible occurred in 1942, ironically as a result of a war in which millions of people were killed. In that year, a United States naval vessel sank while in the harbor at Naples and the containers of mustard gas it was carrying exploded. When the victims who had been exposed to the poisonous gas were examined, it was found that large numbers of the cells in their bone marrow had disappeared and that their lymphatic systems had atrophied. The significance of this was not lost on C. P. "Dusty" Rhodes, the chief of the biological branch of the U.S. Army Chemical Warfare Service, who was on leave from Memorial Hospital Cancer Center, where he was the director. He began large-scale testing on animals of hundreds of drugs similar to the poisonous gas that went down with the ship. These drugs were found to inhibit lymphoid tumors in the animals. The drugs were tested on humans with Hodgkin's disease in 1943, and the subjects experienced temporary remissions.

Around the same time that the beneficial effects of nitrogen mustard

(mustard gas) were so serendipitously discovered, scientists began to realize they had reached an impasse in cancer treatment. Surgery and radiation were local treatments, inappropriate for systemic, disseminated cancers of the blood and lymph systems and ineffective once solid tumors had visibly spread. But more frustrating was the fact that these treatments didn't always cure what appeared to be localized cancer. Scientists theorized, and proved in experiments, that even one or a few surviving cancer cells could result in a recurrence.

Because the preliminary results of the early cancer drugs were so promising, a large-scale search for other drugs that were effective against cancer was begun. In 1955, the National Cancer Institute, an arm of the National Institutes of Health, directed a mammoth screening program. Investigators in England, continental Europe, and Japan participated. Hundreds of thousands of drugs were tested—40,000 (the all-time high) in 1975 alone. This screening continues today, albeit on a more organized, and smaller scale, and eventually the drugs are tested in clinical trials (see "Experimental Chemotherapy" on page 83).

How Chemotherapy Works

Chemotherapy is the only scientifically proven method we have that can reach virtually every part of the body to seek and destroy cancer cells that surgery and radiation can't reach and that even sensitive instruments can't see. Theoretically, it is able to penetrate every nook and cranny because it circulates throughout the body just the way cancer cells do—by flowing through the bloodstream. Once the drug meets up with a cancer cell, it wreaks havoc in a number of ways, which are only partly understood.

Chemotherapy affects the course of cancer by taking advantage of the cancer cell's penchant for constant reproduction. Almost all the drugs used in chemotherapy suppress cancer by somehow altering the cells' ability to reproduce. Since cells are most vulnerable to drug interference during the reproductive phases of the life cycle, cancer cells are more likely to be affected than are the bulk of the body's normal cells, which reproduce at a much more relaxed pace. Thus, the very characteristic that makes cancer so dangerous has proved to contribute to its undoing. In scientific terminology, chemotherapy drugs are either "cell-cycle-specific" (lethal to cells only during a specific reproductive phase) or "cell-cycle-nonspecific" (able to sabotage the cells no matter what phase they are in). Oncologist Ron Bash explains it this way: "In a sense, the inner workings of cells (cancerous and otherwise) are like gearboxes; what chemotherapy does is throw a biochemical monkey wrench into the gearbox causing the machine to grind to a halt—causing the cells to stop working, to die."

When Chemotherapy May Not Work

If chemotherapy works at all, you might wonder why it doesn't work all the time. No medicines, not even those for minor ailments, work all the time. Though cancer is admittedly far more complex than athlete's foot, pimples, and headaches; it may be a bit unrealistic to expect a science that has failed to produce surefire cures for these relatively simple conditions to be able consistently to crack a sophisticated disease like cancer. Since cancer is not a foreign invader like bacteria but an aberration of the body's own cells, it is amazing that anticancer drugs work at all.

The reasons chemotherapy may fail are legion. First of all, there may simply be too many cancer cells growing too rapidly for the drugs to wipe out or even keep at bay. If the goal is to cure, every single cancer cell must die. If even one cell is left behind and manages to proliferate, the cancer will recur.

Chemotherapy may fail because it works best when (1) there are small numbers of cancer cells and (2) they are actively dividing. These conditions are not always present when chemotherapy is given. In experiments, it has been shown that drugs destroy a constant percentage of cells, not a constant number. So if there are 10 trillion cancer cells and 99 percent are killed, 100 billion are still left after the first treatment! After the second treatment, 1 billion cells are left, and after the third, 10 million remain. The proportion of cells killed is the same, but each time a smaller number of cells are killed. The cells that are resting rather than actively reproducing escape the drugs' killing effects. In between treatments, when it is safe, the resting cells resume production and replace the ones that have been killed. Chemotherapy under the best of conditions is a matter of taking two steps forward and one step back, and it is very difficult to make enough progress to kill off every single cell.

Kinetic studies have also shown that as the cancer increases in size— the more cells it contains—the number of actively reproducing cells (the "growth fraction") decreases. The higher the number you start with, the harder and longer you have to work at getting the cell population down, because not only are there more cells to kill, there are more cells that are not vulnerable.

In addition, the tumor cells may not be getting enough of the drug to affect them. Once a drug is injected or ingested, it becomes extremely diluted and weak because it is distributed throughout the bloodstream and the tissues of the body. If a tumor does not have a robust blood supply, the drugs may not reach the cells. In addition, it has been problematic getting drugs at all to the brain and central nervous system because there is a natural protective mechanism called the blood-brain barrier, which prevents drugs from passing through, though there are now ways of getting around this.

Time works against chemotherapy. The body quickly begins to break down toxic substances such as chemotherapy drugs into less harmful substances—another protective mechanism—and then excretes them. Cancer cells and normal cells alike can therefore be exposed to the drugs for just a minimum amount of time. Since many drugs work on cells only during a specific phase of the reproductive cycle, only cells that happen to be in the vulnerable phase will be affected during the time that the drug is viable. Cells in other cycles escape unscathed.

Because the drugs are also highly toxic to normal cells, we are limited in the amounts of the drugs we can tolerate—chemotherapy drugs are said to have a low "therapeutic index." The difference in the amount needed to kill more cancer cells than healthy cells is low; sometimes it is zero. Many promising drugs never get off the drawing board because the amount that would totally wipe out a tumor would also kill the patient.

Another reason chemotherapy may fail is the possibility of drug resistance. A single tumor is usually heterogeneous (composed of a mixture of different cells). Each type of cell varies in its ability to metastasize, its susceptibility to drugs, and its other properties. It is thought that the older a tumor is, the more likely it is to be heterogeneous, thus increasing the probability that some of the cells will be resistant to drugs. In addition, resistance develops as the treatment progresses, just as insects, bacteria, and other unwanted creatures adapt and become less sensitive to pesticides and antibiotics. Eventually all the sensitive cells may be killed, but the sturdy ones remain and continue to grow. There is chilling evidence that indicates that the very things that kill most patients—metastases—do not arise from the random survival of cells released from the primary tumor, as was previously thought. Rather, they are growths of special tumor cells that are particularly heterogeneous, clever, and resistant to the body's own defenses as well as to drugs. It is as if the parent tumor sent its brightest, most athletic children out into the world of the cancer patient's body.

These are the main reasons why chemotherapy is more effective the earlier it is used and after the bulk of the tumor has been reduced by surgery or radiation. They help explain why chemotherapy doesn't always work and why it sometimes works only a little bit, for a little while.

Getting Chemotherapy to Work Better

Researchers have been experimenting with ways to get around the above-mentioned roadblocks and make chemotherapy more effective. Of course, new drugs are always being developed and tested, but drugs already in use could be used differently to squeeze out additional benefit.

One trend is to give more intense doses, but over a shorter period. This may prove to be at least as effective as conventional doses and scheduling but ultimately less toxic to the patient as well as less life-disrupting because of the shortened duration of the therapy.

Another technique is to infuse the drugs continuously at a lower intensity over a longer period of time. With the development of portable pumps, chemotherapy can be administered round the clock, maintaining effective levels of the drug in the blood. This approach offers the possibility that more cancer cells will be killed while reducing the toxicity and avoiding the necessity of long stays in the hospital.

ADMINISTRATION ACCORDING TO CHRONOBIOLOGY

A very exciting approach is based on the principle of *chronobiology*, the study of body cycles that govern our susceptibility to disease and our response to medications. According to oncologist Dr. William Hrushesky, a major proponent and researcher of this approach to cancer treatment, studies have shown that the toxicity and effectiveness of many chemotherapy drugs depend on the time of administration. This effect has been documented for dozens of drugs, and this information is available to any oncologist or cancer patient (see "Timing as a Factor" on page 44). Needless to say, timing can, therefore, have a significant impact on your quality of life and perhaps your prognosis. The problem is hospitals and oncology offices are not set up to treat patients at all hours of the day and night. However, there are portable drug infusion pumps that can be programmed to release chemotherapy drugs, antinausea drugs, and other medications at specific times in specific amounts. Although its use is still uncommon, it is definitely feasible to take advantage of what we know about chronobiology to deliver your particular therapy at the optimum time.

By the way, chronobiology may also change the way breast cancer surgery is done in premenopausal women. Several studies show that breast cancer is less likely to spread and kill when the tumor is removed at a certain time in the menstrual cycle. One study found that premenopausal women who received mastectomies around the time of menstruation had four times the risk of recurrence and death compared with women who were operated on during the middle of the menstrual cycle. Another study found that survival increased from 54 percent to 84 percent when surgery was timed according to the menstrual cycle. This represents a doubling or quadrupling of the ten-year survival rate, simply by paying attention to a woman's body rhythms and scheduling surgery accordingly.

TIMING AS A FACTOR

For information about how the timing of breast cancer surgery can influence prognosis and how chemotherapy treatment can influence the effectiveness and toxicity of chemotherapy drugs, refer to the following sources of information.

- *Circadian Cancer Therapy* by William Hrushesky, M.D. (Boca Raton, FL: CRC Press, 1994).
- "The Application of Circadian Chronobiology to Cancer Treatment" in *Cancer: Principles and Practice of Oncology* edited by Vincent DeVita, Jr., et al. (Philadelphia: Lippincott, 1992).
- "Breast Cancer, Timing of Surgery, and the Menstrual Cycle: Call for a Prospective Trial," by William Hrushesky, M.D., *Journal of Women's Health* 5, no. 6 (Nov. 6, 1996): 555–66.
- William Hrushesky, M.D., VA Medical Center Oncology Department, 113 Holland Avenue, Albany, NY 12208, 518-462-3311, ext. 2792, rpi.edu/~hrushw

HYPERTHERMIA

Hyperthermia is an approach that is based on the theory that fever—that is, heat—is a key element in our biological defense against disease. Laboratory tests have shown that heat can stimulate the white blood cells in the immune system to attack cancer cells, but hyperthermia has been disappointing when used alone. However, it seems that heat also sensitizes cancer cells and makes them more vulnerable to radiation and some forms of chemotherapy, so combining it with these therapies may increase their effectiveness without increasing toxicity. Research is ongoing using hyperthermia devices that heat just the tumor, the region of the body in which the tumor exists, and the whole body.

Another use of heat combined with chemotherapy is called *hyperthermic perfusion.* It involves isolating the circulatory system of an arm or a leg that has a tumor and infusing the limb with a heated chemotherapy solution. Much higher doses of cancer-killing drugs can be given this way, directly to the tumor and to sites where the cancer is most likely to spread, without exposing the rest of the body to the toxic effects of the drug.

Hyperthermia is much more widely used in Europe and Japan than in the United States, where only a handful of cancer centers are doing it. One of them is Duke University, in Durham, North Carolina, where it has been used along with chemo and radiation for ovarian, breast, rectal, and prostate cancer. Duke's Ellen Jones, a radiation oncologist, says they are "very encouraged" with their preliminary results.

Other methods being used experimentally include administering drugs through specific body cavities where tumors occur, and *chemoembolization,* which enables larger doses of the drug to be delivered directly to the tumor and block the tumor's blood supply at the same time.

INCREASING THE DOSAGE

Another way doctors try to get more out of chemotherapy is based on the theory that if a little bit of a drug is good, then more is better. Researchers are pushing the doses of anticancer drugs as close to the edge as possible. They then "rescue" the patient from potentially fatal side effects by either bringing back injured cells or stopping the side effect from happening. For example, Leucovorin is a drug used to block the toxicity of high doses of the chemotherapeutic drug methotrexate. An exciting development in colorectal cancer was the discovery that the immune-stimulating drug levamisole increases the effect of the anticancer drug 5-FU.

The bone marrow, where blood cells are made, is usually the tissue that is most sensitive to chemo. Damaged bone marrow leaves you susceptible to infections, which can be fatal, and to anemia and problems with blood clotting. This limits the doses that can be given and therefore has been a major obstacle to administering high-dose chemo. However, there are now biological substances that help counteract bone marrow damage. When the number of your white blood cells dip too low, your doctor may prescribe colony-stimulating factors (CSFs) to help raise them. When your red blood cells dip too low, you may get erythropoietin (Procrit), another biological material that stimulates your body to produce more red blood cells. This addresses the issue of bone marrow suppression, but does not help with other side effects such as nausea and vomiting, heart damage, and hair loss. Using liposomes (artificial microscopic "fat bubbles") to deliver chemo drugs may help reduce these effects of toxicity as well. These microscopic capsules carry drugs targeted to the tumor, and provide sustained drug levels with less harm to the normal tissues.

Bone marrow transplantation (BMT) provides a dramatic avenue for pushing the dose of chemotherapy very high (five to twenty times higher than conventional doses). After chemo, the treatment team replaces the patient's wiped-out bone marrow with previously harvested marrow. As a result, the immune system cells have a chance to regenerate, and the very high risk of a potentially fatal infection is lowered.

Traditionally, a patient's marrow has been replaced with healthy marrow from a parent or sibling, or an unrelated person. The danger here is that the marrow will be rejected as foreign. As an alternative, the marrow can come from the patient (autologous transplant), but the marrow must be purged of cancer cells as much as possible, or you run the risk of reseeding the cancer. As such, this procedure is rarely done because it is very risky. Recently, stem cells, which circulate in the blood and become mature blood cells with time, have become an alternative to bone-marrow harvesting. The cells are harvested from the blood and reinjected into the blood vessels. Rescue with stem cells is much less painful, requires no hospitalization or anesthesia, and reduces the likelihood of harvesting unhealthy cancer cells along with the healthy blood cells.

BMT is a grueling, dangerous, expensive experience for patient and family alike, but offers the best—or only—hope for some people. This intense form of therapy is fairly standard for some types of leukemia, multiple myeloma, non-Hodgkin's lymphoma, and Hodgkin's disease. It is very controversial for use for other cancers such as breast cancer. For more information, see *Survivor's Guide to a Bone Marrow Transplant* by Keren

Stronach, or contact the National Bone Marrow Transplant Link (1-800-LINK-BMT, or http://comnet.org/nbmtlink).

LOW-DOSE CHEMOTHERAPY

At the other end of the spectrum is low-dose chemotherapy. An increasing number of oncologists and alternative practitioners are suggesting that in some cases "less is more." This approach consists of administering diluted, weakened, or otherwise attenuated doses of chemotherapy, sometimes slowly, over an extended period. The theory is that this kinder, gentler form of chemotherapy may still kill, or at least control, cancer cells, but without wreaking as much havoc on the healthy tissues of the body.

There are oncologists in the United States and in other parts of the world, such as England and Germany, who for many years have been experimenting with low-dose chemotherapy, often combined with natural substances that protect tissues or with hyperthermia, and even with chemotherapy prepared according to homeopathic methods. Burton Goldberg, editor, and the authors of the comprehensive book *An Alternative Medicine Definitive Guide to Cancer* feature several physicians, including oncologists, who offer low-dose chemotherapy. In their book they write, "Low-dose chemotherapy is preferable to what is presently regarded as today's normal dose, and can have a place when used with alternative modalities in the hands of an experienced physician. What needs to be strongly challenged is the prevailing concept that *only* chemotherapy in full strength is a viable way to treat cancer."

This approach is treading a fine line between conventional and unconventional medicine in that doctors are using conventional medicine in an unconventional manner, as the mainstream view is that "more is better."

That may be about to change because new studies show that there is something to this approach. Low-dose chemotherapy has been around in some form for a long time—the first studies I'm aware of go back to the early 1970s. It seems to have had its adherents all along, even among mainstream physicians who reserved it for certain special cases, particularly in people for whom all else had failed. But the success of this strategy has always been puzzling: Why should a tumor that remains unmoved by massive doses of chemotherapy suddenly start to shrink when the patient gets lower doses?

The effectiveness of low-dose chemo may finally have an explanation, and this approach may finally come into its own, thanks to recent research. It has long been known that chemotherapy alone given at lower doses may work where higher doses have not—this gives patients added time, but eventually the tumors return and regrow and the patients die. However, the new studies have added a new ingredient and have shown that low-dose chemotherapy is much more effective when given on a continuous basis along with drugs that inhibit the growth of blood vessels that feed the cancer. It is well known that tumors build their own network of blood vessels, and without these blood vessels, they would starve. This process of forming new blood vessels is called *angiogenesis*. There are drugs that are known to be angiogenesis inhibitors (anti-angiogenetic drugs are being tested alone as anticancer treatment; see "The New Wave of Anticancer Drugs" on page 25).

Dr. Judah Folkman, the "father" of anti-angiogenesis, and colleague Dr. Timothy Brower have a theory for why this regimen works. Traditional chemotherapeutic drugs not only stop cancer cells from dividing and multiplying—the drugs also affect the endothelial cells that line the blood vessels that feed the cancer. The reason that tumors continue to grow on standard chemo doses is that the endothelial cells regrow during the rest periods needed to allow the patient to recover from the toxic effects caused by the large doses of chemo. But, if you lower the dose of chemotherapy, you can give it more frequently because there are fewer side effects. Because there are fewer side effects, you don't need rest periods. Under this gentle but constant bombardment, blood vessels whither and die, and the cancer starves. The endothelial cells do not grow resistant to the chemotherapy because they are normal cells that are stable and do not mutate. However, even then, chemo alone doesn't stop the cancer from growing—it needs the one-two punch of low-dose chemotherapy plus a drug that specifically inhibits blood vessel growth.

This strategy represents a totally new approach to cancer treatment.

Instead of targeting tumor cells directly, this strategy strangles the blood vessels that nourish them. This paradigm shift, in the words of one researcher, "would convert cancer to a chronic, non-life-threatening disease." Dubbed "metronomic therapy" (similar to the constant pulse of the device that keeps musicians on the beat), the drugs are given frequently—perhaps twice a week or even every day, rather than once every three weeks or so. In a variation called "sequential low-dose chemotherapy," different chemotherapy drugs are rotated because evidence suggests that changing chemo drugs every two or three weeks is more effective. Low-dose chemotherapy combined with anti-angiogenetic drugs has brought about dramatic results in laboratory mice and in several human studies. Studies have been conducted at major cancer centers in Canada, Italy and the United States, including Memorial Sloan-Kettering in New York and MD Anderson Cancer Center in Texas—and more are planned or are already underway.

In studies at these and other centers, this approach has shrunk or stabilized tumors in up to 75 percent of women with breast cancer, 60 percent of patients with lung cancer, and 30 percent of women with ovarian cancer. In a study at the European Institute of Oncology in Milan, of women with advanced breast cancer, tumors shrank by more than half in one-third of the patients and remained stable in another 20 percent. In two of the women, tumors disappeared completely. Immediate side effects have been minimal, but researchers are still cautious because no one knows whether there might be toxic effects down the line. And we don't know how long the regression will last. However, because the therapy uses existing chemotherapy drugs coupled with drugs already "on the shelf" that inhibit blood vessel growth (including interferon alpha and thalidomide), doctors are already treating patients outside of clinical trials and without waiting for the results of additional studies.

CHEMOSENSITIVITY ASSAYS

Your oncologist might tell you that a certain drug regimen got a 50-percent response rate. How do you know that your tumor will be in that 50 percent? Well, until recently, you didn't know until after taking the drug and monitoring its results. Now there are tests called *chemosensitivity assays* commercially available, and more are being developed. These tests can help determine which drugs your tumor is likely to be sensitive to, and which they are likely to be resistant to. Many doctors dismiss these tests because when they first were available, they were quite inaccurate. However, they have improved immensely and today the best tests can predict with 75- to 90-percent accuracy which tumors are sensitive and which are resistant to any particular drug.

However, if you want a chemosensitivity assay, you must plan ahead. Most hospital labs are not equipped to do the testing—it must be sent to a special lab. Your surgical team needs to be prepared to send an adequate amount of your tumor to the lab, and it needs to be fresh—not frozen, as is the norm—and delivered in a special package to the assay lab. The lab grows the cancer cells in test tubes and then pretests the drugs by applying them to the different groups of cells. The drugs that are more effective against the samples are used to design the best treatment. It is hoped that tailoring techniques will take some of the guesswork out of chemotherapy, thus saving valuable time and needless wear and tear on the patient. Results take about seven to nine days and cost several thousand dollars. Some labs, such as Rational Therapeutics (see the inset "Chemosensitivity Assay Labs" on page 52) will also test for other substances such as botanicals that potentially could kill cancer cells. Other techniques, such as darkfield microscopy of live blood and electrodermal screening (EDS) may also be used to take some of the guesswork out of chemotherapy. These tests help the physician assess whether chemotherapy is advisable or appropriate in your case. For information about EDS, see the book *An Alternative Medicine Definitive Guide to Cancer,* edited by Burton Goldberg, or call Computronix Electro-Medical Systems at 817-241-2768.

Why isn't every cancer patient and oncologist beating a path to these labs? Well, for one thing, responses in test tubes do not necessarily correlate well with responses in humans. Often, there is only one standard therapy for cancer during the first time it is treated with chemotherapy. That's why Dr. Richard Cohen and many other oncologists feel that tailoring the treatment this way is best saved for people who have had chemotherapy and want to know what other drugs might be useful if the tumor recurs or breaks through in the future. Once cancer recurs, there are usually several choices for second-line treatment.

Also, as of this writing. Medicare and most managed-care plans do not pay for the cost of chemosensitivity tests. Some indemnity insurance companies may pay for part or all of these services. However, at the end of 2000, the tests received a major boost, the impact of which remains to be seen. A Medicare Coverage Advisory Committee concluded that the tests "can aid physicians in deciding which chemotherapies work best in battling an individual patient's form of cancer." The panel's recommendations are being taken into account in developing national coverage policies for the tests, which are currently not covered by Medicare.

OTHER WAYS OF TAILORING YOUR THERAPY

Another way to tailor the therapy is to test the tumor for biomarkers and other characteristics that predict whether the cancer is likely to spread. For example, only 20 to 30 percent of women with small tumors and no positive lymph nodes will see their cancer spread. The standard "yardsticks" for measuring risk—tumor size, tumor grade, and the presence of estrogen receptors—are not sufficiently sensitive tools for assessing their risk. So doctors usually recommend that all women with this diagnosis get chemotherapy—even though up to 80 percent of them won't need it. Researchers from the Chicago Medical Center set to work to solve this problem, and they recently reported that low levels of a certain protein appear to be the single most effective factor for predicting which patients with early breast cancer will need chemotherapy following surgery. According to one of the researchers, this information, along with certain other tumor characteristics, should allow physicians to tailor the therapy to the individual and better predict which women can most safely avoid chemotherapy, while allowing them to increase the intensity of the therapy for women at high risk for metastases.

Another finding is that women with mutations in the BRCA1 gene are more sensitive to certain forms of treatment and resistant to other agents,

CHEMOSENSITIVITY ASSAY LABS

For more information about pretesting chemotherapy drugs before beginning treatment, contact:

Oncotech, Incorporated
15501 Red Hill Avenue
Tustin, CA 92780
714-566-0420
http://www.oncotech.com/

Rational Therapeutics
750 East 29th Street
Long Beach, CA 90806
562-989-6455
http://www.rational-t.com/

Weisenthal Cancer Group
15140 Transistor Lane
Huntington Beach, CA 92649
714-894-0011
http://weisenthal.org/

such as the newly approved drugs paclitaxel (Taxol) and docetaxel. In the future, genetic profiling of patients and their tumors may help individualize therapy in ways we can only dream of.

Still another attempt to tailor treatment and reduce adverse effects is being tried with breast cancer patients. "Sentinel node mapping" is a procedure that allows doctors to evaluate lymph node status by removing and examining one key lymph node. This node, the first draining node, is believed to indicate the status of the remainder of the lymph nodes in the axilla (armpit). The breast tissue surrounding the tumor is injected with a small amount of radioactive material and the radioactive material migrates to the sentinel node, allowing doctors to locate it with a Geiger Counter. The key node is identified and removed surgically and evaluated by the pathologist. If it is found to be negative, no further surgery is required. This not only results in less radical surgery but in some women may be used to determine whether they should have chemotherapy. This technique is currently being performed on selected patients at centers around the country.

CHAPTER FOUR

Getting
the Best Care

It is a rare cancer patient who doesn't panic after the initial diagnosis, who can think clearly and doesn't feel rushed into treatment, who feels well enough to be able to explore treatment possibilities. It is natural to feel overwhelmed and to want to trust and rely on the first doctor you see. But in most cases of cancer, it is not dangerous to take a few weeks to digest the new earth-shattering information. On the contrary, since the quality of chemotherapy varies so greatly, it is wise to take steps to ensure that you get the correct diagnosis and the best treatment. The quality and quantity of your life depend on it. A little effort now can make a big difference later on. But you don't need to make these decisions alone.

In her book *Women's Cancers,* Kerry McGinn, a nurse who was diagnosed with cancer, acknowledges that it takes a team effort to battle cancer. As she notes, in addition to your doctor and nurses, technicians and technologists draw blood and administer imaging tests and radiation therapy. Depending on your needs, there also may be physical therapists, a dietitian, a respiratory therapist, a social worker, office staff, a chaplain, and a mental-health professional, plus complementary therapy professionals, family, friends, and coworkers. McGinn says she felt "shell-shocked" after her diagnosis—vulnerable and overwhelmed. But gathering her get-well team helped her regather her own strength and sense of control. "We were not perfect, any of us," she writes. "We made mistakes, sometimes, failed to communicate, had bad days, or stepped on each other's toes. But at the same time, each person contributed something valuable—the will to get through this, specific chemotherapy drugs, or a care package of paperback mysteries sent with love. Woven together, these strands became far stronger than each alone. A rope? A safety net? A tapestry? . . . A team."

The single most important step you can take is to see at least one qualified cancer specialist and make him or her your main team member. Only a cancer specialist can give you a firm, detailed diagnosis and a clear picture of your options. Once you have accomplished this, you are in a position to evaluate the doctor(s) and treatment(s) and choose whichever suit you individually.

Why a Cancer Specialist?

Most often, suspicion of cancer or the initial diagnosis comes from a family doctor or a specialist in the area in which symptoms are first noted, such as a gynecologist for a breast lump or a urologist for a testicular or prostate problem. These physicians may be very qualified in their particular fields and may have treated cancer years ago. However, in most cases, they are not the best qualified to treat cancer today. Because cancer diagnosis and treatment have become so complex, a special branch of medicine called *oncology* has evolved. Oncology (from the Greek *onkos,* meaning "lump" and *logos,* meaning "study") is a branch of medicine that deals specifically with the study of tumors. A doctor who is specially trained in this field is called an *oncologist.*

Today there are surgical oncologists, radiation oncologists, and medical oncologists (chemotherapists), any and all of whom may be on your treatment team and involved in your overall treatment plan. Oncologists usually refer patients to their colleagues in the other subspecialities when they feel a multidisciplinary approach would be beneficial. For instance, a surgical oncologist may refer a patient to a medical oncologist for chemotherapy. My own experience followed this familiar pattern: My gynecologist examined my breast lump and sent me to a surgical oncologist who specialized in treating breast disease; my surgeon then suggested that I see a medical oncologist for further treatment.

Whereas your primary concern is your chemotherapist, it is to your advantage if all the members of your treatment team are well qualified. The best oncologists are usually board-eligible or board-certified, meaning they have been formally trained in this subspecialty and, if certified, have passed an exam.

Your surgeon, therefore, should be board-certified and should specialize in your type of cancer. If radiotherapy is on the agenda, you should go to a board-certified radiation oncologist rather than to a radiologist whose training is mostly in diagnosis.

And anyone who has been told that he or she needs chemotherapy should be seen by a board-certified or board-eligible medical oncologist who has received two years of formal training in the use of chemotherapeutic drugs.

Hematologists—internists with special training in the area of blood— were the first to use chemotherapy because the earliest cancers treated with drugs were the "blood cancers." Board-certified or board-eligible hematologists with training and experience in cancer still treat the disease. Though they may continue to confine themselves to blood cancers (leukemias, lymphomas, and myelomas), many also treat other cancers. More recently, board-certified internists who are not hematologists have begun specializing in chemotherapy.

I cannot overemphasize how important it is that you see at least one qualified medical oncologist. Chemotherapeutic drugs are highly toxic, and the treatment can be very complex. Their use changes rapidly, and the prescribing doctor not only must know of their availability but also must know how to use them and how to monitor you properly to achieve the ultimate therapeutic effect without severe toxicity. Only a physician who specializes in the use of these drugs is qualified to evaluate a cancer, to choose a chemotherapy protocol, and in most cases to administer or supervise the administration of the drugs. If you like, you can still be seen by your primary physician during your cancer treatment and sometimes even receive some portion of your treatment from him, provided that it is under the guidance of an oncologist.

Where to Find an Oncologist

Comprehensive cancer centers, university hospitals, large medical centers, clinics, community hospitals, and oncologists in private practice all offer chemotherapy. If your primary physician has not referred you to an oncologist, ask him or her for a recommendation or locate a cancer specialist through another doctor you know, your friends or relatives, your local county medical society, the nursing department at a local teaching hospital, the National Cancer Institute (NCI), or the American Cancer Society. You can also contact a hospital directly.

In deciding which of these facilities is best for you, getting the best *treatment* should not be confused with getting the best overall *care;* it is possible to get the most effective, up-to-date technical treatment while other needs go unheeded or unfulfilled. For example, some believe a big cancer center is the place for the seriously ill, but others argue eloquently that these are the very people who should stay closer to home and family. You will need to consider medical, practical, and personal factors. Ask yourself:

- Which offers the most effective program?
- How far am I willing to travel for treatment?
- Will my medical insurance cover the cost? If so, how much? If not, how much can I pay? Am I willing to pay extra to be treated by a doctor who is not enrolled in my medical plan?
- Do I like the environment?
- Do I have a good relationship with the doctor?

The effectiveness of the treatments, the personalities of the doctors, the surroundings in which the treatment is administered, and the cost can and do vary greatly. So does the distance you can travel—be it within your own town, to the next city, or all the way to another state. Fortunately, most chemotherapy is given on an outpatient basis—only the heaviest doses of the most toxic drugs and some highly experimental treatments require hospitalization.

It is a common prejudice that the best place to go for cancer treatment is a big cancer center or university hospital. That is where the famous cancer specialists are, where the most modern technology is available, and where the latest experimental therapies are developed and administered. Yet few people understand what they are or what they have to offer. "Comprehensive cancer center" is a special designation given by the National Cancer Institute to cancer centers that have met certain strict, specific criteria. "Clinical cancer centers" are similar to comprehensive cancer centers in many ways, but they do not have the same status. You can find the centers closest to you by contacting the Cancer Information Service at 1-800-4-CANCER or the National Cancer Institute at www.nci.nih.gov.

At one time, cancer centers *did* offer the very best cancer treatment across the board. However, this is no longer necessarily true. Most cancer patients can get just as good chemotherapy—even investigational drugs—much closer to home. The comprehensive cancer centers are the first to admit this. One of the staff members at Memorial Sloan-Kettering, one of the best-known cancer centers, notes that:

> *Hundreds of physicians pass through cancer centers like Memorial each year to train in oncology and then go out all over the country. We screen patients who call to determine whether they really need to come here or can be diagnosed and treated closer to home. Patients may come in for a diagnosis and we may develop and assign a chemotherapy protocol, but then we try to make every effort to locate local physicians and facilities where they can get high-quality treatment.*

A physician at Memorial says, "People who should come into a cancer center are people with unusual diseases, or people who need a treatment that cannot be offered at another facility."

Cancer centers have physicians and teams who subspecialize in particular cancers. In certain cases, it may be wise for you to contact a cancer center to confirm a complicated diagnosis or to get a second opinion about the treatment of choice.

It might also be advantageous for you to begin your treatment at a cancer center, particularly if you require specialized surgery, radiation, or treatment with technical equipment not available at your local hospital. If you have an unusual or difficult cancer and the standard or the locally available investigational treatment leaves much to be desired, it may definitely be worthwhile for you to travel to see highly experienced specialists.

Dr. Thomas Fahey of Memorial Sloan-Kettering in New York City uses breast cancer as an example. The consensus recommendation from the NCI is that patents whose lymph nodes test positive and *most* patients with negative lymph nodes should receive adjuvant chemo. But only 30 percent of node-negative women will relapse. What's needed is to determine who that 30 percent will be. Some factors, such as the size and location of a tumor in the breast, can be assessed anywhere. But, he says, "There are biochemical and molecular biological factors that may further identify the high-risk women." And for that you probably need to go to a comprehensive cancer center or major university hospital that has a breast cancer center for a detailed workup of the characteristics of your tumor.

Another valid reason for seeking treatment at a cancer center is if it is the only source for a particular experimental program that might help you. You or your local physician can easily find this out through a computerized cancer information service called Physician Data Query or PDQ (see the inset on page 60) and others (see Appendix B: Resources).

University hospitals and large medical centers can offer the same advantages as comprehensive cancer centers: up-to-date experimental treatment by highly experienced cancer specialists and a full range of on-site support services, such as blood transfusions, laboratory testing, and social services. If there are none in your local area, they may have many of the disadvantages that come with being treated away from home: long-distances commutes, which can be disruptive and lonely, and possibly uncomfortable and depressing; the hassle and expense of making travel arrangements and perhaps accommodations for outpatients and/or accompanying family members; and surroundings that are strange and frightening.

Although large facilities have made progress in creating more patient-friendly chemotherapy clinics, some patients still find that the surroundings are too cold and clinical; that the care is on the impersonal side; that

PHYSICIAN DATA QUERY

How do you know your doctor is recommending the most up-to-date treatment? Check the PDQ—Physician Data Query, a service of the NCI's Cancer Information Service. This computer database provides physicians and patients in communities all over the United States with access to the most up-to-date information about all types of cancer, standard and experimental treatment, the prognosis for survival, and physicians who offer state-of-the-art treatment. In some areas, information is available in languages other than English.

Through PDQ you can get descriptions of current NCI-supported clinical studies that are accepting patients, including information about the objectives of the study, medical eligibility requirements, details of the treatment program, and the names and addresses of the physicians and facilities conducting the study.

Although PDQ is available to the general public, in order to get the most out of this service, you must be prepared with detailed information about your diagnosis (such as stage and cell type). In addition, the printout is written in technical terms. Therefore, it is helpful if you and your doctor go over it together and discuss your treatment options. You can access PDQ in a number of ways:

- Through the Cancer Information Service: 1-800-4-CANCER (1-800-422-6237)
- Through the Internet: www.cancer.gov/cancer_information/
- Through the NCI fax service: 1-301-402-5874

they feel like cancer case #342, with outpatients being seen more by the nurses than by the doctors and inpatients being seen by a number of different doctors, including experienced residents, interns, and students.

Community hospitals often supply excellent care for the average cancer patient. The faces seem friendlier, the care more personalized. Some people are more secure being treated at smaller hospitals where they feel there is more compassion, more respect for their wishes, and less risk of becoming guinea pigs or being lost in the shuffle. However, some feel that small hospitals are more likely to have limited or substandard services. They may not offer the treatment plan you need, although they can often follow through with a chemotherapy protocol that has been established by more experienced specialists at larger hospitals, medical centers, or cancer centers. In most cases, adults can be treated in an accredited community hospital under experienced direction.

Medical oncologists in private practice can give you highly personalized care in relatively small, unthreatening, comfortable surroundings. Sometimes they can be more than comfortable. My oncologist's practice was in a lovely brick townhouse. The office was furnished just like a real home—carpet, wallpaper, sofas, chairs, even chamber music tapes that played continuously—and had a lovely garden I could gaze upon before and during my treatment. It was very comfortable, and that made me feel more at ease than a run-of-the-mill doctor's office would have.

Dr. Michael Van Scoy-Mosher, an oncologist at Cedars-Sinai Medical Center in Los Angeles, says:

I personally think that the most personalized care is in a private office. I may be prejudiced, but I've spent six years at three different cancer centers, so I do have a basis for comparison. A patient may be sent to a center for a consultation, but he may be seen and evaluated by an intern. At the very end, the attending physician may only briefly see the patient. What value is that? Mostly there's a difference in orientation. The private practitioner should be concerned only with the patient sitting in the room with him. In a cancer center, there is concern for today's patient, but there is just as much concern with the research that will help the patient who will show up five or six years later. That's fine, but I don't want to be that patient sitting in the room today. It's not the way I would want to be treated, and it's not the way I'd want my mother to be treated. However, certain patients really feel confident only if they are treated in a "Cancer

Center." If I perceive this to be the case, I will recommend a referral there.

Some physicians have a private practice in a hospital and full and immediate access to backup services. Some patients feel safer with physicians in a group practice or in a hospital because this means they are subject to constant review by their peers. At any rate, an oncologist should be affiliated with an accredited hospital in case a patient needs to be admitted. One who was trained at a cancer center and retains his or her ties is more likely to provide up-to-date treatment; private physicians often consult with their fellow specialists at a cancer center and follow through on a treatment program initiated there.

It makes very little sense, then, for the majority of cancer patients to travel very far from home for their chemotherapy treatments. Community facilities do not necessarily provide treatment that is inferior to the treatment you would receive at a large cancer center. And you have the advantage of keeping the disruption of your life to a minimum. (As one health professional asserted, "Patients will do anything to be able to go home at night.")

Your Relationship
with Your Oncologist

Cancer is a frightening disease that may require treatment or monitoring for the rest of your life. The kind of relationship you have with your oncologist can have a great influence on the way you feel about your disease and its treatment. I was very resistant to the idea of having chemotherapy at first. But I found a wonderful oncologist who trained at a comprehensive cancer center and who was kind, was open to questions, spoke regular English (not "medicalese"), and even had a sense of humor. I trusted and liked him, and that made the therapy less scary to start and more bearable as it wore on.

The ideal is to find a crackerjack oncologist who really knows his stuff *and* who treats you like a human being. It is advisable to ask yourself whether your doctor has the unique combination of good credentials, a compatible personality and approach, and the willingness to answer questions. Is he or she a doctor you will be able to stand seeing every week, or every two weeks, or every month for the duration of your therapy? A doctor you will be able to forgive for making you so miserable with such regularity? Good credentials are no guarantee that the doctor will treat the person as well as the disease, that you will get the best treatment and overall care.

In his book *The Facts about Cancer*, Charles F. McKhann describes the special relationship a cancer patient has with the oncologist:

> *It is a long-term association that should sustain you through good and bad, through the uncertainties of the disease, the triumphs of success, or the disappointment of unsuccessful treatment, possibly to the very end of life. A doctor in whom you have real confidence can make everything more tolerable. Your doctor should be compassionate, understanding, and interested in you as a person as well as a patient. If honesty is important to you, insist that you discuss your disease and its treatment openly. For many, however, it is more important to know that the lines of communication are open and that your questions will be answered than to ask actual questions at the time. While it is not essential for good care, it helps a lot to have a doctor whom you really like.*

Most patients would agree with this portrait of the ideal doctor-patient relationship. I know that the relationship I had with my oncologist shaped my attitude and ability to cope. While I was researching this book, my heart went out to patients who said their oncologists fell far short of the mark. Many complained about a coldness, a lack of communication and information, and a lack of respect and concern, about doctors who seem too busy, use technical language, or keep patients waiting very long times without apology or explanation. These failings add insult to injury; chemotherapy is enough of a strain without oncologists adding to their patients' difficulties. One oncologist said to me:

Communicating with patients is an art, and some oncologists can't do it. Sometimes it's a question of doctors lapsing into medical jargon. Most patients don't understand it, and it builds a little barrier between them and their doctors, of which most doctors are unaware. If you don't talk to your patients, you can insulate yourself from their pain. But I think part of the "territory" is accepting the fact that a number of your patients are going to suffer. You have to learn to endure it, too. The justification that some physicians make for their distant attitude is that if you don't achieve that distance, you end up getting very nuts. That's only partly true at best.

My oncologist says he feels "a tremendous outrage" on behalf of cancer patients:

It's a chilling disease. Almost all individuals who have it are inclined to feel shut out from the rest of the world, and to a large extent they are. And because of its nature, taking care of dying patients tends to have a chilling effect on the doctor. It is very easy to be very cold and unable to hear about the aspects of life that are difficult. It's extremely important for the oncologist to be available and willing to hear about that aspect of human existence. There are other people to whom the patient can talk, but it's difficult if the doctor is just writing the prescription and coldly looking at the size of the tumor.

Cancer Care, Inc., a New York–based social service agency, recommends that in addition to medical competence, you look for the following professional and personal qualities in a doctor:

- Has twenty-four-hour telephone accessibility (including coverage for weekends, vacations, and emergencies).
- Allows enough time for you to explain and discuss issues.
- Has reasonable fees and will discuss them with you.
- Keeps a careful record system and a smooth appointment schedule.

- Takes a detailed history.
- Clearly and openly explains your diagnosis, treatment, and condition (if that's what you want).
- Answers your questions in person and on the telephone.
- Does not use medical jargon when speaking to you.
- Is someone you feel you can trust.
- Occasionally indicates that he or she does not know something but suggests referrals to specialists or a consultation with another physician if necessary.

Many experienced patients and professionals point out the importance of entering a partnership with your oncologist in which you regard each other as equals. They also believe that being reasonably knowledgeable about cancer and its treatment is an intrinsic part of coping. It is our right and responsibility to be active, informed participants in the vital decisions affecting our bodies. The more we know, the less of the unknown there is to fear and the better partners we make in the treatment process because we meet our doctors on more equal footing. And as our understanding

SHOULD YOU CHANGE DOCTORS?

Cancer Care, Inc., suggests that you consider changing to another doctor if:

- You are not satisfied with the care you are getting.
- Your doctor repeatedly does not listen to you or answer your questions in a way you can understand.
- Your doctor or the staff members treat you with a lack of respect or don't take your concerns seriously.
- Your phone calls are not returned or the doctor is never available to talk.

about the potentials and limitations of oncology improves, so will our relations with our doctors.

Any relationship is a two-way street. As a patient, you have some responsibility, too. You have to know how to work with the doctor—when to ask questions, how to ask, and how to use his or her time well. Doctors are people like everybody else. You need to work with your doctor in a cooperative, rather than an adversarial, way.

A satisfactory relationship between you and your oncologist can make any chemotherapy plan go more easily and the continual follow-up more pleasant. Honesty, compatibility, mutual respect, an openness and willingness to communicate, trust, confidence—these are the characteristics of any good relationship. They are difficult but not impossible to attain, provided that both parties are aware of their importance and are willing to encourage each other to cultivate them.

The Oncology Nurse

Oncology nurses are becoming more and more involved in all aspects of the care of cancer patients, and many patients will have a nurse or nurses as part of their treatment team. Oncology nurses have specialized training in giving chemotherapy, managing the side effects, controlling pain, and providing emotional support and education to cancer patients and their families. Nurses are often involved in the initial planning of a chemo plan, such as choosing the anticancer drugs and antinausea medications. Since they provide direct care, they are often aware of changes and information that can affect your treatment.

Oncology nurses have become such an integral part of the treatment team that patients may see them more often and for longer periods of time than they see their doctors. Many patients find their nurses to be valuable allies and crucial sources of strength and support, as well as links to their doctors. Oncology nurses can sometimes provide you with a humanizing touch that might otherwise be missing in an oncology practice and so make up for a doctor who doesn't provide you with everything you need.

Is Chemotherapy for You?

Patients usually regard undertaking chemotherapy with *at least* some ambivalence and fear. Having a clear, realistic picture of its goals, the costs versus the benefits, and your alternatives will help you avoid either a distortedly negative picture that may lead to a refusal of beneficial treatment or an overly optimistic or naïve one that may lead you to accept a treatment you decide is ultimately not worth it to you and may lead to disappointment and resentment.

Dr. Michael Van Scoy-Mosher emphasizes:

Chemotherapy is a true cooperative venture. The physician gives the drugs, but the real work is done by the patient. As much as I might sympathize, it is the patient who undergoes the unpleasant therapy. I think whatever it takes—seeing five different doctors, reading in libraries, talking to other people—it's very important that they become convinced that they have made the right decision.

A lot of the bad things you hear about chemotherapy occur because of the ways it's been misused, such as giving chemotherapy to people whom there's no chance in the world that chemotherapy is going to help—give them chemotherapy for a couple of months, make them bald, make them sicker, and they die anyway. You know what the family of the patient says later? "That chemotherapy—it's the worst thing in the world. It killed my brother—he was bald, he was sick." It's hard to separate out the effects of the cancer from those of chemotherapy anyway, but the next time someone in that family gets cancer, they say they will never take chemotherapy. So I have to undo all of that if they've had a previous experience.

These patients bear him out:

I had a fear of chemo. I knew people who had had it, and I had seen the horrors of chemo. They just faded away, they became skeletons.

But now I realize that there's chemo, and then there's chemo. I just thought everybody got the same thing and reacted the same way.

I didn't like the idea that they were going to be putting poison in my system. I was upset about losing my hair—all my life it's been my pride. I already had gum problems and now they were telling me I might have mouth sores. As soon as the doctor left the room, I had this terrific outburst of crying. I cried and cried and really got it out of my system. And then I started to get hold of myself. If I didn't have it, and God forbid something happens a few years from now, I'm going to say to myself, "You know you had a shot at this and you didn't take it." It took me forty-five minutes to decide that I was going to take the best shot I had.

Others accept the doctor's advice without question, without finding out what they are getting into:

My regular medical GP, the surgeon, and the oncologist had a conference and decided I should have chemo. I was kind of stupid in a way. When they suggested I have it, I said, "Oh sure," not knowing what chemo was like. I knew nothing about it. I figured if other people have gone through it, it can't be that bad.

The decision to undergo chemotherapy cannot be made intelligently, confidently, and wholeheartedly unless you have gathered enough information to allow you to assess the risks versus the benefits for *you,* in your particular circumstances. Your doctor is your *primary* source for medical information and advice. But it should not be left up to him to make the final decision—or to provide all the information you might need in order to make the choice. Dr. Van Scoy-Mosher, for instance, finds that:

In very controversial uses of chemotherapy some patients want me to make the decision for them. Much as they try to pin me down, I won't do it. All I can do is spell out the arguments for and against a treat-

ment. Often they'll leave the office more anxious than when they came in; but the important issue to me is that they've made their own decisions. And in the long run, patients who have made their own decisions do quite well with those decisions. I know that a year or two from then, they'll feel good about it.

Dr. Richard Gralla, formerly of Memorial Sloan-Kettering, says:

For me, I have to talk to my patients a little bit to find out what their outlook is. I have to tell them what we have available and what their alternatives are. I can give my advice, what I would do if I were they. But ultimately the choice comes to them. Some people say, "I want this treatment if it's a one in a thousand chance." Some people say that a three out of four chance of benefit is not good enough. But that's their individual philosophy. I can just tell them their alternatives and help them make that decision.

What's really important is that people have to understand that when a cure is not possible, then improvement of quality of life becomes a major goal. Some people say they want their quality of life, not their length of life necessarily, to be improved. Usually the two go hand in hand. It is rare to get one without the other, and I think a lot of people don't realize that. If you have improvement in time, usually you have improvement in quality of life during that time.

The Goals of Chemotherapy

In the early days chemotherapy was considered a last resort to be used only in terminal cases when all else had failed to cure a cancer. When it was used so late in the disease, there was every reason for pessimism, for the chances were indeed slim that drugs—or anything—could save anyone at the eleventh hour. Chemotherapy then was highly experimental, and there were relatively few drugs to experiment with. No wonder it usually failed to perform the hoped-for miracles that surgery and radiation had also failed to perform, and it was said that the treatment was worse than the disease.

Although progress has been in baby steps, we know more about how and when to administer chemotherapy drugs, how much of them to give in what combinations and for how long, what side effects to expect and what to do about them, and what kind of response to expect. For instance, we now know that chemotherapy works best when used as early as possible, when the tumor burden is small. The increasing success of chemotherapy is due in large part to the big push toward giving it much sooner than was previously thought advisable, even when there is no detectable spread. However, there are also drugs that are effective even in the more advanced, metastatic cancers.

Today chemotherapy is being used to achieve goals that are both more optimistic and more realistic than those in the past. It is being used to:

• Cure some cancers outright.
• Induce long-term remissions in others.
• Decrease the likelihood of a recurrence or spread after surgery or radiation (adjuvant chemotherapy) in potentially curable cancers.
• Slow the growth and alleviate symptoms such as pain (palliation) in incurable or recurrent cancers.
• Shrink large tumors to operable size.
• Make radiation more effective.
• "Buy" time in order to be able to follow up with alternative or complementary therapies.

According to the 1997 National Cancer Institute's SEER Cancer Statistics Review, the overall cancer survival rate for all forms of cancer had increased from 35 percent in the 1950s to 59 percent by the mid 1990s. The survival rate used is the "relative survival rate"—the percentage of people who can expect to reach the five-year mark, or are curable. This rate has been adjusted to take normal life expectancy into consideration and to factor in deaths from other causes, such as heart disease and accidents. "Nonserious" cancers—nonmelanoma skin cancer and *in situ* cervical cancer—are highly curable and are not included. (For the most up-to-date statistics, go to the SEER Web site at http://www.nci.nih.gov/ statistics/)

This sounds like progress, but since this is a book about coping with chemotherapy, I would be remiss if I didn't include a discussion of the un- certainties and controversies surrounding the treatment. It's no secret that chemo has had its critics, and not just among the proponents of alternative therapies. Many mainstream scientists disagree with the National Cancer Institute's estimate that conventional treatments now cure over half of American patients and that this figure continues to rise thanks to advances in treatment.

For example, in 1986 a report coauthored by John C. Bailar III, a bio- statician and epidemiologist who worked for twenty years at the NCI, was published in the *New England Journal of Medicine*. The authors found that mortality rates hadn't improved since the 1950s; that statistical im- provements in the number of "cured" patients were largely due to earlier diagnosis, not treatment advances; and that the most significant advances have occurred only in relatively rare forms of cancer. The report con- cluded that "some thirty-five years of intense effort focused largely on im- proving treatment must be considered a failure." Ten years later, Bailar still estimated that the latest statistics really reflected a "flattening out" of the age-related cancer mortality rate, not a true drop.

In 1987 the U.S. Congress's General Accounting Office (GAO) re- leased a study of the years 1950 to 1982 that basically confirmed Bailar's conclusions. "Progress has been made," the report said, "but not as great as that reported." The GAO did not challenge the data on survival rates but did question their interpretation; it cited earlier detection as a factor, plus changes in the way data were compiled as reasons why the amount of "true" progress appeared inflated. Dr. Vincent DeVita, Jr., who was direc- tor of NCI at the time, replied that the figures did not reflect recent treat- ment advances that would become evident in the future. Chemotherapy seems to have had stunning results in some cancers, such as Hodgkin's disease and childhood and testicular cancer.

Then, in 1990 a West German biostatician named Ulrich Abel, who had worked for ten years helping cancer doctors conduct research, evalu- ated chemotherapy studies published all over the world. He found that overall there is no conclusive scientific evidence that chemotherapy appreciably extends the lives of patients suffering from the most common cancers. Another of his findings relates to the definition of success. In most clinical trials, it is defined in terms of the "response rate." Most patients interpret this as a "survival rate" when it actually means that the tumor has shrunk partly or completely, which doesn't necessarily correlate with a longer survival time.

And in 1993, the *Journal of the National Cancer Institute* published its review of the overall effectiveness of chemotherapy. The authors found that chemotherapy benefited only 7 percent of patients—it resulted in a "durable response" in 3 percent and a "significantly long survival period" in 4 percent. The latest evaluation of the death rate from cancer was published in June 2000 in the *Journal of the American Medical Association*. In this analysis, the National Cancer Institute found that any overall increase in survival rates is mostly due to earlier cancer diagnosis, rather than to advances in treatment. Since the five-year survival rate is computed from the moment of diagnosis, early diagnosis makes it look like people are living longer—but in fact, they are only learning that they have cancer earlier. Of course, some experts disagree with this conclusion, but if you, like me, find these criticisms, findings, and issues disturbing, I encourage you to discuss them with your oncologist in relation to your individual disease and prognosis. And you need to better understand what chemo can or can't do for you.

TO CURE CANCER

In cancer treatment, no word is more controversial than the word "cure." This is so because in the first place, it is difficult to cure cancer; in the second, it is difficult to know when it has been cured. Even when doctors are reasonably sure that a cure has been accomplished, the nature of the disease makes it difficult to confirm this with the certainty with which one can proclaim, for instance, that a case of bronchitis has been cured. With cancer—a varied, capricious, tenacious disease—it's not quite so simple.

Part of the problem is that cancers grow at different rates. Their progress is unpredictable. They may grow back slowly or astoundingly fast after a seemingly successful course of treatment has been completed. Take, for example, the frequently heard term "five-year survival," which is often equated with a cure. Some patients believe once they have passed the five-year mark, they are cured once and for all. Others are under the impression that even though they have been disease-free all that time, their disease will recur after five years are up.

In actuality, once some cancer patients pass this benchmark and are without symptoms, they *can* breathe more easily because the chances for a recurrence are sharply diminished. However, while this is true for *some* cancers, it is by no means true for *all*. With some, it takes less time to start talking about a cure.

In the case of some cancers, such as leukemia, Burkitt's lymphoma, and testicular cancer, two years is enough time to pronounce a cure. With others, such as breast, thyroid, and bladder cancers, and melanoma, eight to ten or more years must pass before we can begin to entertain thoughts of a cure. However, even with these stubborn types, the chance of a recurrence decreases with each passing year. Statistically, patients who survive for five years after diagnosis have, on the average, an 85-percent chance of surviving for twenty years. Five-year survival rates, then, have some meaning for some cancers and are useful when one is talking in terms of general averages. It is not an arbitrary cutoff date, but neither is it some universal magic number.

Compounding the growth-rate problem is the newness of much of the treatment. How do you know if someone is cured if the therapy is only five years old? If even a single cancer cell escapes treatment, it may reproduce and form a recurrence somewhere—perhaps twenty years down the line, perhaps five years and one day down the line. Modern organized, scientifically controlled chemotherapy is just twenty years old; some forms are only a few years old when they reach patients, and newer experimental therapies have even less of a track record.

Therefore, doctors would much rather stick to terms such as "no evidence of disease" (NED) and "remission." NED or full remission means that the patient has no cancer that is detectable using the techniques that are currently available. Since a person can be alive after five (or ten) years and still have (undetected or detected) cancer, these are much more cautious, though more accurate and realistic, terms that are usually used for several years after treatment.

Most chemotherapy given with an intent to cure widespread cancer is aggressive, high-dose, and highly toxic. The side effects can be severe, and complications requiring hospitalization are more common. However, many people feel the risks are worth it. For them, the time lost to chemotherapy—usually a year or less—is a reasonable price to pay for the chance of living out a normal life span.

TO PREVENT OR DELAY A RECURRENCE OR SPREAD

Chemotherapy is being given earlier and earlier in some types of cancers, before metastases are detectable. When the drugs are administered soon after surgery, or radiotherapy has eradicated the bulk of the tumor, the chances are high that the drugs will be able to mop up the microscopic stragglers left behind. The goal is to wipe out the small numbers of circulating cells before they have time to mature and grow into secondary tumors. Thus, a recurrence is at least delayed; time may prove it to be prevented altogether and the patient cured.

The concept of adjuvant chemotherapy began to be tested only in the early 1970s. But since then evidence has been accumulating to show that it does work in several cancers—mostly children's cancers such as Wilms' tumor and osteogenic carcinoma. Many women have also responded to adjuvant chemotherapy for breast cancer.

Adjuvant chemotherapy should be given only to people whose disease has been carefully diagnosed and who have a high risk of recurrence, and only when there are drugs available that have been proved effective against their type of cancer. This is the case with breast cancer when there are more than four positive lymph nodes—a woman has a 75-percent chance of a recurrence within ten years even though a mastectomy or lumpectomy plus radiation removed all detectable traces of cancer—and in osteogenic sarcoma, which has an 80-percent chance of recurring with lung metastases within a year after surgery. However, the encouraging results of adjuvant chemo studies with these cancers suggest that other cancers may respond as well because it is now suspected that microscopic colonies of cancer cells are present in the majority of cancer patients with solid tumors.

Historically, in breast cancer, adjuvant chemotherapy has been given to women who are at high risk for recurrence because the cancer has entered their lymph nodes. But 30 percent of women who have no lymph node involvement will also have a recurrence, and recent studies show that some of these women may also benefit from adjuvant chemotherapy. But it makes little sense to treat every breast cancer patient so that a few may gain. Although some tests do exist, we need to develop better ways to determine who among these groups has the highest risk of a recurrence and therefore the greatest chance of benefit. As mentioned earlier (see "Other Ways of Tailoring Your Therapy" on page 51), there have been improvements in determining whose breast cancer is likely to spread, although this information doesn't seem to be widely disseminated and used.

Adjuvant chemo is being given in an increasing number of cases, but the practice is controversial because we can't say with certainty who will benefit and because it may prove to be more harmful than beneficial: In some cancers, patients have actually done worse, and the cancer recurs earlier and with greater frequency than in patients who have not had the drugs.

The decision to undergo adjuvant chemotherapy is in some ways harder to make than that for other types of chemo. The chances are overwhelming that the micrometastases are there, but there's always a chance that there is no spread or that the body will be able to control the remaining cancer cells naturally. This is chemotherapy as an insurance policy, and it is difficult to justify at the time because there's no concrete proof, except for past experience and statistical probability, that cancer is still there. The patient feels well, there is no discernible disease, and he or she may undergo all those side effects for nothing. Dr. Van Scoy-Mosher is well aware that it presents quite unique and troublesome issues:

I find adjuvant chemotherapy for breast cancer is one of the most interesting and challenging things in the world to give. Because the questions that come up all the time are: How do you know it's needed? How do you know it's working? The only news in adjuvant chemotherapy is bad news. As long as I find nothing, that's good news.

I make it clear to patients that I don't know if they need it— there's no way of knowing because the surgery might have cured them to start with. And as years go by and the patient remains fine, I'll never know whether that's because of the therapy or whether she would have been fine anyway. And if that bothers me, I can imagine how it would make the patient crazy: The therapy's a drag, you get sick, maybe you didn't need it. At some level, you're going to have to take this on faith: that my educated guess is the right one.

The decision may be less agonizing for women with small tumors. Research published in 2002 suggests that women with breast tumors smaller than a centimeter in diameter do better in the long run if they do not have adjuvant chemo or tamoxifen. The authors of the study, conducted at UCLA, questioned 760 women who were an average of 6.3 years past their initial diagnosis. Questions related to quality of life issues, such as physical and social functioning, body image, and sexual desire. They found that women with very small tumors who received adjuvant treatment experienced long-term decline in physical functioning compared with women who did not receive the extra treatment. They concluded that the risk of a long-term physical decline caused by the treatment outweighed the possible benefits in these women, who are at such a low risk of having a recurrence. Because of these subtle costs of adjuvant chemotherapy, it may not be advisable for every woman with a tumor less than one centimeter in size to have adjuvant treatment.

A medical psychologist at Long Beach Memorial Medical Center adds:

People who undergo this type of therapy have a great will to live. They also have some advantages. They know that they will not be on these drugs forever. It is not an infinite process. They know that their disease is fairly local or in an early stage. I think it really helps to tackle something like chemotherapy knowing that your chances of getting well are so great. The decision to choose chemotherapy is much different for people with advanced disease. They must hope for disease control and palliation.

TO CONTROL CANCER

Even when a cancer isn't cured, it may be controlled for a time by chemotherapy. The goals here are to stop or slow down the growth of a tumor or shrink it at least partially (partial remission) and to alleviate any pain, bleeding, obstruction, or other symptoms of the cancer (palliation). As a result, some patients feel better and live longer.

Although, as we have seen, cancer can be a curable disease, the idea of controlling cancer so people can still live with it reflects one current medical view of cancer as a chronic disease. By definition, a chronic disease is not curable; however, it is treatable, and people don't usually die from it right away. Dr. Charles Vogel of the University of Miami's Comprehensive Cancer Center explains:

When one speaks about incurable cancer, as in the case of some metastatic disease, that's a chronic disease. But even with people who have had a recurrence, though we usually can't cure them, we can maintain these people's normal lifestyles, without hospitalization, for three, four, five, eight, or ten years. This isn't commonly realized even by my medical colleagues. There is a gestalt that equates cancer with imminent death. When we talk about chronic disease, we talk about people with arthritis, congestive heart failure, emphysema, multiple sclerosis. You can't cure these, but you can give people drugs and keep them functioning. Many types of cancer fit into that category.

When chemotherapy for palliation is offered, it is crucial to weigh the severity of the symptoms against the toxicity of the drug and the expected response rate to the drug. Also considered are the patient's age and general health, the cost of treatment, and where it will be given. When cure is not a realistic hope, the minuses may outweigh the pluses. It may not be worthwhile to begin or continue treatment if a few extra months of life are spent feeling nauseated, vomiting, and being away from family and friends.

A CLEAR UNDERSTANDING

Cure, preventing or delaying recurrence, and palliation—these are the main goals of chemotherapy, and it is important that you understand the difference. As Dr. Thomas Hakes, a physician at Memorial Sloan-Kettering in New York, says, "When you're trying to decide whether to go on chemotherapy or not, you should have a clear understanding of what you are trying to accomplish. People often have unrealistic expectations."

After asking your oncologist what the goal is in your case, you can also ask what the likelihood is of achieving that goal. The response rate varies from treatment to treatment; the average rate at which patients respond to a specific treatment is based on a statistical analysis of past experience, and this rate differs in different treatments. For example, the cure rate may be 50 percent or more, as in Hodgkin's disease or metastatic testicular cancer; or there may be a 15-percent chance of temporary improvement, as with metastatic melanoma. Awareness of such response rates and of what is meant by "response" can be useful when one is deciding upon a treatment.

But beware of the doctor who tells you how long you have to live; even though the doctor may be correct statistically, patients and their cancers are highly individual. Statistics are based on average figures for a group of patients with the same type and stage of cancer who get the same treatment. To get this average number, patients who lived much shorter periods of time and those who lived much longer were included. While statistical comparisons are valuable for comparing overall results of treatments, no one can ever say with certainty at which end of the spectrum any one particular patient will fall. Dr. Philip Schulman, an oncologist at North Shore University Hospital in New York, feels that "percentages simply don't mean anything. Each individual is either 100 percent or zero percent. Nobody wants to gamble with his or her life, and that's what percentages are."

Other Factors

Whether you're a gambler or not, percentages are not the only issue. Dr. Van Scoy-Mosher enumerates some of the many other factors that influence patients' decisions to have chemotherapy or not:

You have to consider the cancer and the stage, the symptoms or problems with cancer they are having, what kind of longevity they are likely to have, the question of them getting much sicker from the cancer—these are medical issues.

There's a real dilemma in evaluating the cost-benefit ratio: What's the realistic goal of this therapy—what am I likely to do for the patient as opposed to what am I likely to do to the patient? How do you balance those two things? Is a little longer life, but a sicker one, worth it? Or is just the chance of a longer life worth the certainty of a lot of side effects?

Then there is a whole set of issues related to the individual person—age, psychology, expectations, family structure, which is something very important—some are under a lot of pressure from their family to take chemo. You have to blend all these.

It's a complex decision to make in some patients; other situations are fairly clear-cut to me. If a person has advanced Hodgkin's disease, I know realistically I can probably cure him with chemicals. Assuming he wants to live, I don't see a big dilemma there. If there's a person with breast cancer with positive nodes, I am quite convinced that chemotherapy is a good idea and will recommend it very strongly. Then there are the marginal situations where chemotherapy may or may not help for a short period of time. Here's when you have to consider the other factors. Then there are other situations where I think chemotherapy is far more likely to make someone worse than better. The decision not to give chemotherapy is easy in those patients. What's harder is telling them.

Chemotherapy, for instance, is not for anyone whose diagnosis has not been confirmed via biopsy, whose tumor has not been staged and graded via X rays, scans, and other diagnostic tests. In addition, chemo may be too much of a strain on you physically and mentally if your general health is weak. Poor nutritional status or digestion, liver or kidney problems, infection, and other conditions may preclude, postpone, or modify the treatment with chemotherapy.

As an oncologist who specializes in treating lung cancer says:

Chemotherapy works best in people who are not greatly disabled by the cancer. There's a certain point beyond which I don't believe chemotherapy is a good choice for a patient. If there's a chance that it will do more harm than good, I try to talk with the patients and their families and explain the situation. If they insist—"I really want the treatment"—I can say, "We can try to get you up to the point where you're strong enough for chemo—use antibiotics, nutrition, pain medicine. Then maybe yes. But I'm not comfortable giving you this, I don't think it's a good idea."

Sometimes I'm criticized by my colleagues outside this hospital because in general I will not treat people's lung cancer with drugs unless they are capable of being an outpatient. If somebody's bedridden, then they're usually too sick for drug therapy for lung cancer. This is not the case with some other cancers such as leukemia or lymphoma. But you have to know the patient and find out what his or her philosophy is. Everybody's different, both in terms of outlook and physical condition at the time of presentation.

To help you make this all-important decision, you can refer to any one of several comprehensive books on cancer care. I have listed several in the Bibliography and Suggested Reading Section (Appendix C). You may also find it helpful to go to a medical library and read articles about your type of cancer that have been published in professional journals within the last three years. These articles may be difficult for the average person to understand, but they will provide the names of doctors and institutions that specialize in your type of cancer that you can contact for advice.

Ideally, you should discuss the therapy and its ramifications with one or more people who are close to you and who will be involved in your life while you undergo the treatment. They are the ones who can help support you during treatment if and when you need it. Together with a few health professionals whose judgment you trust—nurses, social workers, your family doctor—they can form a network of helpers who can offer to gather facts about alternative therapies, including alternative chemo protocols, support services, side effects, and economics. They can also help sort out conflicting information, evaluate and "translate" technical information, and participate in your making decisions based on that information.

I decided to have chemo because it seemed to be my best chance to continue to live and be well—to be cured. Even though I knew that there would be side effects and that chemo was no guarantee, it was still the lesser of two evils. People decide to have chemo because they believe it will give them something they need and want. What it gives in return might be a cure, it might be a few extra years of life or a more comfortable life, or it might only be hope that makes life bearable. Whatever the reason, it is a positive choice, a vote for life, which seems more precious because it is being threatened, and a vow to fight to the best of your ability to enjoy your life for as long as you can.

There are people who are alive today because they decided that the risk of chemotherapy was worth taking. Others have lived beyond expectation, long enough to accomplish important goals such as completing the writing of a book, seeing a daughter graduate from college, or enjoying the birth of a grandson. Even those who were not cured were perhaps able to share a few more precious moments with people close to them, buy extra time to come to grips with their illness, take care of business, or say good-bye.

Elenore Pred is a prime example. Seven years after an initial diagnosis of breast cancer, she suffered a recurrence. Chemotherapy kept her alive far longer than expected—more than three years. It allowed her extra time with her grandchildren and time to become an advocate for breast cancer patients. She founded Breast Cancer Action, an education and advocacy organization. In a little over one year, Elenore and her organization became nationally prominent in the effort to get medical policymakers to pay more attention to the disease. Although toward the end, as toxicity took its toll, Elenore felt that those years on chemo was "a hell of a way to

QUESTIONS TO ASK
ABOUT YOUR CHEMOTHERAPY PROGRAM

This checklist of questions is based in part on suggestions from the National Cancer Institute. The questions are a good starting point; you may have others of your own.

- Why do I need chemotherapy?
- What are the pros and cons (benefits and risks)?
- How successful is this treatment for the type of cancer I have?
- Are there other treatments for my type of cancer?
- When will my chemotherapy begin?
- Who will be giving me the treatments?
- Where will I receive my treatments?
- How long will I need chemotherapy?
- What drug or drugs will I be taking?
- How will the chemo be given?
- How will my lifestyle change?
- Will I be able to work while I have chemotherapy?
- What kinds of tests will I need?
- What are the possible side effects?
- Are there any long-term side effects?
- What should I do if I have side effects?
- Are there any side effects I should report right away?
- May I take other medicines while I'm having chemotherapy?
- May I drink alcohol, such as wine, beer, or cocktails?
- Are there any foods I should avoid?
- Is there anything I should not try to do during treatment?
- How much will the treatment cost? How will payment be handled?

live," she also realized that it allowed her to make a difference and leave behind a powerful legacy.

Is Standard or Investigational Chemotherapy for You?

Mainstream medicine offers two tracks: standard therapy or experimental therapy. Most people opt for standard therapy, but there may be compelling reasons to explore what experimental therapy has to offer.

STANDARD CHEMOTHERAPY

It has been estimated by the National Cancer Institute and other cancer organizations that 250,000 to 400,000 people receive chemotherapy each year. Most of them receive the standard therapy for their particular form of cancer: the drug or combination of drugs that has been proved to be the best treatment available "off the shelf." All drugs used in standard treatment have been tested to the satisfaction of the Food and Drug Administration and approved for use. The medical profession is confident that it knows enough about the side effects so that these drugs pose an acceptable amount of risk in relation to the benefits they offer. You don't need to sign a formal consent form for standard therapy; the physician simply tells you what the known possible risks and benefits are, and if you accept the treatment, you begin soon afterward.

However, standard therapy does not work for every cancer patient or may have only a minimal effect; in some cancers, no effective standard therapy exists. These patients are usually offered new experimental chemotherapy that may be more effective.

EXPERIMENTAL CHEMOTHERAPY

Each year approximately 40,000 to 45,000 people receive experimental, or investigational, treatments. That's a small fraction of the estimated

400,000 people who undergo chemotherapy each year. Formal experiments are called *clinical trials;* in effect, they put new, promising treatments on trial. If one proves itself to be as effective as or more effective than any standard treatment, it, too, becomes standard. And if a treatment is at least equal to other established treatments but is toxic in a different way, it becomes an alternative standard therapy useful for some patients.

There are many kinds of clinical trials. They range from studies of ways to prevent, detect and diagnose, control, and treat cancer to studies of the psychological impact of the disease and ways to improve the patient's comfort and quality of life (including pain control). There are also studies of support therapies, such as the impact of support groups. However, most trials evaluate innovations in treatment: surgery, radiation, chemotherapy, and immunotherapy either alone or in combination.

In chemotherapy, studies are needed to test each new drug individually, to test drugs in new combinations, to test using standard drugs in new ways, and to directly compare two types of treatments, each of which is known to be effective. The development and widespread use of a new drug is a long, complex, expensive process involving testing cancer in test tubes, laboratory animals, and humans. Human testing itself goes through three phases.

Participating in an investigational trial gives patients an opportunity to receive state-of-the-art treatment—imperfections and all—that would not otherwise be available and that can make a vast difference in their prognoses. Though these studies can vary tremendously in their risk to the patient, there is always an implied double benefit: Both the patient and the discipline of medical oncology can gain. In addition, some feel that a patient gets better all-around treatment in a clinical trial because there are strict criteria for control. The diagnosis must be specific and confirmed, the staging complete, and the required laboratory tests done. Patients are thoroughly monitored during and after treatment. This is true even if a patient is randomized—assigned by chance—to a standard therapy.

As a result of investigational chemotherapy, some people are helped, some are cured, but many are not helped. Some get sicker because of the drugs, and some even die because of them.

Experimental chemotherapy is given by "investigators"—physicians who are usually highly trained and qualified to specialize in cancer care and who conduct studies. They must have access to laboratory and hospital support facilities. If the therapy is very new and highly experimental, it may be given only at comprehensive cancer centers or university hospitals. Recently more and more investigational therapies have become available from physicians at community hospitals or physicians in private practice. These physicians would not normally have enough patients of their own to complete a study. To overcome this deficit, cooperative oncology groups have been established. Doctors who are members participate in cooperative studies that include patients in other cities with similar cancers. Your local physician can make arrangements for you to be included in a study.

Costs are a major concern of patients and their families. In some cases, patients undergoing investigational therapies are treated without charge. However, different arrangements and policies exist at different institutions, and of course, insurance coverage varies, though experimental therapy is often not covered. Patients should freely discuss what costs are involved in their cases ahead of time. Not everyone who applies will be accepted. You must fit the eligibility criteria as to type and stage of cancer, general condition, and previous treatment.

An institutional review board (IRB) at the institution must first approve federally funded and federally regulated clinical trials where the study is to take place. IRBs, designed to protect patients, are made up of scientists, doctors, clergy, and other people from the local community. An IRB reviews a study to see that it is well designed with safeguards for patients and that the risks are reasonable in relation to the potential benefits.

Anyone who enters an investigational study must sign an "informed consent" form. These vary from institution to institution and from group to group, but in general the form tells the patient the known possible side effects and the possible benefits to be expected from the treatment.

If you are contemplating investigational therapy, the informed consent form should be only a jumping-off point for healthy discussions between you and your doctor. Study it carefully. It may not contain all the information you need to make your decision. If you want to know more, ask your doctor. He or she should be willing to explain the treatment thoroughly and honestly tell you what benefits you might derive. In all cases, be sure there is no alternative therapy that you might prefer. Ask about what is already known about the drug—whether it has worked for other cancer patients and what the rare side effects might be. Find out how many people with your type of cancer have received the therapy and how many have responded. Knowing that others were helped by this treatment might influence your decision, no matter what the risks. Remember, you have the right to refuse this treatment or to discontinue it at any time.

You might want to consider experimental therapy simply because it's better than doing nothing. If you are the type of person who refuses to give up, who will try anything to live longer, investigational therapy may provide you with more than a physical therapy—it can help you psychologically. Some patients' motivation is the emotional satisfaction they derive from knowing that they are helping others who might benefit from the therapy in the future.

Trials usually have three phases, which pose three questions: Is it safe? Is it effective? Is it better than standard treatment? In general, the further along the investigation is, the higher the likelihood that you will benefit.

In *phase I*, the chances of benefit are small. Usually very little is known about the drug. Therapeutic effect may be seen in phase I, but since doses may be below the ideal therapeutic range, positive results often do not occur even with drugs that later prove to be effective. An estimated 10 percent of patients respond to phase I drugs. A doctor who offers a patient a phase I investigational drug is saying in effect: "We know of nothing that will help you. But we have a new drug that might. It might also make you worse, and you might die sooner than you would without it. But if you take it, I will be watching you very carefully to try to prevent anything really bad from happening." Some of these adverse reactions may not be predictable from the animal studies—mice, rats, dogs, and apes do not react to the drugs exactly like human beings. These preclinical studies usually do reveal liver and kidney toxicity, but they may not alert investigators to possible damage to the central nervous system, heart, lungs, and skin in humans.

Toward the end of a phase I trial, some encouraging data might have

QUESTIONS TO ASK ABOUT A CLINICAL TRIAL

If you are thinking about taking part in a clinical trial, the National Cancer Institute recommends that you ask these important questions:

- What is the purpose of the study?
- What does the study involve? What kinds of tests and treatments will be given? (Find out what is done and how it is done.)
- What is likely to happen in my case with or without this new research treatment? (What may the cancer do, and what may this treatment do?)
- What are the other choices and their advantages and disadvantages? (Are there standard treatments for my case, and how does the study compare with them?)
- How could the study affect my daily life?
- What side effects could I expect from the study? (There can also be side effects from standard treatments and from the disease itself.)
- How long will the study last? (Will it require an extra time commitment on my part?)
- Will I have to be hospitalized? If so, how often and for how long?
- Will I have any costs? Will any of the treatment be free?
- If I am harmed as a result of the research, what treatment would I be entitled to?
- What type of long-term follow-up care is part of the study?

EXPANDED ACCESS OR "COMPASSIONATE" USE

It can take from three to twenty years to develop, test, and get approval for a new cancer drug. That's a long time for a cancer patient to wait. Patients who elect to take part in clinical trials at least have a fifty-fifty chance of getting a new—and possibly more effective—drug. But what about people who don't fit the criteria for the investigational new drug protocol? What if you are suffering from a terminal cancer and treatment with an investigational drug is your only chance to extend your life? Should you be able to get that drug anyway? Cancer activists believe you should, and like the AIDS activists before them, have convinced the FDA that it should "fast track" promising new drugs as well as make them available to people outside of clinical trials. In 1996, the FDA announced that it intended to speed up the approval process for anticancer drugs. In streamlining the process, cancer treatments would become available sooner and benefit more people.

"Compassionate use" is also part of the plan. Also called "expanded access," this term applies to an unapproved drug outside a clinical trial. These are experimental drugs already approved in other countries but still being studied in the United States. It allows cancer patients in the United States to gain access to new drugs by participating in expanded access protocols. Another possibility is the individual treatment IND (investigational new drug), in which a patient gets a drug even if it has not been tested for efficacy against that patient's particular type of cancer. IND is expanded access for one person. Expanded access protocols are initiated by the drug company and usually occur when they have too many single-patient INDs. To apply for an IND, you call the drug company. If the company says yes, your doctor gets in touch with the company. Then your doctor and the company call the Food and Drug Administration (FDA) to get permission. According to an FDA representative, it takes the FDA only about twenty-four hours to approve an IND. When considering applying for compassionate use, remember it is extremely rare for a single drug to make much difference in a person's prognosis. But hope and belief are very important aspects of cancer treatment, and so the FDA tends to be rather liberal in its approach. However, the FDA recognizes that its obligation is for people to be treated safely, and it also usually insists that you be first treated with standard therapy even if studies show first-line treatment isn't very effective. As Robert Irwin, founder of the Marti Nelson Cancer Research Foundation, pointed out in his presentation to the FDA in 2000, "Patients should always be given every chance to fully understand the risks and uncertainties of treatment, but I do not think an individual should be denied a chance for benefit because another person, or group of people, considers the risk to be too high and essentially makes the decision for the patient." He continues, "Policies that facilitate access have the potential to make a life and death difference to many families one person at a time."

come in about the drug, and you might be able to find out if the drug has helped anyone else, particularly with your type of cancer. In addition, more will be known about the range of therapeutic dosage. This bit of knowledge can significantly shift the odds in your favor.

In *phase II*, the outlook is better. At least most of the side effects and dose limitations are known from phase I. Still, it is usually uncertain whether the drug is effective in human cancers, let alone which types are most likely to respond. So the chances that you will benefit are still rather small. However, it is possible that someone with your type of cancer did respond to this drug. In the early stages of a phase II study, there may be some positive data from phase I, and in the later stages of a phase II, there may be some good news from the previous studies done in this phase. So ask your doctor—if you happen along at the end of a phase II that has shown good responses to your type of cancer, it could mean a dramatic difference in your prognosis.

A doctor who offers a patient a phase II drug is saying: "We have very little standard therapy that can help you. We think we have a drug that might work in your type of cancer, we're pretty sure it won't harm you severely, and we have a very good idea of what to watch out for."

Phase III trials are usually the safest of all. By the time a drug reaches this point, it has gone through enough testing so that doctors know which cancers respond to it, how much they respond, and what the side effects are. You are offered this treatment only if it has already been proved effective in your type of cancer.

If you are offered phase III treatment, your doctor is saying: "We have standard drugs that we know will help you. But we think we have something that may be even better. The investigational arm of the study consists of a recipe (protocol) that we have a tremendous amount of confidence is just as good as the conventional arm and that we think is better. This study compares the two treatments and we think will prove that the new drug is better." So with phase III, the patient is not taking much more of a gamble than if he or she took conventional therapy.

The most comprehensive listing of cancer clinical trials is the National Cancer Institute's PDQ database, which contains close to 2,000 cancer clinical trails. (See page 60 for more information.) Visit http://clinicaltrials .gov/.

For information about clinical trials that are not funded by NCI, go to www.veritasmedicine.com (affiliated with Harvard and Tufts), or www .emergingmed.com (financed by investors and venture capitalists), or www .Centerwatch.com.

Getting a Second Opinion

As cancer care has improved, it has gotten more complex and sophisticated. If you have any lingering doubts about your diagnosis or the recommended treatment, you should definitely consider getting a second, and perhaps even a third, opinion by consulting with another expert in the field. Be sure to find out from your oncologist how much time you have to decide—some cancers do not require immediate treatment, but a delay in others could alter your prognosis dramatically. So ask how fast the cancer is growing. If it is slow growing, you have more time to research and make a decision; if it is growing quickly, you must act quickly, too.

Consultations are especially important at the time of diagnosis. Many oncologists routinely send biopsy slides to a second pathologist, and it's a good idea for you to ask whether yours has done this. Biopsies examined in small communities by a lone pathologist are prime candidates for second opinions at larger institutions such as cancer centers, major medical centers, and university medical centers. The finer points of a diagnosis can dictate crucial differences in your prognosis and treatment. Other possible motivating factors for getting a second opinion are dissatisfaction with the therapeutic effects of your treatment, the side effects and the way they are handled, and an irreconcilable doctor-patient personality conflict.

Training, capabilities, and philosophies vary greatly; no one can expect every doctor to have learned everything in his field, even if he is a specialist. Some stay more up-to-date than others do by attending seminars and conventions and reading many journals; some have a more aggressive approach to disease than others. Some have sub-subspecialties, such as bone cancer, breast cancer, or lung cancer. None of the treatments is fun. You want to be sure to get the maximum return on whatever effects you suffer, and a consultation helps you do that. Remember to ask your insurance company if they pay for second opinions—many of them do. Richard Bloch's Cancer Hotline provides an extensive listing of institutions that offer multidisciplinary second opinions (1-800-433-0464 or www.blochcancer.org). A useful Internet site is http://www.guideline.gov for the National Guideline Clearinghouse (NGC), which offers treatment recommendations based on the latest scientific evidence. It is a comprehensive database of evidence-based clinical practice guidelines and related documents produced by the Agency for Healthcare Research and Quality (AHRQ) (formerly the Agency for Health Care Policy and Research [AHCPR]), in partnership with the American Medical Association (AMA) and the American Association of Health Plans (AAHP). The NGC mission is to "provide an accessible mechanism for obtaining objective, detailed information on clinical practice guidelines and to further their dissemination, implementation and use." For second opinions regarding alternative therapies, see the Resources section (Appendix B).

Often a situation is not clear-cut, or new therapies are being developed. Dr. Thomas Hakes specializes in treating breast cancer at Memorial Sloan-Kettering and gives a lot of second opinions. "Often there are no real right answers or best answers," he says. "Rather, there are several possibilities." How often does he disagree with the first opinion? "I'd say 40 to 50 percent of the time I agree exactly; about 25 percent of the time it's not exactly what I would do, but it's still acceptable; and 25 percent of the time I disagree completely." According to David Bognar, author of *Cancer: Increasing Your Odds for Survival,* "Of patients seeking second opinions at one major cancer center, 70 percent made changes in their treatment."

Going for a consultation also gives you time to think, reflect, and digest—time that is invaluable for the coping process. Many health-care professionals, including oncologists themselves, recognize the advantages of hearing someone else's views at any point during treatment.

Though justifiable, asking for a second opinion is not always easy. An oncology nurse at New York's Memorial Sloan-Kettering points out that "there's a certain gut feeling you have about a doctor. If you like him and trust him, you may be reluctant to see someone else. It's hard to break in a new doctor." For some patients, such as this one, the idea never occurs. "This whole thing was rather new to me—though I suppose it is to everybody. I never thought about my alternatives. I just trusted my doctors and did what they told me."

Other cancer patients, no matter how they long for a confirmation or consultation, are timid about suggesting it. "I don't want to hurt my doctor's feelings," they say, or "I'm afraid my doctor won't treat me if I go see someone else." This lung cancer patient, for example, was very unhappy with the treatment her oncologist, who was affiliated with a top cancer center, was giving her:

"I was so violently ill—I thought dying couldn't be worse. So I went to a large cancer center for another opinion. My doctor was very angry with me. But I said, 'Doctor, I *need* this.' Finally he agreed to forward my records. The panel at the center told me the way I was being treated was *the way*, if I was to survive this. That put my mind at ease; it was the best five hundred dollars I ever spent."

Most oncologists, however, encourage their patients to tap another expert's thoughts. Dr. Michael Van Scoy-Mosher is one:

I might want to hear what another doctor has to say. Somewhere early on, I bring it up with the patients, just so they don't view it as an insult to my ego. I really like my patients to know that they can do that. The other thing I do is ask that they let me guide them a little bit about where to get that second opinion. I want to be sure it's from a reputable, well-respected oncologist. They also must understand that when you seek another opinion, you risk actually getting another opinion—and that you will then have to reconcile the conflict.

Though you may find a good oncologist locally, he may not have access to all the benefits of the explosion of knowledge in the cancer field. He should, however, make sure that somehow *you* do have access. Most smaller local hospitals have tie-ins with nearby larger centers. The key is for you to be able to discuss the need for expert consultation with your doctor and have his willingness to cooperate.

If you do go for a second opinion, the names of consulting physicians may be obtained and their credentials and affiliations checked out by using the same channels and methods suggested for finding a first physician. In addition, your first physician may be more than happy to recommend other specialists. Many people also find that participants in a support group can recommend good physicians.

If you are hesitant about broaching the subject with your doctor, enlist the aid of a relative or friend. They can supply moral support or courage when you explain your need to your physician or perhaps do the explaining for you. A concurring second opinion will strengthen your physician's conclusions and make you feel more secure, confident, and at ease with the treatment. Belief in the treatment seems to have a strong effect on how well you do with chemotherapy. If your doctor is offended by the suggestion to get another opinion, get another doctor.

I remember when my oncologist outlined the course of the chemo he planned for me. The next week, when I came back to start the treatment, he told me he'd found that an older protocol for adjuvant breast cancer chemotherapy was more effective than the one currently in vogue. It called for slightly different drugs and a different schedule, and it lasted nine months rather than the twelve months the other therapy stipulated. I was glad about the relative brevity of the plan, but I also felt a vague uneasiness about the therapy. I wondered: Is there yet another therapy that's even more effective? In spite of this, I never went for a second opinion. It wasn't until I researched this book that I inadvertently got a belated "second opinion" from one of the oncologists I interviewed. He confirmed that my oncologist "knew what he was doing," and I breathed a huge sigh of relief. Three years is a long time to wait for that kind of reassurance, no matter how slight your doubt.

When calling for an appointment, make it clear that you are interested in a consultation; arrangements will have to be made for your records and test results to be forwarded. Although the consulting physician could end up treating you if you prefer, you are not obligated to stay with the last doctor you see.

What if you receive two differing opinions about the diagnosis or treatment plan? You could consider breaking the tie by getting a third opinion and going along with the majority opinion. Another alternative is to ask the two differing doctors to discuss your case and perhaps come up with a solution they both agree on.

TREATMENT OUTSIDE THE U.S.

The ultimate in second opinions would be to consult with a clinic in Europe or possibly Japan. Cancer medicine is practiced differently in other parts of the world, with greater leeway for alternative therapies and combining them with standard treatments. For example, they may combine hyperthermia with low-dose chemotherapy drugs, anti-cancer herbs such as mistletoe, and natural immune boosters. For information about reputable clinics outside the U.S., contact the resources for alternative therapy listed in the Resources section (Appendix B) of this book. When speaking with alternative proponents and consultants, make sure that they have personal and current knowledge of the clinics they recommend. Ralph Moss, M.D., for example, regularly visits the clinics he refers patients to. When consulting a clinic, ask the same questions you would ask a conventional U.S. oncologist about results, side effects, and so on. And also find an oncologist stateside that will work with you and your outside clinic to provide follow up and local care.

CHAPTER FIVE

Coping with Chemotherapy

Dr. Michael Van Scoy-Mosher believes that "it's very important for most patients to have an understanding of what the therapy is all about, what its purpose is, what its goals are—and to have a certain attitude about it that the therapy is more an ally than an enemy. It is the disease that is the enemy."

Barbara Blumberg, formerly a public health educator at the National Cancer Institute, thinks it's important for people to keep in mind the reason why they're doing the chemotherapy—that it's for the ultimate good. "You have to be goal-oriented because the way to that goal is not that wonderful.

Psychologist Lari Wenzel says:

People who want to know as much as possible about their disease and treatment, why they are experiencing side effects and that these side effects can be controlled—those people tend to do well because their attitude and approach allow them an active role in fighting their disease. People should try to retain their lifestyles as much as possible so that they are not identifying themselves only as cancer patients undergoing chemotherapy, but rather thinking that this is one event among many that is taking place in their lives. People who are able to work, even part-time—if they can retain their work identity and family identity—tend to cope better.

Patients have their own theories about coping, too:

When you're so very sick, you go through all these emotions. You're angry and sorry for yourself at first. And then you say, "Hey, I'm not going to let this get me down." I just made up my mind I wasn't going to have to worry about who was going to raise my daughter. I was going to do it myself.

I guess everybody handles it in his or her own way. There's no set answer. If you're religious, you pray. If you're not, you turn to an inner strength. But behind all of us, there has to be some stirring, some push. Because we're all afraid. When you're told you're going to die, you'll put yourself through anything to be able to live.

It wasn't easy, but you learn. Friends would pitch in when my wife wasn't there to help me. We all worked together. Somehow, you just do it.

The mind has to really take over the body. If you let what they are doing to your body really sink in and go to your head—chances are you won't make it. I just stopped thinking about my body being systematically poisoned, the fact that I was agreeing to it, paying for it, and even putting some of it in my mouth myself.

With the admirable resilience, adaptability, and ingenuity that characterize the human race, most patients do manage to adjust to living in what has been called chemotherapy's "twilight world" of not being really sick but not being really well, either. In spite of the side effects great and small, physical and emotional, many people find that they are able to live fairly normal, satisfying lives while on chemotherapy. They continue to work, play, eat, socialize, go to school, take care of their households and families, and even travel pretty much as usual, at least most of the time.

In most cases, chemotherapy is only a temporary way of life, but it is still a life that must be lived. Regardless of your prognosis, you can have a rich, enjoyable, and rewarding life if you make every moment count. Even if you decide to give up certain "bad habits" in order to clean up your act and live a healthier life, why not substitute other pleasurable activities that don't harm your health (I'm thinking massages and movies). There is no reason to deprive yourself unnecessarily. Every avenue should be explored that will help you live fully within your real—and not your imagined—limitations. It may take some extra effort and planning by you and those who care about you; adjustments and perhaps some substitutions may have to be made. You may need to set up new priorities. But there is usually some way to do the things that are most important to you. There is more to life than cancer and chemotherapy.

If you find you are particularly bothered or concerned about a side effect, refer to the sections on side effects in Part Two and the section on complementary therapies in Part Three. Be sure to report your side effects to your doctor, who should have some suggestions that may help. For example, it's quite common to have a few days after a treatment when you feel more or less out of commission and simply have to take it easy. No one should expect to maintain a full schedule of activities when saddled with nausea, vomiting, or just plain overwhelming weakness. Eventually, a certain rhythm will take hold; you may learn to dread this part of the cycle or actually welcome, in some strange way, the quiet days. Should your life be too disrupted, nutritional support, household help, physical activity, or psychosocial counseling can often help alleviate your troubles. Remember that schedules can be adjusted so your worst days coincide with the times you least mind having to take it easy, be it weekends or workdays, and most dosages and drugs can be adjusted, too.

My ability to cope was certainly helped by a relatively good prognosis, a supportive husband-to-be, a compassionate and optimistic oncologist who added nutritional therapy and encouraged me to exercise, the ability to continue to work and keep my sense of humor, and the means to escape reality for a few moments by focusing on something other than chemotherapy.

We all learn to cope because we have to—the alternative is much worse. We choose chemotherapy because no matter what price we pay—in time, money, side effects, and emotional energy—the benefits are greater than without it. Whether chemo gives us a cure, a few extra years, or only hope, our will to live is what gives us the wherewithal to find and utilize whatever inner and outer help is available. Outside support makes it easier and removes some of the strain, but nothing can make chemo go away completely. The stubborn daily reality of chemo always remains.

I knew I was going to be on chemo for a specific period of time, that it would at some point be over. Like other people in this situation, I needed to figure out how to just "get through" this period on drugs even if I hated the treatment. For those who will be on chemo for an undetermined length of time, perhaps for the rest of their lives, the task is different. They must somehow integrate chemo into their lives, learn to live with it, to not only "tolerate" it but "embrace" it, as one counselor put it.

Making peace with chemo is no easy task, although it is easier for some than for others. It probably doesn't help to hate chemo, to think of it as the enemy. The experiences of two different women, each with advanced breast cancer, illustrate this point. Both were on long-term chemo with a drug whose color was bright blue. One of them had many clothes and home furnishings in the same bright blue because it had been her favorite color. But while on chemo, she began to associate the color with chemo and the side effects it caused. She began to enjoy the color less and less, even hate it, because she hated chemo. All the blue things in her life were negative reminders. The other woman associated the blue with chemo, too, but in a positive way. She knew the drug was keeping her alive and well. She went out of her way to surround herself with clothes and household things in bright blue to serve as a reinforcement, a positive reminder that the drug was doing her good.

Ultimately it is something within ourselves that allows us to make that extra effort to forge a certain relationship with chemo. Chemo for me seemed very much like life itself, only more so: a great challenge and a great adventure. I had my ups and downs, but I learned to take one day at a time. I tried not to expect the worst, not to think too much about the bad things that might happen—only the good ones.

Getting Information

Being well informed is widely recognized as essential to the coping process. Most people fear the unknown more than anything; the fantasies they conjure up are often far worse than the real thing. A reasonable amount of information can put anxieties to rest or at least into perspective. Since your oncologist knows the most about your particular case—your disease and its treatment—he or she should ideally be your primary source of information. Yet what patients want to know and what their doctors think they want to know rarely coincide.

Dr. Michael Van Scoy-Mosher thinks that as a general rule, doctors tend to underestimate their patients' needs for information and understanding of their disease and its treatment. He feels they don't supply patients with nearly enough information and hesitate to bring up touchy issues on their own.

It's up to you to ask for more information if you want it. People are often hesitant to pose additional questions once they've gotten an initial explanation or as the therapy wears on. There are many reasons for this: They say they are still in shock from the diagnosis, or they don't know what questions to ask, or they forget to ask, or they feel too shy and intimidated, or they don't want to look like fools, or they don't want to "waste" time asking silly questions of a busy doctor. Faced with an authority figure who knows more about us than we know about him, who has the power to cure, to heal, to relieve us of our pain, or to make us feel sicker, we can feel as though we were children who should be "seen but not heard."

You should not feel guilty about taking up a lot of the doctor's time— that's what the doctors are there for. Taking up time *unnecessarily* is another matter, so it is best to come prepared. When you are asking questions, there are several procedures you can follow so that your queries are more effective. You can educate yourself by reading up on your disease and its treatment (your doctor can refer you to specific volumes and periodicals, or your librarian can). You can contact local branches of national cancer organizations such as the American Cancer Society and the National Cancer Institute's Cancer Information Service. They will give you information over the phone and send you booklets and articles pertinent to your disease. It is difficult to retain huge amounts of new information; at a time when your mind is under a lot of pressure, it is impossible. You can overcome this problem during visits to your doctor by bringing a pad and pencil and jotting down notes, or you can bring along a small cassette recorder and tape the whole conversation. Bringing a friend or family member with you is another possibility. They can remember things you don't, act as your health advocate by thinking up questions that you might not have, and pose questions you may not have the nerve to ask.

Many cancer patients and professionals suggest that you write down your questions as you think of them during the visit or during the time between visits. Some suggest you send a copy to your doctor ahead of your next visit so he or she can be prepared, and your concerns can be kept as part of your records.

I didn't start writing down questions until well into the therapy for fear of feeling foolish. Finally, I decided it was more foolish not to. When I whipped out my list, my doctor just quipped, "Oh, a shopping list," and didn't bat an eyelash.

Your Chemotherapy Plan

The chemotherapy plan (also referred to as a protocol, program, or regimen) is like a cooking recipe that specifies the drugs, the baseline doses of the drugs, and the scheduling of the treatments. Cancers as well as people vary in their responses to different plans, so in choosing a protocol, the oncologist tries to match your disease and general condition with the possible effectiveness and side effects of the thousands of available protocols. The plan he or she chooses and how it is implemented play a crucial role in how well you cope.

As you have seen, your chemotherapy may be standard or investigational; in addition, it may be a single drug (single-agent chemotherapy), or your cancer might respond best to a multitude of drugs given simultaneously or sequentially (combination chemotherapy). You may be getting high-dose chemo, which is generally reserved for systemic cancers such as leukemias and lymphoma or for metastatic disease that has a good chance for a cure or remission. Or the chemo may be conventional-dose or low-dose, which are used for adjuvant chemo and for palliation. The actual dose you get is usually calculated according to a formula based on body weight or total body surface area. Using the body surface area is more reliable because it tends to fluctuate less than body weight.

How Much Leeway?

Every effort is made to adhere to the established program as closely as is feasible because past experience shows that the treatment works best that way. An investigational protocol must be followed to the letter because it is a test, or else the results of the trial will be inaccurate. (However, a patient may be taken off a study and still receive some type of chemotherapy.)

But chemotherapy is not an all-or-nothing proposition. The goal in chemotherapy is to administer the "maximum tolerated dosage." This is the delicately balanced point at which as many cancer cells as possible are being killed without sacrificing too many normal cells. Too little of the drug, and too few cancer cells are killed; too much of it, and too many normal cells are killed. When too many normal cells are affected, the therapy becomes too toxic and side effects become intolerable and possibly dangerous.

Everyone comes to chemotherapy with a different set of physical characteristics, and everyone reacts in a unique way. The art and science of giving chemotherapy well in part consist of knowing when and how to change a protocol so the patient is getting the best care. An oncologist will make changes in your treatment if the side effects are too debilitating or the drugs are not working well. Initially, a set protocol may be used intact, or drugs may be dropped and/or added. For instance, certain drugs may be toxic for you if a key organ is weak or malfunctioning. Your liver and kidneys process and excrete anticancer drugs, so those organs are particularly stressed. But problems with other organs may mean that your doctor will have to give you less of a drug than it is standard practice to give, drop it from the plan entirely, or simply keep a very close watch on organs that he or she suspects may be dangerously affected.

You usually begin chemotherapy within a month after diagnosis. Thereafter, your treatments are paced carefully. Unless you are getting continuous low-dose chemotherapy, the drugs are given intermittently, in cycles, with enough time between treatments so that normal cells can reproduce and replace their lost sister cells in sufficient numbers to maintain an acceptable level of function. However, you can't leave so much time between treatments that the cancer cells can recoup their losses.

Consequently, you should try to make your treatments as scheduled, if possible, on the exact day stipulated by your protocol, and to continue it for as long as your oncologist recommends. As with the drugs themselves, the timing and length of the therapy may be fine-tuned according to your response, your side effects, the goals of the treatment, and the availability of alternative treatments.

Chemotherapy protocols given with an intent to cure or bring about complete remission usually have a predetermined end date. They can last three months, six months, nine months, one year, two years, or three years. Experience has shown that on the average this is the minimum amount of time required to get the sought-after results, with acceptable side effects, in the greatest number of people.

Where the goal is partial remission or when the protocol is investigational, the therapy is more open-ended. Chemotherapy may be relatively brief, a long constant haul, or an on-again, off-again proposition for the remainder of the patient's life. Your doctor may switch drugs, doses, and schedules regularly in an attempt to prolong a comfortable, productive life.

In cases of discernible disease, chemotherapy is given for as long as the drugs can be seen to be affecting the tumor and you are not suffering from severe side effects. The way you feel and various tests tell your doctor how well the drugs are working: Is the tumor still growing; if so, how fast? Has it stopped growing? Is it shrinking? Is it gone?

If your tumor continues to grow or "progress," most oncologists will take you off chemotherapy or switch to a different group of drugs no matter how well you tolerate the first group. They feel that if it continues to grow despite various different drugs or combinations of them, chemotherapy is probably doing more harm than good; you are probably wasting your time, energy, and whatever health you have left. In some cases, a tumor whose growth has slowed down is an acceptable response and you may continue to be treated with chemotherapy, provided that the side effects are tolerable. In others, a stable tumor (one that has stopped growing but is not shrinking) may be the criterion for continuing.

If the tumor responds so well that it actually shrinks (partial remission), chemotherapy may be continued until the tumor either no longer responds (that is, shrinks) or begins to grow again; at this point you may get drugs, if possible, to which the tumor is not resistant. If you are in full remission with no detectable disease, chemotherapy may be continued on a maintenance basis or stopped—it depends on the cancer. Long-term remission can indicate a cure, but many remissions do not last forever; when the disease recurs, chemotherapy may be started again with the same or new drugs.

How much leeway to take in a chemotherapy regimen is one of the greatest dilemmas facing the oncologist and one a cancer patient faces, too, if he or she is an informed partner in the decisions concerning the treatment. Doctors often treat patients who are vomiting, who feel sick, whose blood counts are slipping, and who are on the edge of developing any number of possibly serious additional ailments. How much toxicity is too much? At what point do you reduce, postpone, alter, or stop treatment even though you know it probably lessens the chance for a cure or a remission? A heart-to-heart discussion with your doctor should enable both of you to plan a treatment program you are comfortable with. Together you must take personal factors into consideration, such as whether you need to keep on working or keep your household together.

In these cases it is not advisable for your doctor to prescribe drugs that would knock you off your feet. You have to balance your emotional need to stay alert, capable, and "up" with the physical need to take strong chemotherapy to treat your cancer. There usually are a few choices to make.

If you suffer from immediate debilitating side effects and need to stay well and alert because you are continuing to work, you can often schedule your appointments for a weekday evening or for a Friday. If weekends are important to you, you can have your treatments early in the week. Both these strategies will usually allow time for the worst of the immediate side effects to wear off in time for you to live your life pretty much as planned. Because work was important to me, I got my treatments on Fridays. That way I could moan and mope over the weekend, when the side effects were the worst. By Monday, I'd be ready to face the world again.

Itinerant chemotherapy patients can stay on schedule, too, with a little ingenuity. When I took a trip related to my work, I didn't miss a shot (as much as I would have liked to). I told my oncologist my itinerary, and he located a lab in one city and an oncologist in another and gave me my drugs to tote along. I had two blood tests and one treatment away from home under his long-distance guidance. Two weeks later, I got off the plane and had my next treatment, right on schedule.

Methods of Administration

Chemotherapeutic drugs may be given in any of several different ways, depending on the dose, the preferences of the doctor and the patient, and the type of cancer. The drugs may be introduced into the body in the following ways:

- Orally (PO)—pills, capsules, or liquids taken by mouth.
- Intravenously (IV)—injected into a vein, either fast (IV push) or slow (IV drip or infusion).
- Intramuscularly (IM)—injected into a muscle.
- Subcutaneously (SQ)—injected underneath the skin.
- Intra-arterially (IA)—injected into an artery.
- Intrathecally (IT)—injected into the spinal fluid.
- Intracavitarily (IC)—injected into the pleural cavity of the chest or into the abdomen.
- Topically—applied directly to the skin, in the mouth, or into the vagina.

Most chemotherapy is given either orally or intravenously; many protocols combine both methods. When given orally, it enters your bloodstream via the digestive system; intravenous medication enters the blood directly via a vein. Once in the bloodstream, the drug diffuses throughout the body and goes to every cell of every organ supplied with blood by the capillaries. The other methods are generally reserved for special conditions to increase the drugs' effectiveness, reduce the side effects, or both. For instance, a great deal of effort has been made to give drugs intra-arterially, by regional perfusion. This method allows spot treatment of tumors in which very high concentrations of drugs circulate only in the region of the tumor. When it is used in cases such as arm, leg, neck, or head tumors or liver metastases, the results of this method compare favorably with those of intravenous administration, with fewer side effects to the rest of the body. Intrathecal injections directly into the spinal fluid are another example. They are an attempt to overcome the blood-brain barrier and are often used in cancers, such as leukemia, that tend to spread to the central nervous system.

ORAL CHEMOTHERAPY

Some cancers are treated solely with oral chemotherapy. In many other protocols, oral drugs are used in addition to the injections. Your plan may call for you to take oral medication—pills, capsules, or liquid a few days every month or every day throughout the therapy. Since the pills, capsules, or liquid can be taken over the course of the day, oral administration allows a steadier supply of the drug to be circulating in the body.

Oral chemotherapy is particularly useful for patients who have "bad veins" making it difficult, very painful, or impossible to have IV chemotherapy. However, it leaves the accuracy of the dosing up to the patient, and the pills themselves can have a horrible taste that stubbornly refuses to be disguised. One patient comments:

> *I took six pills a day, and they tasted so bitter. I can still taste them now, five years later. My oncologist suggested putting them in applesauce, but I don't like applesauce. I tried jelly, but that didn't work. I knew that people wrap pills for animals in cooked meat or bread, so I tried wrapping pills in pieces of soft bread, but they stuck in my throat. I'll never forget the taste.*

Following these simple procedures will make pill taking easier: It is better to stand rather than to sit. For some reason, the pill goes down more easily when standing. Take a sip of water or another liquid to lubricate the throat to prevent the tablet from getting stuck. Then take a sip of liquid along with the pill and tilt the head back to swallow. Wash the pill down with a hefty chaser of more water. It is important to remember to lubricate the throat first. In one study, X-rays revealed that medications stick in dry throats despite up to forty swallows and additional gulps of water. If you still have trouble, you might try coating the pills with a bit of margarine or butter before taking them. This reportedly makes the pills slippery for easier swallowing and eliminates any bitter aftertaste.

If you are taking oral medication, it helps to establish a schedule related in some way to your other activities. For instance, coordinate your pill taking with certain meals or with a favorite TV or radio show. Or a family member or neighbor may be able to remind you. Ask your doctor, nurse, or pharmacist to help you set up a workable schedule. Some drugs are best taken on an empty stomach, others on a full one. Some should not be taken just before bedtime. If you are taking a number of drugs by mouth, take care not to mix them up and to take each one at the proper time. If you are following a very complicated schedule, it may help to set out your medication for one day in a special container or to keep a written record of your tablets. Another aid is to hang a large calendar near the location of your pills and mark large X's on the dates you are to take your pills. If you are taking several pills, use a different color pen to mark each bottle of medication.

If you miss a dose, check with your doctor about how to proceed. Sometimes you should take a missed dose as soon as possible; sometimes you should not take the missed dose or double up on the next dose to make it up but continue as usual with the next scheduled dose.

Even though you may experience side effects from oral chemotherapy, you should not stop taking it or reduce the dosage on your own. Check with your doctor. He may prescribe different drugs, reduce the dose of your present drugs, prescribe additional drugs, or make suggestions that will alleviate the side effects.

Chemotherapy pills are very strong medications. As with all drugs, keep your chemotherapy pills out of the reach of children and do not transfer them to another drug container that might cause confusion and accidental dosing.

INTRAVENOUS CHEMOTHERAPY

For many drugs, intravenous (IV) injections are the preferred—or only—way for the drugs to enter your body. Drugs are usually given intravenously because they reach more parts of the body that way or because they are easier or cheaper to manufacture in that form. Some drugs are absorbed only when they are given by injection. Some may be too irritating or unstable to be used in oral form.

Chemotherapy is most often injected into veins in the lower arm or hand because they are usually the most accessible and convenient. Sometimes veins in other areas of the body are used when these are not usable.

If you don't have any good, accessible veins or if your good veins have been "used up," there are ways of avoiding the need to stick those veins again and again. A catheter, a port, or sometimes a pump may be surgically implanted, usually under local anesthesia.

An indwelling catheter is a thin plastic tube that is temporarily implanted under the skin and extends into a vein in the neck, chest, or abdomen. The catheter provides access for injections or slow-drip infusions. Catheters are also used to administer other drugs, such as antibiotics, antinausea medicines, antipain medicines, or nutritional formulas. With proper maintenance and cleaning, catheters can stay in place for weeks or months.

A port (Portacath or LifePort) is a small disk-shaped chamber placed under the skin. Most often, it is implanted in an area on the upper chest, near the shoulder. The port is attached to a catheter that is placed in a vein or artery. Drugs are then injected through the skin into the port, which then empties into the blood via the catheter.

There are also ambulatory pumps, which may be internal or external (worn inside or outside the body). The pump is filled with a drug or drugs, which are then slowly and steadily infused into the body. Pumps are becoming quite sophisticated, and some can be programmed to deliver several different drugs in a specific sequence. Dr. Richard Cohen, a San Francisco oncologist, has seen how portable pumps are "changing people's lives—they don't have to go to the hospital and treatment is less costly. In addition, now we can control certain cancers that couldn't be controlled at all, with less side effects."

There are two methods of giving an intravenous injection of chemotherapy drugs: push and drip (infusion). The push is the fastest and simplest, but the method used for certain drugs on different people depends on which works best and which is least painful. Drugs given by the drip method are usually those that are deactivated very quickly; the drip method ensures that a certain level of these drugs is maintained in the body for a long time to increase the number of cells killed. Sometimes a drug must be given slowly in a diluted form because it pains the patient or results in adverse effects when it is given quickly.

An IV push takes five to fifteen minutes, depending on the number of drugs, the size of the needle, and the ease with which the needle can be inserted into the vein. If you are getting combination chemotherapy, your doctor or nurse will insert a single needle into a vein and one by one feed a succession of drugs through the same needle to spare the vein from repeated piercings.

An IV drip takes longer—up to twelve hours for a single drug. For this technique, a bottle of the drug hangs from a pole. A thin tube connects the bottle to the needle and allows the drug to drip slowly at a steady rate into the vein. Patients who are on a protocol involving several drugs given by slow IV drip stay in the hospital for several days, and the IV needle remains in the vein for the duration of the treatment, with each drug administered in succession. Thanks to the aforementioned pump, more and more IV drip chemotherapy is being given on an outpatient basis.

The sensations felt during the actual chemotherapy injection depend on the skill of the oncologist or oncology nurse who administers the injection, the nature of the drugs, and the size and condition of the vein. A psychological component enters into it, too—in some people, fear and apprehension can make an unpleasant sensation feel worse.

Knowing this, I tried to relax as much as possible when the moment came. Eventually the treatments became less painful, less shocking, almost routine and normal. My oncologist had a skillful, gentle technique and used a tiny needle; still, a needle is a needle, and I never got used to it completely. I looked away when he made the injection, especially when he was having trouble. Even though the pain was minimal compared with the surgery I'd been through, I couldn't stop a few tears from forming just the same—at that moment, I'd feel sorry for myself all over again, and I'd think, "Isn't it bad enough? I don't need this."

Some fortunate patients are endowed with huge, ropy veins, close to the surface of the skin. They never realize how lucky they are until chemotherapy enters their lives—"God may have given me cancer, but at least He gave me good veins." At the other end of the spectrum are the unfortunate ones with truly "bad veins"—small, thin-walled or tough-walled, or buried below the surface. If your veins are in this category, you will probably be advised to have an indwelling catheter or port implanted surgically.

A good oncology nurse or doctor will do everything possible to make a vein more accessible to treatment and spare the patient discomfort. They may use ultrasmall needles and look for veins in odd places. Some try wrapping the arm with warm towels or running warm water over the area to get the veins to come closer to the surface. Dr. Ronald Bash formerly of Einstein Medical Center recommends that his patients exercise, since this pumps up the veins: "It makes a modest difference, but that's often enough. This is especially so in women undergoing chemotherapy for breast cancer, and who are getting injections in only one arm." My oncologist specifically recommended that I squeeze a rubber ball as often as possible to "pump up" the veins, but any exercise helps.

The drugs themselves—and the imagination and sensitivities of the patient—also impart unique sensations at injection time. A lot of the sensations are minor, localized, and temporary. Some patients say they feel a burning at the injection site; others feel a coldness or a warmth that spreads throughout the body and lasts for several minutes or more. Others feel an overall tingling, a chill, or a kind of "high." Some say they can "taste" their drugs within a few seconds of the beginning of the injection. I'd joke around and say, "Mmm—strawberry," and name another flavor every time. For other patients, the taste is no joke. For example: "That metallic taste would hit my mouth shortly after the infusion began. If I live to be a million, I will never forget it. It's just bad. We tried using mints, which were somewhat effective, but not really. And it was one of those long-lasting things."

Some of these reactions are predictable, but others are not. Always tell your chemotherapist or nurse about any sensations, no matter how silly they seem to you at the time. Occasionally the drug may leak into the surrounding tissue; this can be a serious side effect of chemotherapy and is called extravasation.

Your First Treatment

Some patients look forward to their first treatment because it signifies help for their disease. They are relieved that something can be and is being done. Some experience an element of curiosity or excitement; many, however, approach their first "shot" with a good deal of anxiety and fear.

My doctor had warned me about vomiting and tiredness after a treatment and had told me that my hair might fall out later. These were only possibilities; I had no idea whether I would have them, and this uncertainty was kind of exciting and horrifying at the same time. When the treatment was over, my husband and I rode the bus home. The anticipation was excruciating, but as the hours passed, I began to feel only a little queasy and spaced-out, a little tired. That was all! Hardly the vision I had had of hanging out over the toilet bowl for hours. The next day I still felt crummy, tired, and cranky.

Many people experience minimal side effects as I did, but the initial experiences vary, just as the overall experiences do:

> *I was petrified to go for my first treatment. My doctor gave me the injection and had me lie down. Five minutes later he came back and asked, "How are you feeling?" I felt fine and went home by subway alone, having sent my future husband, Larry, back to work. I thought if this is the way it's going to be, what's the big deal? About three hours later, I felt every ounce of energy drain from my body.*

Larry helped me get into bed, and from that moment on I proceeded to throw up for four days.

They started me on my first round of chemo while I was still in the hospital recovering from surgery. The resident on the case came in trundling a whole sack of little chemicals. Vile yellow colors, an ugly brown thing . . . some of them were so-called antinausea drugs which knocked me out for the better part of the first day. That first day . . . it was miserable. Feeling totally out of it, weak from the surgery, vomiting in spite of the antinausea drugs, my wife sort of floating in and out of my consciousness. My surgeon recommended that I hire a private duty nurse, and I thank God we had a health plan that allowed it—having someone there around the clock that first day really made a great deal of difference in my case.

I thought: I'm going to go into this office and I'm going to see all these awful-looking people sitting around with all white faces. I thought they would all be dying of cancer, and it would be depressing seeing all those people. But it didn't turn out like that at all.

My doctor didn't tell me much about the side effects. So I wasn't terribly nervous—I didn't have that fear. When I started throwing up violently that night, I was frightened to death. I called him on the phone and said, "If this is the way it's going to be every time, I can't go through with it!" It wasn't, though.

Since there's no way for you to know exactly what the initial chemo treatment is going to be like for you, the best course is to be as generally prepared as possible for every eventuality. Your preparation should include a basic grasp of what is going to happen before and during the injection, what will be expected of you, what the surroundings will be like, how long the injection will take, and what the immediate side effects might be. There is some dissension among the ranks as to how much detail a doctor should go into when describing the possible side effects of a particular set of drugs.

But if you are being treated as an outpatient, you should at least find out whether the side effects might affect your ability to get back home and function for the rest of the day. It is probably unwise in most cases to plan to put in a full day's—or evening's—activities after your injection. Though most drugs don't cause vomiting until hours after administration and you may not feel any immediate effects at all, it is better to be safe than to be caught by surprise feeling sick in the middle of Main Street. In addition, you should be able to contact your doctor or a knowledgeable nurse in case anything occurs that you might need help with (as should be the case throughout your therapy).

Cedar-Sinai's Dr. Van Scoy-Mosher acknowledges that anxiety is a problem with some patients:

> *What I've seen to be useful is for patients who are feeling particularly anxious to talk with another patient who had the same therapy. Patients can ask their doctors—I often arrange for this. Even if the patient had gotten sick with it—just to talk to somebody who had it a while ago or is having it and is still functioning, is doing okay, can relieve a lot of anxiety.*

Many hospitals have instituted—or are in the throes of instituting—some kind of group orientation meetings or workshops to deal with the ins and outs of chemotherapy. While these can prepare you generally, they usually include a large variety of patients, cancers, and treatments and so may not be specific enough. Your doctor or nurse is still the best source for nitty-gritty information about your chemotherapy plan. In addition, a patient volunteer—someone who has been through it—can share valuable firsthand experience. Your doctor, nurse, or hospital may also give you drug information cards that list the side effects and remedies or other printed matter such as booklets to reinforce whatever you have been told.

An oncology nurse at a large cancer center says:

> *Patients should have some knowledge, something in their hands, because they forget by the time they get home. They get bombarded with so much, and by the time they come for chemotherapy here,*

they're tired, they've been waiting for the doctor, the doctor has seen
them, they may not like what was said to them or the way it was said
to them, they may have gotten bad news, they may be worrying
about the kids coming home from school, or feeling angry . . .
they're just not concentrating. They should have some form of writ-
ten instruction.

Most oncologists advise against the patient's going alone for any treatment, but this is especially important for the first treatment, when the immediate side effects are more up in the air than at any time during
treatment. A familiar presence—a spouse, parent, adult son or daughter,
friend or neighbor—can allay a lot of anxiety. He or she can also run interference, help deal with red tape, ask questions for you, and perhaps retain more information than you can at this time. From a purely practical
standpoint, another person can keep you company during long waiting periods and accompany you home or take over any driving that is necessary.

Handling the Side Effects

Without a doubt, it is the side effects that have given chemotherapy a bad
name and worry people the most. Dr. Richard Gralla feels that the media
help paint an unfair view of them.

People are misinformed, and some extra anxiety has been built up
because of that. A magazine article once said that the cancer patient
had to face the "twin horrors" of cancer and chemotherapy. That
doesn't help people. A lot of things have been done, especially in the
last few years, to make the side effects easier to take. Response to
treatment can greatly reduce the symptoms of cancer and bolster a
person both physically and emotionally.

On the other hand, playing down the side effects, or sugar-coating the
experience, paints a false picture that can be just as harmful. A women's
magazine quoted a noted breast cancer specialist as saying, "The vast ma-

jority of patients should experience chemotherapy as no more than an inconvenience in their lives." Although some women do breeze through, this is patently untrue of the "vast majority," and it does these women a vast disservice to tell them that this is so far from the norm.

To a certain degree, your side effects can depend on you—your attitude and overall health—and on your doctor. A positive attitude full of hope and confidence can make side effects less noticeable and more tolerable. A strong, healthy young body may withstand the rigors of some drugs better than a weakened or older one. A good doctor-patient relationship helps, too: Sometimes it seems that the way a patient feels about the oncologist has a great deal to do with the severity of the side effects and how well the patient can cope with them. In the hands of a competent, caring physician or health-care team and with the judicious use of the support services and therapies, the side effects picture is much better than it used to be. Today the side effects of chemotherapy are preventable or treatable or have the potential to be made more bearable.

Coping with side effects begins with an understanding of what they are, which ones you can reasonably expect to get, which ones are serious, and what you can do about them. Ideally, your oncologist will be able to help you in all these areas.

Some physicians and nurses feel that giving patients information about side effects increases the likelihood that the patients will develop the side effects or will increase their severity. However, there have been several studies conducted by Marilyn Dodd, an oncology nurse and the author of *Managing the Side Effects of Chemotherapy and Radiation* that have shown that this is not the case. She found that patients who were fully informed did not report more side effects and that they were more active in taking care of themselves than were patients who were not well informed.

The science and art of medical oncology consist of treating the patient's cancer and treating the side effects caused by the treatment. Doing both well takes a lot of time and skill, as Dr. William Grace, chief of oncology at St. Vincent's Hospital in New York, explains:

Good care of patients is attention to detail. It's like anything else: If you are concerned about your patients, you make every effort

to assure that they don't get too sick from the disease or the ther-
apy. Good care is labor-intensive, feeling compassion, having good
ideas, and common sense. It means you have to do a lot of fine-
tuning. When the doctor-patient exchange is fruitful, medication
can be given carefully and effectively in high doses without unac-
ceptable toxicity.

No two people are exactly the same, and no two will react exactly the same to the same drugs, just as no two tumors will. In Part Two, I discuss the most common side effects and provide information about managing them. In Appendix A, I list the anticancer drugs that have been approved by the FDA along with their side effects. A glance at this list can be terrifying and misleading unless you remember this very important point: These are the side effects that *might* occur; they are not the ones that necessarily *will* occur. And as you will see, there are many ways that you, your doctor, and your support system can work to prevent or alleviate those which do occur.

A few of the side effects listed for the drugs in your chemotherapy plan are very common and happen to some degree to nearly everyone who takes them; others are less common; and still others are quite rare. Side effects can sometimes occur in only a fraction of a percentage point of the total number of people who take the drugs. Some side effects may be only temporary or intermittent, or they may persist for the duration of the treatment, linger after treatment is just a memory, or never go away completely. They may be severe or slight, serious or minor, annoying or devastating. Sometimes there is confusion about whether a condition is actually the result of chemotherapy.

Oncologists are therefore put in a very tough position when their patients ask about side effects. People want to know what side effects they are going to get; they want to know what they can expect. Dr. Thomas Fahey of Memorial Sloan-Kettering in New York expresses the frustration of all oncologists when he says:

One of the things that's so frightening about it is that you can't sit
down with a patient beforehand and say, "Look, this is exactly what

you can expect. And since this is what you can expect, this is what we're going to do about it." It's so variable. I think it's probably not a good idea to present all the possible terrible things that can happen to people before they get chemotherapy because they may not get any of them. The patients should know, however, that certain side effects of chemotherapy are experienced to some degree by most patients who receive these treatments, and although they are variable, they are not unexpected. These could include stomach upset, hair loss, loss of energy, and blood count depression.

You don't dwell on what the side effects are but say that if there are side effects, we can anticipate them, and there are methods we can use to make them minimal. For example, now you can really reassure people that you can virtually stop nausea and vomiting. The newer antinausea drugs are very effective.

In addition, it is usually impossible to say exactly when side effects will occur and how long they will last. Some may occur within a few minutes or hours after the treatment. These include nausea and vomiting, extreme tiredness or weakness, dizziness, diarrhea, and constipation. These typically last a few hours to a few days and then, like a bad dream, are over. In some cases these side effects can plague the patient in milder form for some time. Sometimes a patient experiences a severe reaction with the very first treatment. At other times, it can take many treatments until toxicity has built up. Reactions may be more severe after some treatments, almost negligible after others. Emotional states, too, can vary, with some reactions not taking hold for months until the reality and drudgery of chemotherapy set in.

Dr. Fahey says:

For some patients the hair loss is the worst possible thing that could ever be inflicted on them. Others, that doesn't bother at all. . . . It's the fact that they have to keep coming back to an institution or an office and being reminded that they have cancer. The chemotherapy is a continual reminder of the disease, the treatment must be given on a certain schedule, and their lives become so ordered around the

schedule that that's the worst part of it. Then there are others who
say they just feel crummy, that it makes them feel sick, nauseous.
Some describe it as depression; I'm not sure it is a psychological de-
pression, I think it's a physical depression. Chemotherapy depresses
the whole body, and that's the most disturbing thing to them.

Sister Rosemary Moynihan, former assistant director of social service
at Memorial Sloan-Kettering, says:

Chemotherapy is not like other medicine. It has a mystique built up
around it, and people have all sorts of fears about what will happen.
They have a lot riding on this, but there are so many uncertainties
and ambiguities. Most people feel anxious about receiving chemo-
therapy. What will it feel like? Will I be able to tolerate it? How will
I cope? Will it work? They expect to feel bad, but if they don't, does
that mean it's not working? It's important for people to talk about
these feelings, clarify misconceptions, and find someone to walk
them through that initial treatment.

Your oncologist will be giving you tests and physical exams regularly
to keep tabs on your condition. These tests, though bothersome, reveal
valuable clues about what is going on inside your body and are an integral
part of the chemotherapy treatment. Many of these tests—scans, X-rays,
lab tests—are also used during the initial diagnosis; during chemo, tests
involving the blood are used with the greatest frequency and regularity.

Some of these tests reveal how well the drugs are working; others indicate how much damage is being done to normal cells (toxicity). Using the
results of the tests, the oncologist decides whether to switch drugs, increase the dosage, decrease the dosage, change the schedule, or continue
the therapy at all.

Complete Blood Counts

Blood counts are the bread-and-butter tests of chemotherapy. The blood is composed of various types of cells that are produced in the bone marrow, spleen, and lymph glands. Both cancer and chemo can affect the composition of cells in your blood. A complete blood count (CBC) shows how your blood compares with the normal amounts of these cells and blood substances. Below are the normal ranges.

- *White blood cells* fight infection (4,500–10,500).
- *Red blood cells,* or erythrocytes, carry oxygen and waste (4.5–5 million).
- *Platelets,* or thrombocytes, help clot the blood (200,000–350,000).
- *Hemoglobin* is contained in the red cells and is responsible for carrying oxygen (13–16 g/100 ml).
- *Hematocrit* is the percentage of red blood cells (38–46 percent in women and 40–54 in men).
- *Differential* is the ratio of mature cells to immature cells (100).

Your oncologist will order a CBC for you at least every time you are due for a treatment. Many oncologists feel that weekly tests are best even if you don't have weekly treatments because real trends are more easily discernible the more data there are to go on and because a low count may require attention immediately. Very low counts may require transfusions of blood products. If your count drops too low, your oncologist will hold back on your treatment, usually by reducing the dosage or postponing the treatment.

Blood tests may be performed in your oncologist's office if there is a lab on the premises or at a hospital, clinic, or independent laboratory. Blood may be drawn from a vein separately or through the intravenous needle or catheter used to administer chemotherapy if you are getting an IV drip and/or are being admitted as an inpatient to a hospital. Blood may also be taken from a finger prick—to spare veins for chemotherapy injections, oncologists sometimes order blood to be drawn only by this method.

After some time on chemo, I became adept at guessing when my blood count was down. I'd be feeling pretty down—tired, with no pep and a gray face—and sure enough, it was down. So my doctor would pull back a bit on the drugs, and I'd start to feel better. My count would creep up, and he'd be able to blast away again. I think I found the blood tests more loathsome than the chemo injections. My technician had to use the finger prick each time because I had only one good vein in one good arm—the other arm was off limits because of the mastectomy. She'd say "Ready?" and then make a quick jab and then squeeze and squeeze. I'd scrunch up my face each time—that somehow made it more tolerable. Between the blood tests every week and the chemo every other week, I felt like a pincushion. Over nine months of therapy, I was stuck a total of at least sixty times. In spite of all the jabbing, some patients manage to keep their senses of humor, as did this one who told me, "Every Wednesday I had a blood test for lunch. I called the nurse my little vampire."

Biochemistries and Other Tests

The bulk of chemotherapy's side effects is due to toxicity to the rapidly reproducing cells in organs such as the blood-producing bone marrow. But as Dr. Richard Gralla points out, "When you look closely at a variety of drugs, it's not the bone marrow that is the major limitation, it's other organs." This second group of vital organs includes the lungs, heart, liver, kidney, bladder, and nerves. Damage to these organs may be quick, dramatic, and difficult to predict or slow, insidious, and easy to miss. Sometimes these organs need to be pushed only a little before the damage becomes irreversible. The danger to these organs may be great or small, depending on the drugs, the doses, and the health of the organs to begin with. New drugs and high doses pose especially high risks. Your oncologist will order tests to monitor the condition of these organs if you fall into the high-risk category.

With Adriamycin, for example, the dose-limiting toxicity (the side effect that limits the amount of drug that can be safely given) affects the heart; with cisplatin, the kidneys and auditory nerves are in jeopardy; with the nitrosoureas, the kidneys and lungs may be damaged; high doses of Cytoxan can affect the bladder. The danger of harming these organs is why it is necessary to give tests such as an echocardiogram for the heart, hearing tests, blood chemistry tests, liver function tests, and pulmonary function tests periodically and sometimes daily for a period of time.

Tumor Markers

Tumor markers (also called biological markers) are substances that either are contained within cancer cells or are released by them into the bloodstream. Some of these are chemicals that normally occur in the body but whose levels are higher when cancer is present. A few of these tests have become fairly standard. Many more have recently been developed and are being tested. So far, none of these tests is perfect. They are not foolproof in detecting all types of cancer. Though they are not the last word, they are useful tools in monitoring and detecting cancer growth and regression, especially in the early detection of recurrences or metastases. Among the alphabet soup of biological markers for which your blood may be tested are CEA for colorectal cancer, CA 15-3 for breast cancer, CA-125 for ovarian cancer, PSA for prostate cancer, and Alpha-fetoprotein for testicular cancer.

Reporting Your Side Effects

But lab tests and physical exams are only one component of the ongoing monitoring process. It also consists of the feedback you give your oncologist. Doctors and their nurses should be accessible and willing and able to give you the time you need, but they are not mind readers.

When your doctor asks you how you feel, be honest. You may fib to your friends and family if you feel it's necessary to put up a good front, but you should never lie to your oncologist about your condition. Don't say you feel fine when you feel lousy. It is not your responsibility to make him or her feel good and be pleased with your condition. It is your responsibility to do all in your power to help your oncologist help you; and help cannot be forthcoming if he or she hasn't a clue. Bravery can make you very sick, so don't tell your doctor what you think your doctor wants to hear—tell her what she *needs* to hear.

The sooner you report a side effect, the sooner it can be treated. Even if it's not "serious," there's no reason you should suffer even the slightest unnecessary discomfort, worry, or danger. In addition, what seems unimportant or insignificant to you could lead to something serious or be an indication of other already serious troubles.

Dr. Michael Van Scoy-Mosher says:

> *There's no question that patients are very symptom-conscious. I think one thing the physician can do is make the patients feel welcome to call with what they know are often minor complaints. One minute on the phone can sometimes head off two weeks of anxiety.*
>
> *Sometimes when patients call up with certain complaints, I try to explain to them why I don't think that's important. I don't just say, "Don't worry about it." It depends upon the patient—for instance, if he or she has a backache today, and tomorrow the shoulder aches a little bit, and next week the rib aches, that's not something to worry about.*

Many side effects can indeed wait until you see your doctor or nurse during your next scheduled treatment. Some, however, may indicate that you are seriously ill and should be treated right away.

I have included a list of possible signs of side effects that can be serious enough to require immediate treatment. If you are unsure or worried, speak up instantly. Speak to the doctor or nurse on the phone; your problem may be able to be settled right then and there. If not, your doctor might want you to make an appointment or admit you to a hospital. If you cannot reach your doctor, you can get in touch with the physician who is covering for him or her. As a last resort, you can go to the emergency room of the nearest hospital to which your doctor has admitting privileges or to the hospital at which you are receiving treatment as an outpatient. Not all cancer centers have emergency rooms, and clinics do not have inpatients at all. If you do go to a hospital with which your oncologist is not affiliated, he cannot treat you while you are there; you will be treated by a staff or house physician.

Your oncologist has several approaches available to alleviate the side effects you may develop. One is to change the timing or the way chemo is given—this works for a few side effects, such as nausea, tiredness, phlebitis, and heart toxicity. For example, there is evidence that cisplatin is much less toxic when given in the evening rather than in the morning and that Adriamycin is less toxic when given in the morning rather than in the evening. Another option might be to suggest nondrug therapies such as nutrition, exercise, and psychological therapy or counseling. A third approach is to reduce the dosage or frequency of treatment.

SIDE EFFECTS THAT SHOULD BE REPORTED IMMEDIATELY

You may be hesitant about reporting adverse symptoms to your doctor, especially if they seem minor. Some symptoms, however, should be reported right away, as they may be clues to further problems. Notify your doctor immediately if you experience any of the following symptoms during chemotherapy:

- Fever over 100° F.
- Bleeding or bruising.
- Rash or other allergic reaction (swollen eyelids, hands, or feet).
- Shaking and chills.
- Pain at the injection site.
- Unusual pain anywhere, including headaches and joint pain.
- Shortness of breath.
- Severe diarrhea or constipation.
- Bloody urine.

This course is usually taken only if the side effect is serious—that is, life-threatening—such as a low blood count as opposed to nausea, and if no other effective method exists to relieve it. The last tactic, to prescribe additional symptom-relieving medication, is sometimes preferred when the other methods are ineffective or because reducing the chemo drugs reduces the drugs' effectiveness to too great a degree. (Doctors may, of course, use any combination of these methods.) Fortunately, medication usually works just as well on conditions caused by chemo as on those due to some other reason.

Medication is useful, for instance, in controlling pain that might otherwise ruin your sleep, your appetite, and your social life. If you are nauseated and vomiting, an antinausea drug may help you maintain a better nutritional status and boost your morale. Insomnia can wear you out, but the short-term use of sleeping pills will help you get the rest you need to face the next day and help your body replace the tissue being damaged by chemotherapy. If you are anxious or depressed about your disease and its treatment, a tranquilizer or antidepressant can help restore your sense of well-being and relieve stress that may be detrimental to your prognosis and your quality of life. Erythropoietin (Procrit) can help restore your blood counts so you are not totally wiped out by fatigue.

Drugs such as these can bring welcome relief, but they can also impose their own set of distressing side effects. They may not, but if they do, these in turn can be treated. For instance, narcotics used to control pain often cause constipation, which in turn can be alleviated by laxatives, enemas, stool softeners, and a change in diet. Antinausea medication is usually sedative, but this can be dealt with by changing the schedule of medication.

Though it is generally wise to keep any additional drugs to a minimum and though some people may prefer to try nondrug methods first, drugs do have their uses. Just as strong drugs are needed to fight cancer, other drugs may at some point be justified to keep us going. When symptoms are severe or acute or don't respond well enough to nondrug measures, the stress and discomfort caused by the unrelieved symptom may be more harmful than the drug that relieves them. It is reasonable to be concerned about drugs you don't need, but drastic times call for drastic measures, and you shouldn't hesitate to call upon modern medicine for help. Part of living with cancer entails living in the here and now—and not being overly concerned with what a drug might do in some undefined future. The benefits of taking additional medication, especially if it's temporary, may far outweigh the risks.

I had a prescription for Compazine, but I never took it. My nausea wasn't bad, and I figured that since I was being pumped up with all those other drugs, why take more unless I really had to? I did eventually take something for a week or so to help me get to sleep. And then I also took an antidepressant for about a month. But it made me feel dizzy, so I stopped. By that time I was over the big depression, anyway. As my doctor said, "We have to use whatever we need to get you through this."

Dr. William Grace believes that you should "use whatever pharmacology you have to so a patient may lead as normal a life as possible." He notes that some of his patients have discovered that Dexatrim counteracts some of the fatigue related to chemo; some doctors even prescribe Dexedrine for this same purpose in selected patients. He says:

You have to remember that in small, careful doses, it's safe, and that chemotherapy patients are not drug abusers—they are quite normal people for whom a little bit of Dexedrine goes a long way. These people don't easily become drug-dependent. When they finish the chemotherapy course, they don't want any more Dexedrine or other medicines that made the therapy more tolerable.

You should be aware that both over-the-counter (OTC) and prescription drugs can affect you more than usual or interact dangerously with chemotherapy drugs. Common aspirin, for example, can compound the problem of slow blood clotting. Chemotherapy patients are usually advised to switch to aspirin-free analgesics and to learn to read labels carefully since many OTC products contain aspirin. Even diuretics and antibiotics can interact with your chemotherapy regimen.

Always inform your chemotherapist about any drugs you may be taking and keep him up to date on any changes. Other drugs that may interfere with chemotherapy include anticoagulants, blood pressure drugs, anticonvulsants, barbiturates, cough medicines, sleeping pills, tranquilizers, and birth control pills.

Alcohol is not usually thought of as a drug, but it is one, so some thought should be given to its use during chemotherapy. Usually, the chemotherapy patient is able to drink some alcohol—one or two glasses of wine or beer a day. Occasionally, however, no alcohol is allowed because it can aggravate the side effects of some drugs. In addition, consumption of huge amounts of alcohol can cause liver damage and vitamin deficiencies. Not only can chemotherapy cause the same thing to happen, but a well-functioning liver is crucial in detoxifying the anticancer drugs, so be sure to ask your doctor about alcohol consumption. I'm not exactly a lush, but I do like wine when I go out. When I asked if wine was permissible, my doctor said, "Sure, go ahead, have some fun." But I began to notice that even a glass or two made me more tired the next day. I was feeling tired enough from my chemo, so I stopped the booze altogether. Later, my surgeon told me this was quite common. (Still later, evidence cropped up that alcohol consumption may increase the risk of breast cancer.)

Other common medical measures that may be called upon to support the chemotherapy patient and limit the short- and long-term effects include the various blood products. When the blood count falls too low, transfusions of red cells, platelets, or leukocytes may be required together or individually. Some new therapies are adding substances that stimulate blood cell growth such as colony-stimulating factors.

Treating the Whole Person

There is more to progressive, caring chemotherapy than simply giving a passive patient the right anticancer drugs in the right amounts, and there is more to minimizing side effects than supplying patients with yet more drugs. Though a sound, disease-oriented treatment is paramount and symptom-relieving drugs have their place, you can't treat a disease completely and humanely in isolated technological splendor. It is becoming increasingly obvious that having chemotherapy affects you totally; there-

BEFORE STARTING CHEMOTHERAPY

Are you ready? Undergoing chemotherapy is much like running a marathon. The better prepared you are, the better the race you can run. You'll most likely do better and have fewer unwelcome surprises if you do the following:

- Trust your doctor(s). And if you have doubts, trust your feelings.
- Believe you are doing the right thing for *you.*
- Get a second opinion of your diagnosis and treatment plan.
- Build up your strength and resistance by eating well and getting appropriate exercise and sleep.
- Have your support system in place.
- Understand what your medical plan covers and requires.
- Know which drugs you will be getting and which side effects to expect or be on the alert for.
- Prepare your family, friends, and coworkers for possible changes in your energy level, appearance, and moods.
- Know whom to call with your concerns.
- Have a dental checkup, cleaning, and any necessary dental work completed before your first chemotherapy treatment.
- Set aside a file folder, box, or loose-leaf binder in which you can keep all papers relating to your treatment, important phone numbers and contacts, your personal journal if you are keeping one, notes of conversations with your health-care professionals, lists of questions, and printed Internet articles or other research.

fore, you need to be treated as a whole person. Medicine, in the narrow sense of using drugs to treat disease, cannot begin to determine and fulfill your physical, psychological, social, and spiritual needs, but broadening its scope to include nondrug support therapies can. "Good medicine" can help you keep your life at the highest quality possible by taking care of the rest of you while the chemo takes care of the cancer.

In Part Three, I include suggestions for a wide variety of steps you can take and methods you can utilize to get through chemotherapy as unscathed as possible. They include commonsense measures, medications, and "complementary therapies" such as emotional help from family, friends, and professionals; stress management and reduction; diet and nutrition; and exercise. Which ones you choose, to what degree you utilize them, where you find them, and how they fit in with your chemotherapy program depend on your individual reactions to chemotherapy, your needs, your style, and your own resources. For some patients, these therapies play a major and integral part in keeping body and soul together.

My oncologist, who looks to both traditional and nontraditional sources of support for his cancer patients, believes:

> The most important thing in medicine is to individualize. Each person needs something slightly different. You can't just use the cookie-cutter system. An oncologist has to use the very finest that is available at the present time. That includes a continuing search for protocols that have been demonstrated to be of validity in doses that have been shown to be valuable; it includes very careful attention to the known side effects and known toxic effects of the medication; and it includes their application in a program that involves a certain amount of building and strengthening of the body as well as simply destroying.

Through all your emotional and physical experiences, your oncologist is the central figure around whom everything else seems to revolve. Your doctor, then, is the most natural person to whom you turn for support. In an ideal world, he or she would be able to treat all your related needs or recommend people who can. In reality, doctors are somewhat limited in their methods and patients often look elsewhere for help—to a primary-care physician or nurse or to someone outside the medical mainstream. It's best to inform your oncologist of any additional therapies you are undertaking. Make it clear at the outset that they are being used as supplementary therapies to, not in place of, chemotherapy. Even if your oncologist does not endorse a particular therapy (chances are getting better that he or she will), it is important to reveal everything there is to know about your health practices. Some practices—such as the more extreme diets—may actually do more harm than good. But if a therapy does do good, your doctor may pass the information on to other patients.

When used as supplements to chemotherapy, support therapies can be thought of as a form of "insurance" and a means of improving the quality of life that is being eroded by the drugs. In addition, these therapies can help fill the gap between the cold technical approach sometimes offered to the patient and the warm, human approach the patient really needs. Perhaps their greatest value, however, lies in the way they enable you to play a more active role in your treatment, to feel a sense of control rather than playing the part of a passive patient leaving your life totally in the hands of the doctor and the drugs. Chemotherapy need not be a spectator sport. Dr. Ernest Rosenbaum writes in the introduction to his book *A Comprehensive Guide for Cancer Patients and Their Families:*

> *When you are an active participant in your medical care and rehabilitation, you can maintain a sense of control over your disease and your therapy. Only you can take responsibility for your state of mind, nutritional status, and physical fitness. The act of taking responsibility is in itself an important factor in maintaining self-esteem, a feeling of independence, and faith in your ability to cope. It is a critical part of therapy.*

PART TWO

Coping with Side Effects

This section is probably the reason that most of you have bought this book. Everyone is concerned about side effects—more accurately called adverse effects—of the drugs they will be taking, or are already taking. I don't blame you—after the effectiveness of the drugs, this was my next biggest concern. While I had heard about the nausea and vomiting and the hair loss—two of the most common adverse effects—I was totally in the dark about all the others, including the likelihood that I would go through menopause at age thirty-one. This was a surprise (I could not for the life of me figure out why this should happen, or what to do about it), but even more devastating was the extreme fatigue. And the emotional side effects—including the "chemo blues"—were also a surprise.

Fortunately, both physical and emotional side effects are receiving greater recognition and attention, even among conventional medical professionals. Be sure to tell your doctor about any effects that may be a result of your treatment regimen; there are medications he or she may prescribe for you or over-the-counter medications you can try. In addition, you may be able to reduce and prevent certain side effects by building up your strength and body reserves before you begin chemo through good nutrition, herbs, exercise, nutritional supplements, and mind-body techniques. Of course, you may also want to continue with these during the chemo to prolong their protective, mitigating effects.

CHAPTER SIX

The Physical Effects of Chemotherapy

While chemotherapy can be lifesaving, it brings with it a litany of side effects for many. Here in Part Two, I present an A-to-Z listing of common adverse physical side effects of chemotherapy and what you can do about them. As you'll see, there are many physical measures to take to minimize and alleviate physical side effects, but don't overlook the mind-body connection. Pay attention to your mental state and perhaps practice one or more of the mind-body techniques included in Chapter 7 on emotional side effects.

Appetite Changes and Weight Loss

Loss of appetite (*anorexia*) and the resulting weight loss are of primary concern during chemotherapy. Often it is complications caused by malnutrition that lead to other illnesses and possibly death, especially in advanced cancer patients. Losses of five, ten, fifteen, and even more pounds are common. If you have lost more than a few pounds, try to follow my recommendations below to minimize or prevent further loss if possible because chances are you'll feel healthier and stronger physically and psychologically if you maintain your normal weight.

CAUSES OF APPETITE LOSS

Anorexia is one of the most difficult side effects to treat because it can have so many contributing causes. These include psychological and emotional factors, the disease itself, and its treatment. For example, depression, fear, and anxiety may be causing you to lose your desire for food. These emotions can begin to take their toll early on: Patients who have been told that they might have cancer have been known to lose between five and ten pounds while waiting for a firm diagnosis! After diagnosis, emotions continue to affect the appetite, and they don't stop during the ups and downs of treatment or if the disease recurs.

Side effects of chemotherapy such as mouth sores (see MOUTH, GUM, AND THROAT PROBLEMS), diarrhea (see DIARRHEA), constipation (see CONSTIPATION), malabsorption, lethargy, sleep disturbances (see SLEEP DISTURBANCES), and alterations in the ability to taste and/or smell food (see TASTE CHANGES) also play their parts. The comedienne Gilda Radner wrote in her memoir, *It's Always Something*, "Eating was very unpleasant. I craved salty things because I could taste them. I ate what I ordinarily wouldn't eat. I wanted cheeseburgers, cheese, and pickles. Lettuce and vegetables tasted like plastic . . . bland foods tasted like something they weren't . . . a carrot tasted like a ceramic kitchen magnet."

Other factors that influence appetite and eating are changes in lifestyle such as isolation from other people and reduced physical activity. In addition, conditioned responses from nausea or pain caused by the treatment make the idea of food less appealing. Physical problems related to the location of a tumor (in cancers of the head, neck, esophagus, stomach, or bowels) can affect the ability to eat; surgery and radiation to these parts can cause difficulty in swallowing, dry mouth, pain, and problems with digestion and taste perception. The tumor itself, rapidly dying cells, or toxicity to organs such as the hypothalamus or liver can release chemical messages that interfere with your appetite.

If you are overweight at the start of your therapy, you might not mind the expected weight loss! However, as explained in Chapter 8, it is important to keep nourished. In addition, weight loss can set off harmful chemical reactions in the body or may be interpreted as a sign that the disease is advancing. Health professionals do not like to see their patients lose weight at this time. Lisa Logan, clinical dietitian at Denver Presbyterian Hospital, says, "The last thing I usually recommend for cancer patients is weight loss, no matter how much they weigh when I assess their conditions." Dr. Ronald Bash agrees: "Oncologists get scared when they see their patients losing weight. It's a bad sign in cancer. And you never know when a patient is going to need his or her weight."

WHAT YOU CAN DO

There are many practices that can help you increase or maintain your appetite and/or the amount of food you eat. Many are simple tips or tricks, some involve behavior modification, and others rely on special products or foods to boost nutrition.

Eat More and Better

- You may need to change the meaning of food in your life. Instead of eating to satisfy your taste buds or your hunger, you may need to eat foods that seem tasteless and eat at times when you are not really hungry. A good deal of pleasure may be missing, but eating good, nourishing food is an integral part of your treatment.

- If possible, consult with a dietitian and/or nutritionist who will explain what a balanced, nutritious diet contains and help you plan your daily menu. Take a few sample hospital menus home with you as examples when planning your own meals after you have been released. It may be advisable to add vitamin/mineral supplements to your diet to supply the nutrients that you are missing.

- Drink plenty of liquids and emphasize those with high nutritional content, such as milk (use soy, oat, rice, or nut milks if you have a problem digesting cow's milk), milk shakes, and juices. Fruit nectars are high in calories and are delicious.

- If you are also suffering from appetite-depressing side effects such as pain (see PAIN), stress, fatigue (see FATIGUE AND WEAKNESS), mouth sores (see MOUTH, GUM, AND THROAT PROBLEMS), taste blindness (see TASTE CHANGES), constipation (see CONSTIPATION), and diarrhea (see

DIARRHEA), try relieving them by using the methods recommended in this book.

- Eat in a relaxing, pleasant atmosphere with soft music, good company, and perhaps a glass of wine. It is helpful if friends and family members encourage you, but they should understand that it is unwise to try to force you to eat at this time.

- What you eat is as important as how much you eat. Although you should eat the foods you like, it may be wise to stay away from your favorite foods when you don't feel like eating. Patients often develop an aversion to foods eaten when ill and then find them undesirable even when they feel well. When you're feeling ill, it's better to stick with nonaromatic cold or room-temperature foods about which you have neutral feelings, such as juices, Popsicles, and gelatin desserts.

- Try to include as many highly nutritious foods as possible, especially between treatments, when your appetite is better. That's the time to indulge in your favorite foods, too. Patients have told me that they often make up for lost time by gorging on pizza or cheesecake after the nausea subsides. Donna Park, former assistant director of nursing, ambulatory care, at New York's Memorial Sloan-Kettering, thinks that "people are too strict with chemotherapy patients sometimes and insist that they eat something nutritious when they have no appetite for it. I'd rather they eat something that is maybe less nutritious but at least gets eaten. At least it has calories. So what if a patient eats ice cream three days a week?"

- Arrange to have your biggest meals whenever your appetite is at its best—this is usually in the morning, but it may be different for you.

- If you are too tired to shop and cook, ask friends and relatives to help out. During your "up" periods you can cook and freeze food portions that you can easily warm up and eat during your "down" times. Or rely on nutritious convenience foods such as creamed soups or "Lite" frozen dinners.

- Exercise before a meal can perk up a flagging appetite. Do simple range-of-motion exercises, walking, or anything you like and can manage for at least five to ten minutes a half hour before meals.

- Studies show that cancer patients can require up to hundreds of additional calories and twice as much protein as noncancer patients. However, many high-protein foods—meat particularly—are often repulsive to cancer patients. Unfortunately, many high-protein foods are also high in fat, which chemotherapy patients may have trouble digesting and are of questionable value health wise. Many professionals, nevertheless, advise patients to try to add high-calorie, high-protein (and, often, coincidentally high-fat, high-sugar) foods and food supplements to their diets and usual recipes. These foods include butter, peanut butter, cheese, eggs, powdered milk or protein supplements (found in health food stores) added to milk, juice, shakes, other prepared dishes, instant breakfast or granola bars, or eggnogs and milk shakes. Other sources of low-fat protein can be found by combining plant proteins with each other and with small amounts of fish, poultry, milk products, or meat. Vegetable protein made from soybeans can be added to ground meat dishes—this lightens them by reducing the fat content without sacrificing the protein.

Take Nutritional Supplements

If you experience severe weight loss—5 percent or more of your total body weight—you become a "candidate" for nutritional supplements. There are commercially prepared high-protein, high-calorie food supplements available in liquid or pudding form. These "formulas" are available in drugstores and from home-health care suppliers and can be used as substitutes for regular food or in addition to it. "These do tend to have an unpleasant aftertaste," admits Lisa Logan. "So I try to make them more palatable for the patient by adding ice cream, fruit, milk products, and eggs, which mask the flavor and boost up the nutrients." Other possible additions include flavoring extracts, fruit juice, and carbonated beverages. These preparations are low-residue, however, and can lead to constipation. Sometimes freezing liquid supplements and eating them like ice cream or blending them in a milk shake makes them more palatable.

In advanced cancer patients, when there is pronounced weight loss, weakness, and malnutrition, *hyperalimentation* may be used. The patient is fed with liquids containing vitamins, minerals, protein, fat, and other substances through tubes inserted into the gastrointestinal tract or the veins.

Up to 4,000 calories can be taken in this way by patients who badly need them and whose condition can improve remarkably because of this therapy.

Take Certain Medications

Anorexia and cachexia (wasting away syndrome) often go hand in hand. However, sometimes people on chemo lose weight even while eating plenty because they are not absorbing the nutrients in their food. There are some medications that don't necessarily stimulate the appetite, but make the most of what you do take in. We're learning how certain drugs can help fight cachexia from studies done with AIDS patients. "Megace, a progestrone, is used in high doses to produce weight gain in patients who are losing too much weight from chemo, radiation, or the cancer process itself," says Dr. Richard Cohen. "This is useful weight gain—both fat and muscle."

Hydrazine sulfate, which has been studied in the United States and many other countries worldwide for many years, is another interesting compound. Studies show that it can reduce wasting away caused by cancer, and some studies show it may reduce tumor size by starving cancer cells while leaving normal cells alone. Hydrazine sulfate was on the American Cancer Society's "Unproven Cancer Cures" list for many years. Although it is no longer on this list, its use is still controversial in the United States and the FDA has not approved it for this purpose. However, if you are dropping weight, you may want to ask your physician to obtain it through the FDA's compassionate use program from a compounding pharmacy in the United States.

Many people have noticed that medical marijuana reduces nausea and vomiting (see NAUSEA AND VOMITING). Many chemo patients and non-chemo patients alike have noticed that marijuana improves appetite and restores a zest for eating (aka "the munchies").

Bladder and Kidney Problems

Cyclophosphamide (Cytoxan) can cause acute noninfectious (hemor-rhagic) cystitis, or a bladder infection. Since 70 percent of this drug is excreted by the kidneys, the bladder is given plenty of exposure, and it is thought that the cystitis results from the drug acting directly on the mucosa that lines the bladder. Chronic bladder irritation can cause scar tissue to form, and as a result, the bladder is able to hold less, and you need to urinate more frequently. The symptoms of this relatively rare complication of therapy are painful; frequent urination, urgency of urination, low back pain, and blood in the urine.

The onset of the symptoms may occur as early as twenty-four hours after the first drug dose or may be delayed until several weeks after the end of the treatment. Acute symptoms usually go away when the drug is stopped, but slight bleeding may persist for months. Treatment for noninfectious cystitis that is not severe consists of medication; when it is more serious, surgery may be necessary. The same symptoms of noninfectious cystitis may indicate infectious cystitis, which may be treated with antibiotics.

Other drugs given to treat cancer can act on the kidneys (renal toxicity). These include cisplatin, dacarbazine, daunorubicin, doxorubicin, lomustine, methotrexate, the mitomycins, and mithramycin. Kidney damage can be serious and sometimes is severe and leads to fatal kidney failure. However, it may be reversible if caught early enough. Symptoms include headache, swelling of the body, and flank pain. (Doxorubicin in the system creates red-colored urine, which lasts only one or two days and is not serious.)

WHAT YOU CAN DO

- For bladder problems: Cystitis seems to appear to be more of a danger in those who receive large doses of cyclophosphamide intravenously, who are on prolonged therapy, or who do not drink enough fluids. If you are receiving this drug, you should drink as much liquid as possible—at least two quarts a day, most of which should be in the form of water, but some of which can be other beverages such as herbal tea, mineral water, soda, and juices or in the form of Popsicles or Jell-O.

- For kidney problems: As is the case with bladder toxicity, drinking large quantities of liquids can prevent these problems from occurring or at least minimize them. In some cases and with some drugs, large doses of vitamin C, mannitol, or sodium bicarbonate have been used in an attempt to further minimize the risks. Renal function may also be affected by the remnants of dead cancer cells that pass through the kidneys. Drinking plenty of liquids usually forestalls any problems, but your doctor may also prescribe allopurinol to prevent problems in patients with leukemia and lymphomas, where large numbers of cancer cells are destroyed. Your doctor may prescribe dieuretics and hydration to prevent kidney damage from cisplatinum.

Blood and Bone Marrow Effects

Your blood cells are manufactured in the bone marrow and reproduce rapidly and frequently and so are quite vulnerable to chemotherapy drugs. Almost all the drugs used in cancer chemotherapy affect these cells. The drugs that depress, or lower the activity of, the bone marrow are called *myelosuppressive drugs.*

The bone marrow produces three types of cells: the white blood cells, which help fight infections; platelets, which help clot the blood and control bleeding; and the red blood cells, which carry oxygen to the cells of the body. Low blood counts, therefore, affect you in three main ways: too few white cells (*leukopenia*) make you more vulnerable to infection; low platelets (*thrombocytopenia*) mean your blood will have trouble clotting properly; and low red cell counts (*anemia*) leave you tired, weak, and listless. All three counts can and do drop simultaneously; this is called *pancytopenia.* Your body has an enormous capacity to churn out new blood cells but not a great enough one to completely forestall the side effects. As a result, it is likely that you will have blood-related side effects to some degree. Blood counts generally are at their lowest level seven to ten days after a treatment, and at this point, called the *nadir,* you are at the greatest risk of developing complications.

WHAT YOU CAN DO

Since low blood counts are expected in most chemotherapies, your oncologist will periodically order blood tests, called complete blood counts (CBCs), to use as the main guide in determining whether there should be any changes in the dosage and/or scheduling of the drugs. If the counts dip too low, your treatment will be cut down or held back until the counts return to safer limits. If you experience severe myelosuppression, you will be watched closely, perhaps in the hospital.

In some cases, your doctor may prescribe drugs such as antibiotics, colony-stimulating factors (CSF), or transfusions of blood cells. But there are many precautions and special steps that you can take both to minimize the side effects and to prevent complications from setting in. (See BLOOD-CLOTTING PROBLEMS, FATIGUE AND WEAKNESS, and INFECTIONS.)

Blood-Clotting Problems

When your platelet count drops, the ability of your blood to clot is reduced. Because there are other coagulation factors in the blood, most of which are produced by the liver and are rarely affected by chemotherapy, the blood will still be able to clot eventually, but the process will take longer than usual.

WHAT YOU CAN DO

- Your oncologist will know from your blood test whether your platelet count is low. In between blood tests you should watch out for signs yourself: red dots in the skin (*petechiae*), an abundance of black-and-blue marks, unusual bleeding from the nose or gums, or blood in the urine or bowel movements. You should bring these symptoms to the immediate attention of your physician.
- When your platelet count is low, you should take precautions to protect yourself from any physical trauma that could cause bleeding.

Take it easy and avoid dangerous situations such as contact sports, heavy physical labor, or any violent jarring activity that could cause you to bleed in your joints. Wear protective gear during gardening and cooking and other potentially hazardous activities. Be careful with knives, scissors, and razors. Even blowing your nose forcefully can damage delicate blood vessels and cause bleeding. Use a soft-bristled toothbrush and avoid flossing if you find that your gums bleed easily. Sometimes switching from a wet razor to an electric razor is advised.

• Your doctors will probably advise you not to take aspirin because it further diminishes the blood's ability to clot. Use an aspirin substitute such as Tylenol or Datril.

• If you should injure yourself in spite of taking precautions, help the clotting process along by putting a clean cloth or paper towel over the wound and applying pressure for five or ten minutes. Elevate the affected part if possible, and use ice or cold water to constrict the blood vessels. Since a low platelet count is often accompanied by a low white cell count, take careful antiseptic measures to help prevent infection. If the bleeding hasn't stopped after twenty minutes, consult your doctor.

Breathing Problems. *See* LUNG PROBLEMS.

Cardiac Toxicity. *See* HEART PROBLEMS.

Constipation

Overall, constipation occurs less frequently in chemotherapy patients than does diarrhea. This condition, which is characterized by infrequent bowel movements; hard, dark, small stools; or straining, is uncomfortable and can be dangerous. The abdomen becomes distended, and you suffer from cramping, a decrease in appetite, and possibly fecal impaction. Oddly enough, constipation can lead to diarrhea when it increases the bacterial growth within the intestines. The result is explosive diarrhea occurring around the hard stool.

Constipation in chemotherapy patients may be due to a lack of fiber in the diet, the use of narcotics to control pain, antidepressants, diuretics, tranquilizers, a lack of exercise, and emotional stress. Often these are contributing factors to constipation caused by a group of drugs called the vinca alkaloids: vincristine and vinblastine. Vincristine, for example, has been reported to cause this side effect in 30 percent of those who get the drug. These drugs are toxic to the nerves. This leads to a sluggish or paralyzed bowel because the muscle contractions (peristalsis) that move food through the bowel do not occur.

Constipation from chemotherapy may occur within twenty-four hours of treatment, but it may not be obvious until several courses of treatment have been received. Numb or tingling fingers and/or toes usually accompany this side effect, when it is due to nerve damage. It appears to be minor but is an early warning of neural drug toxicity, a potentially serious and nonreversible condition when allowed to progress.

WHAT YOU CAN DO

Be sure to tell your physician if you are experiencing constipation. He or she may want to test you to see if there is nerve damage and adjust your drugs accordingly. You make need to take laxatives, suppositories, enemas, or stool softeners until the condition eases or reverses. Thereafter, or if the condition is slight, the following measures may help alone or be used in addition to occasional treatment with the harsher measures listed above. (The continual use of laxatives can be habit-forming. They irritate the digestive tract and make it difficult to have normal bowel movements without them.)

- Eat high-fiber (bulk) foods: fresh fruit and vegetables—raw or cooked but still crisp—dried fruit such as prunes, whole-grain breads and cereals, nuts, popcorn, and bran. Add bran to your diet gradually—start with two teaspoons a day and slowly work up to two tablespoons, then up to four or six. Too much fiber too soon can cause cramping, gas, and diarrhea.

- Avoid raw fruits and vegetables if your white cell count dips below 1,800.
- Drink plenty of fluids, which the fiber will absorb, keeping stools soft.
- Liquid or powdered acidophilus ("friendly" bacteria), available in health-food stores, is another natural way to keep "regular."
- Coffee, tea, and alcohol tend to stimulate the intestines—but don't overindulge.
- Get more exercise—walk, do isometrics.
- Set aside enough "bathroom time" to give sluggish bowels a chance to move.
- Take measures to alleviate depression or anxiety. A hot bath relaxes you all over, including the sphincter muscle.
- Avoid cheese, refined grain products (white flour), and chocolate because they can be constipating.

Cough.

See MOUTH, GUM, AND THROAT PROBLEMS and LUNG PROBLEMS.

Diarrhea

Diarrhea, to one degree or another, is a common complaint among chemotherapy patients. It occurs when bowel movements are more frequent, loose, and fluid than usual. You may have cramping, flatulence (gas), bloating, and sore, irritated skin around the rectum. Diarrhea is not merely uncomfortable and embarrassing; it can disrupt your lifestyle and lead to weakness, malnutrition, dehydration, and chemical imbalances because nutrients and water are not properly absorbed by the body.

The anticancer drugs that are prime culprits in this side effect are the antimetabolites and the antibiotics. These drugs kill the rapidly dividing cells that line the intestines. This causes a reduction in the production of the food-digesting enzymes normally present in the intestines, irritation, swelling, and an overproduction of mucus. Neither food nor water is absorbed, and since intestinal activity is stimulated, the food is passed along to the outside world before it is fully digested.

WHAT YOU CAN DO

If you suffer from three or more loose bowel movements a day, consult your physician. He or she may suggest that you adopt an all-liquid diet for a few days to give the bowels a rest and then gradually add some low-bulk, "binding" foods. Your doctor may also prescribe antidiarrhea medication such as Kaopectate or Lomotil.

Foods to Avoid

Experts usually advise that you avoid the following foods because they tend to encourage diarrhea—they are high in fiber or irritate or stimulate the gastrointestinal tract in other ways.

- Whole-grain bread and cereal.
- Nuts, seeds, coconut, and popcorn.
- Fried, greasy, fatty foods; pastries; and potato chips.
- Fresh and dried fruits and fruit juices (see exceptions below).
- Raw vegetables, cooked vegetables that are gas-producing, dried beans, and peas,
- Strong spices and spicy foods such as chili powder, pepper, curry, garlic, horseradish, olives, pickles, and relishes.
- Chocolate, alcoholic beverages, coffee, regular tea, tobacco, and carbonated beverages (unless they have been allowed to go flat).
- Milk and milk products (see also MILK INTOLERANCE.)

Foods to Emphasize

The following "binding" foods are low in residue or fiber, are easily digested, and tend to be soothing to the digestive tract.

- Soft high-protein foods such as cottage cheese, cream cheese, mild soft cheese, eggs, custards, and creamy peanut butter.
- Mild high-protein foods such as fish and poultry; low-fat meats such as veal, lamb, and some cuts of beef—broiled or roasted rather than fried.
- Cooked cereals such as cream of wheat and farina.
- Some fruits such as bananas (high in potassium), applesauce, peeled apples (contain pectin, an antidiarrheal), apple juice, grape juice, and avocados.
- White bread or toast.
- Macaroni, white rice, noodles; and baked, broiled, or mashed potatoes.
- Some cooked vegetables such as asparagus tips, green beans, carrots, peas, spinach, and squash.
- Nutmeg (added to dishes sometimes slows down the digestive tract).

Additional Measures

In addition, you should:

- Include rest periods during the day if you find you are very tired.
- Drink plenty of fluids to replace the water lost through diarrhea; sip slowly.
- Add foods high in potassium—bananas, apricot and peach nectars, potatoes, broccoli, halibut, and asparagus—to replace the potassium depleted during fluid loss. If the problem is severe, your doctor may prescribe a potassium supplement.
- Eat small, frequent meals, slowly—this is easier on the digestive system. Foods served at room temperature or slightly warmer are advised, since very hot or very cold foods can stimulate contractions of the digestive tract.
- Cleanse the rectal area after each bowel movement if it becomes sore from frequent evacuation. Use warm water and a nondrying, nonirritating deodorant-free soap such as Dove, Basis, or Castile. A healing salve such as Desitine or A & D ointment, or a local anesthetic such

as Tucks will give you comfort, as will frequent sitz baths or sitting in a tub of warm water.

Eye and Vision Problems

Though the problem is long ignored and still rarely recognized or acknowledged, many chemotherapy drugs have the potential to affect your eyes or vision in a variety of ways. Cataracts, retinal problems, blurred vision, altered color perception, excess tearing or dry eye, conjunctivitis, glaucoma and increased eye pressure—these and more have been linked with various chemotherapy drugs. Drugs most often associated with ocular effects include busulfan, corticosteroids, mitotane, chlorambucil, tamoxifen, cisplatin, cyclophosphamide, nitrosoureas, and methotrexate.

WHAT YOU CAN DO

Fortunately, these ocular toxicities may be reversible if your oncologist recognizes them early on and reduces or discontinues the drug that is responsible.

- Have a baseline ophthalmologic exam before beginning chemotherapy.
- Tell your doctor of any changes—burning, tearing, or blurry vision—you notice while on therapy and have your eyes compared to the baseline exam.
- For some symptoms, such as dry eyes, over-the-counter or prescription eye drops may help.

Fatigue and Weakness

For many chemotherapy patients, ever-present tiredness is the toughest side effect to contend with. This feeling of "general malaise," as the textbooks call it, though hardly life-threatening, is the side effect that is nevertheless most likely to turn your life upside down. A constant lack of energy is what keeps you from living a more normal life, from doing all the things that you want or need to do, from feeling like yourself.

I am normally full of energy, the instigator of escapades (or easily talked into them), but on chemo I did a lot of staying at home. This state of not being quite myself was probably the most demoralizing side effect I had to live with. You think, "Who is this person?" The tiredness of chemo is not an ordinary tiredness and is rather hard to describe. It's more oppressive than coming home from a rough day on the job or staying up all night. I'd hear other people complain, "I'm so tired," and think, "If you only *knew!*"

Sometimes it felt like the day before a cold or the flu arrives: a vague, all-over dragginess, like a car running on the wrong fuel. Mornings were usually the worst. I'm not a morning person to begin with, but some days it was so hard to get started that my husband had to help drag me out of bed even though I knew that I would probably feel better once I was up and about. Other times it seemed I spent whole days sluggishly moving, dreamlike, through air as thick as water, my limbs made of lead, the very cells of my body made of stone. Chemo sometimes deprived me of the energy to walk, to drink, to hold a pencil or a conversation, so overpowering was the heaviness in my mind, my bones, my guts, and my soul. The day after a treatment, I'd find myself facedown on a friend's couch or under the covers of my bed, unable to do anything but complain.

Eventually, I discovered that on these low days quietly moaning to myself actually helped. It sounds silly, but there was nothing specific I could do to actually change the way I felt, and moaning at least allowed me to express my misery and functioned as some kind of outlet. Who knows? Maybe the inner vibrations became a kind of chant that helped the healing process.

When the weakness was bad, it was very bad; when it wasn't, it was bearable. I did manage to continue to work the whole time I was on chemo—I completed one book in progress, wrote another, and delivered the finished manuscript the same week I wrapped up my chemo. I continued a modified exercise regimen. And I did socialize and have fun—went to dinner, parties, dances, movies, and so on—but I coordinated these outings with my "up" periods, those times when I felt nearly normal, and then I was almost hyperenergetic, as if to make up for lost time.

Though individual, my experience was not unique. Fatigue tends to come and go in cycles, with the worst days usually occurring right after a treatment, the listless feeling may never really disappear completely. This is how one person describes it:

It was like they were shooting an A-bomb into me that blew me away every time. The two weeks I was off chemo I spent getting myself back on my feet again. But I never really had the chance to say, "Gee, I feel great"—by the time I got to feel human again, it was time to go back. It would have been nice to feel what it was like to be normal again just for a minute.

Another patient recalls:

I was exceptionally tired while I was on chemo; I had been the type of person who took on two jobs and worked sixteen hours. When I was on chemo, I worked one job and would come home and have to take a nap if I was going to be able to cope with the evening's activities.

I was more tired than usual. In the afternoons I almost always had to lie down and take a nap. Then I was able to get right back into everything. Right back into my painting, right back into the choir, right back into the other activities I enjoyed before.

And another:

I used to come home from work and clean—I don't do it anymore; I have help once a week. Now I clean in the morning when I have most of my strength, because when I come home in the afternoon I can't do it. I wake up an hour earlier just to get the house straightened out so at least when I come home, everything is neat and clean.

According to a 2001 editorial published in the *British Medical Journal,* "A consensus is emerging among patients, caregivers and oncologists that cancer related fatigue is the most important untreated symptom in cancer today . . . Though the problem is real, it is rarely discussed and seldom treated." Donna Park, former assistant director of nursing, ambulatory care, at New York's Memorial Sloan-Kettering, says, "I think the biggest thing that people complain about is being tired." But in spite of the expected tiredness, people, especially women on adjuvant breast chemotherapy, are encouraged to "carry out their current lifestyles." However, she adds, "As health professionals we had at first underestimated the impact of this treatment on patients' daily lives."

Ms. Park's observations are confirmed by a study published in 1997 in *Seminars in Hematology.* When patients and doctors were surveyed, nearly 80 percent of patients experienced fatigue, with 32 percent experiencing it daily, and 32 percent reporting that it significantly affected their daily routines. Oncologists believed that pain affected their patients lives more than fatigue (61 percent versus 37 percent), but patients said fatigue affected their lives much more than pain (61 percent versus 19 percent). A follow-up study offered more confirmation: when patients were asked which symptom most affected quality of life, fatigue won by a landslide (60 percent), with nausea coming in a distant second (22 percent), followed by depression (10 percent) and pain (6 percent). These and other studies are signs that fatigue will be getting the attention it deserves. In addition, the Oncology Nursing Society and a lung cancer advocacy group cosponsor a Web site devoted to cancer-related fatigue, and April 6 has been declared Cancer Fatigue Awareness Day.

Much of the anxiety about the tiredness is related to the issue of working. Showing up at the job every day like everybody else can be a real problem about which not much can be done specifically, unless you have an understanding employer, terrific insurance, and an undemanding job or can make your own hours. Still, many people who need to continue to work do manage to muster enough strength to get there and get through the work-day. (See "Getting Through the Work Day" on page 156.) So much of our identities and sense of accomplishment are tied up with what we do, and it is this, combined with the necessity of earning a living, that drives us to get up and out in spite of the gargantuan effort it sometimes takes. One patient recounts:

> *I got very tired when my blood count went too low. The lack of energy . . . I'm back to my normal habits now, but it took a while. I'm not one to sleep beyond seven or eight hours, even on my day off; on chemo I'd stay in bed until ten. Usually I'm at work by seven-thirty every morning; on chemo I got calls at eight-fifteen asking, "Are you coming to work today?" Twice that happened. Then I got myself two alarm clocks.*

Being able to continue to work during chemotherapy can be a major emotional and social support in helping you cope. Work gives you the opportunity to reach out beyond yourself, to have a broader identity, to feel able to master things. If you have the type of job where you have to look good and be on top and be present at odd hours—that's tough turf. Or if you have a job that is physically demanding, if you operate heavy machinery, or are in sales and always have to be "up" and "on," or are in a high-powered executive position—that's difficult, too. But if you have a job with flexibility, where your appearance doesn't have primary importance and you can have one day up and one day down, you do better.

Overwhelming tiredness can affect your social and home lives, too. Friends and family members may not realize how tired and awful you feel; without any outward signs or symptoms, this is a side effect that others easily forget or are skeptical about. They may mistake your lack of enthusiasm for laziness or as a sign of depression or unsociability.

Fatigue is largely due to anemia, or a lack of oxygen-bearing red blood cells. The cells of your body literally become starved for oxygen and function suboptimally. Feeling dizzy, chilly, short of breath, and having a tendency to become upset more easily than usual are also indications of anemia. Fatigue is also somehow related to low white cell counts, although no one is sure why. It may be that your weakened immune system is using up energy to battle infections. (See INFECTIONS.)

Fatigue may also be caused or contributed to by the accumulation of waste products that are produced when large numbers of cells are killed by chemotherapy, a poor diet, lack of sleep, and the emotional stress of coping with cancer and chemotherapy. (See Chapter 7.) Factors such as boredom, pain, and a lack of exercise may exaggerate the feeling of listlessness. Advanced cancer itself can make you tired.

Additional signs of fatigue are irritability, tearfulness, decreased ability to make decisions, withdrawal, apathy, feelings of hopelessness and helplessness, impaired concentration and memory, inability to think clearly, increasing insomnia, lack of appetite, and thoughts of suicide. Your body, especially your arms and legs, may feel heavy, or you may have less desire to engage in normal activities like eating or shopping. These are all serious impediments to living a full, enjoyable life.

WHAT YOU CAN DO

Most patients assume that fatigue must simply be endured. In the survey mentioned on page 152, when patients complained of fatigue to their doctors, most of the doctors had no solutions, or recommended rest (which can be one of the worst things you can do). As an oncology nurse put it, "There's no simple, easy solution to tiredness." It is important for you to make the effort to keep contact with the people you care about and to continue to do the things you like and need to do. Explain to people that you still want to spend time with them, but maybe not as often, or for as long, or in doing the same things you used to. You may need to learn how to get around the fatigue by, for instance, making some changes, setting priorities, and taking naps. There are many ways to help you lessen, prevent, and learn to live with fatigue.

Adjust Your Activities

At first I'd lie around the apartment in the evenings being so *bored* and miserable. I was used to an active life, but I had to save what energy I had for work during the day. How much can you read? How much TV can you watch? About three months into the chemo I decided this would be the perfect time to do something I'd always wanted to do: learn to play a musical instrument. It was just active enough, kept my mind busy, and really gave me a sense of accomplishment. Here are some other ways to adjust activities to cope better with fatigue:

- Plan your days' activities and take advantage of ways to save your energy either by figuring out easier means by which to do them yourself or by getting someone else to do them. Sometimes your family or friends will be glad to pitch in, sometimes not. Outside household helpers can make all the difference during times when you just can't do what's needed—and some social agencies will help pay for this service. Many patients dislike asking for help from anyone, friend or stranger, but sometimes having help is the only way to get things done:

  I didn't do much housework at all. If you could have seen my place, you would have said, "Oh, I see how she managed." I didn't do the dishes until hours after dinner was over. My mother was a great deal of help, but the rest of my family did not cooperate in this area. Someone came in to help once in a while.

  I was so debilitated that my husband and daughter were assuming some household responsibilities, and we had someone come in during the weeks I was on chemo. You spend two or three days a week throwing up and it's gonna knock you out.

  The worst part is the lack of energy. Needing the care of other people. It is embarrassing. It makes me feel old. People do things for old people. If you're independent, as I am, you're used to doing things for yourself—and it's hard. I feel guilty when others do the work for me.

- Set reasonable goals and priorities; conserve energy for those tasks you must or prefer to do yourself. One expert advises patients to "carve out those activities and interests that are most important for you to continue. That may be work, it may be taking care of your children, it may be communicating and socializing with certain

GETTING THROUGH THE WORK DAY

Lack of communication between you, your employer, and your coworkers regarding your treatment-related fatigue can often lead to confusion, mistrust, and anxiety. Here are some pointers on dealing with fatigue at work.

- Talk with your employer and your coworkers ahead of time to dispel any uncertainty or uneasiness they may feel. The more they know and understand about cancer treatment–related fatigue, the better they can support you.
- Let your employer or supervisor know that, to the best of your ability, you would like to remain a productive worker while you are taking your cancer treatment.
- Be realistic with yourself and your employer about your work goals during this time. You may need to reassess and reprioritize and make some changes to manage your fatigue, such as setting realistic work priorities on a day-to-day basis, and adjusting your workload and routines as necessary.
- Discuss with your employer or supervisor possible ways to make adjustments in your workplace responsibilities in order to minimize the impact of cancer treatment–related fatigue on your ability to do your job effectively. These include flexible scheduling to take advantage of peak energy times, a change or modification in your current job responsibility, and learning a new job skill that might be less physically or mentally demanding.
- Know the provisions of the Americans with Disabilities Act and the Family Medical Leave Act so that you understand your employee rights. Become familiar with your own company's policy regarding sick leave, disability, flexible scheduling, and work retraining options.

- Utilize the Job Accommodation Network at 800-ADA-WORK (800-232-9675) as a resource for you and your employer. The Job Accommodation Network is a free service that helps employers make special arrangements like flexible hours for employees who need them.

—Adapted from the Oncology Nursing Society's Web site, team@cancerfatigue.org.

friends. Even if you can't do it at your normal level, try to maintain at least some level or one aspect of that activity—it's an important dimension of continuity."

- Keep safety in mind—accidents tend to happen to those who are tired or weak. Perform as many day-to-day activities as you can. The activity is beneficial and helps you maintain a sense of normality, independence, and self-esteem. Speaking of patients with advanced diseases, an oncology nurse says, "One of my pet things is that when people come into the clinic they're a little bit short of breath and tired. So I say, 'Please use a wheelchair.' For them it's like giving in. And I'll say to them, 'Don't waste your energy here. Save it. Wait till you get home.'"

- Rest when you are tired, especially before and after a chemotherapy treatment. Avoid trying to do too much after a chemotherapy treatment—pace yourself. No one should expect you to be Superman or Wonder Woman. Many patients find that short naps in the afternoon work wonders. On the other hand, the Oncology Nursing Society warns, "Rest and sleep are important, but don't overdo it. Too much rest can decrease your energy level. In other words, the more you rest, the more tired you will feel."

- Get more sleep—deep, restful, uninterrupted sleep if possible. You may require more hours of sleep than you used to, so don't go by the old days. Go to bed earlier and/or get up later, whichever is more convenient. To help yourself sleep, you may want to take a tranquilizer or a sedative. Alternatively, there are a variety of herbal and homeopathic products on the market that many people find help them relax and fall asleep without adding their own side effects such as daytime fatigue. Many patients also find these tips helpful: Maintain a regular bedtime schedule and ritual; keep your environment quiet and calm, without distractions; use relaxation techniques; and try to find the cause of any sleep-disturbing anxieties and fears and alleviate them.

• Begin a mild exercise program that may be intensified eventually. Walk, do errands, and do light work around the house. In the right amounts, exercise energizes you—it doesn't tire you out. In a study published in 2001, women on adjuvant chemotherapy for breast cancer demonstrated that exercise can have dramatic effects on energy levels. Among those who exercised, only 6 percent were able to continue to go to work, as compared with nearly 20 percent of those who did not exercise.

• Begin or resume a favorite hobby or activity to alleviate boredom. It's best to have some degree of productive work or employment while you are on chemotherapy because it makes life more fun and keeps you from dwelling on cancer, chemotherapy, and how crummy you feel. The Oncology Nursing Society recommends that to restore energy, you "do activities that you enjoy and make you feel good." They suggest "nature activities such as bird watching or gardening, listening to music, or visiting with friends and family, or looking at pleasant pictures" and recommend you try to do these activities at least three times per week.

Nourish Your Body

• Check your diet to make sure it is nourishing. You may need to increase your intake of protein and carbohydrates or take nutritional supplements. Some doctors may recommend iron or vitamin supplements to help build up your red cell count.

• Make sure to drink plenty of fluids to prevent the accumulation of cellular waste products, the by-products of chemo.

Take Appropriate Medications

- Ask your oncologist about erythropoietin (Procrit), which helps boost red blood cell counts and thus reduces fatigue. Erythropoietin or EPO is a hormone naturally produced by your body, and Procrit is the synthetic form. It works so well that it has become a popular drug with healthy endurance athletes because the extra oxygen carried by the blood delays their fatigue and improves their performance.

- Ask your doctor about other medications to get you through this time, and adjust medications that might be robbing you of sleep. Dr. William Grace of New York City's St. Vincent's Hospital says: "Some patients use Dexatrim to counteract some of the fatigue. There are even some patients for whom we prescribe Dexedrine for chemotherapy-related fatigue. If you give it carefully, in small doses, it is safe, and many patients are able to continue working and lead more normal lives."

- If you are taking glucocorticoids, such as prednisone, which will keep some people on a little bit of a high, Dr. Grace recommends that you take this medication in the morning. "This way, they don't get the same 'high' and insomnia they usually get if they take it at night." Also be aware that when you take steroid drugs for a long period of time, you often get tired when you stop taking them. This is because the drug has caused your adrenal glands to stop producing enough cortisol. There are medications that can replace the cortisol your body no longer makes.

Flulike Symptoms

While on chemotherapy, you may feel like you have the flu—an all-over achiness in your muscles and/or bones, possibly a fever and chills, fatigue, nausea, or a feeling of general malaise. You may indeed have caught an infectious virus, since your immune system is likely to be compromised. However, some drugs used in chemotherapy can themselves cause these symptoms to appear when no infection is actually present. Any of the antibiotics can give you flulike symptoms, as can cytarabine, dacarbazine, thiotepa, and VP-16-213. Vincristine and vinblastine can give you an all-over achy feeling. So can the new biologicals. (See "The New Wave of Anticancer Drugs" on page 25.)

WHAT YOU CAN DO

These symptoms are temporary and usually pass within days of treatment. They should respond to the usual nostrums prescribed for the flu: Tylenol, fluids, and rest. See also FATIGUE AND WEAKNESS, and INFECTIONS.

Gastrointestinal Effects

Clearly, many of chemotherapy's side effects occur in the gastrointestinal system. The most common are nausea and vomiting (see NAUSEA AND VOMITING), loss of appetite, and weight loss (see APPETITE CHANGES AND WEIGHT LOSS). In addition, chemotherapy can cause bloating (see WEIGHT GAIN/WATER RETENTION/BLOATING), constipation (see CONSTIPATION), dehydration, dental problems, diarrhea (see DIARRHEA), dry mouth, esophagitis (a sore, irritated throat) (see MOUTH, GUM, AND THROAT PROBLEMS), heartburn, indigestion, milk intolerance (see MILK INTOLERANCE), pain (see PAIN), stomatitis (a sore, irritated mouth), swallowing difficulty, taste blindness (see TASTE CHANGES), and weight gain (see WEIGHT GAIN/WATER RETENTION/BLOATING). In addition, drugs can change the way in which nutrients are absorbed, metabolized, utilized, and excreted.

The gastrointestinal (GI) system, which includes the mouth and teeth, throat, esophagus, stomach, intestines, and rectum, is lined with cells that reproduce rapidly. These cells are therefore prime targets for anticancer drugs. Chemotherapy drugs also affect other organs that in turn influence the activity of the organs of the gastrointestinal tract. In addition, psychological factors such as fear, anxiety, and depression can affect both the digestive process itself and the way you feel about food, as can disruptions in your lifestyle and daily routine:

I still cook for the family, that doesn't bother me. But a lot of times I'd rather not eat at all, just go to bed instead.

I'd go to the cafeteria for lunch, get a bowl of soup, and think maybe I could eat. Once one of my coworkers came by and said in a friendly way, "Hello, dear." I don't remember what was on his tray, but whatever it was, the smell just made me jump up and run out because I thought I was going to vomit. He didn't know I was on chemo, and when I later explained, he said, "That's all right. It's just that nobody ever turned green in front of me."

I could only eat light breakfasts the days of my treatments. I was so worked up psychologically—knowing what I was going to go through a few hours later—that if I looked at food those mornings it would make me sick.

A change in eating habits and preferences can affect your life in many ways. I think what bothered me most about the change in eating habits was first that I love food and second that eating is such a social event. I had to choose restaurants very carefully and eat differently from usual. Thanksgiving was especially trying, since my mother makes a huge, scrumptious dinner. All that food—that rich food. Friends and relatives eventually understood that I couldn't eat that much and that plain food was the best for me. But it still made me feel guilty and like the odd man out. It was like being on a reducing diet and feeling sick at the same time—it wasn't really by choice that I couldn't join in the gastronomic fun. One of life's greatest pleasures was taken away from me.

WHAT YOU CAN DO

The side effects can alter both the amounts and types of food eaten as well as the way the body handles the nutrients that are being ingested. Patients on chemotherapy can easily become malnourished to one degree or another. However, a well-nourished patient has been shown to tolerate treatment better, respond to treatment more favorably, recover from individual treatments more rapidly, maintain desirable weight, feel better, and remain more active. (See Chapter 8.) It is ironic that at the very time a patient needs to be highly nourished, he or she is undernourished because of the therapy.

Sometimes the toxicity to the gastrointestinal system is so severe that your chemotherapy plan may be modified, but since the toxicity is usually not at a life-threatening level, oncologists generally are reluctant to do this. Luckily, there is some headway being made in understanding, alleviating, and preventing many of these side effects through watching what and how the patient eats. Many of the suggestions can be carried out by the patients themselves, their families, and their friends. (A dietitian, nutritionist, or nutrition-oriented physician or nurse can give a nutritional evaluation and more individual advice.)

Living conditions and the presence or absence of friends and relatives can make a big difference in how easily you are able to overcome your side effects and maintain a healthful diet. If you are being treated as a hospital inpatient, you are assured on the one hand of having food of at least a minimum level of quality and quantity. On the other hand, you forfeit a certain amount of control over what and when you eat. Mealtimes can be quite lonely, sterile affairs because most hospitals do not have communal dining areas. Meals are served in large portions, three times a day, but most chemotherapy patients do better with small, frequent meals. Hospital food is notoriously unappetizing, and it may also be of a different type from what you are used to: Very few institutions take into consideration the ethnic backgrounds and cultural preferences of their patients. It is not surprising that malnutrition has been found in 30 to 40 percent of hospital patients and that the percentages are even higher in cancer patients. Friends and relatives can be especially supportive in this area by bringing in some of your favorite foods (after checking with hospital authorities) and by scheduling their visits around mealtimes so you have company while you eat.

If you are being treated as an outpatient or by a physician in private practice, you may be living at home or staying at a hotel, motel, or rented apartment or with friends or relatives. In these cases, you should be able to have a certain amount of control over your food and its preparation—possibly over whole meals or parts of them and/or between-meal snacks. It is important to buy and prepare wholesome fresh foods instead of settling for poorly prepared fare such as "fast foods." Friends and family members can help out here, too, whether or not they normally are responsible for preparing the meals in your family.

The National Cancer Institute, among others, has published booklets that deal specifically with gastrointestinal problems that result from cancer and chemotherapy. Many contain additional tips to those suggested here, plus recipes for special diets such as bland diets, blenderized foods, high-protein diets, low-fat or low-fiber diets, and liquid diets.

Hair Loss

If you are average, your scalp contains 100,000 hairs, 10 to 15 percent of which are in the resting stage at any given time. Most hairs are therefore in the growing stage, which makes them unwitting targets for the effects of many of the most commonly used chemotherapy drugs. In addition to the drugs, a faulty diet and severe stress—particularly from illness, surgery, and emotional trauma—can affect the health of your hair and scalp.

Depending on your regimen, you may lose all or some of the hair on your head, including scalp, beard, mustache, eyebrows, and eyelashes. Your body hair may eventually thin out or disappear completely from your arms, armpits, legs, and groin. Though far from dangerous medically, losing your hair (*alopecia*) can be devastating psychologically.

Being bald on top of being sick is a terrible blow to our self-image; it can plunge some of us into the depths of depression or make those who are already depressed even more so. Feeling anxious about our appearance is a daily insult to our quality of life; it can even jeopardize our prognosis by causing us to doubt the wisdom of continuing with chemotherapy. Hair can mean so much to some people that the mere prospect of losing it is enough to make them refuse to begin chemotherapy even if it might save or extend their lives.

Patients' experiences with hair loss and their reactions to it vary greatly. Some say they feel naked, ugly, sexless, and vulnerable, that being bereft of hair is a constant reminder of their cancer. A professional who had been designing wigs for nearly forty years and also had devoted much of her own time to fitting cancer patients, told me that "losing the hair is so devastating because cancer is so often not really visual, and it can be ignored or denied. But being bald is very visual, a tremendous psychological problem." She told me about a woman in her thirties who came into her salon. "She was completely beyond herself, saying, 'I want to die, I want to die.'" Another businesswoman client of hers found the hair loss a greater blow than the cancer; she quit her job and refused to talk to friends. An elderly gentleman felt like a freak; he became a recluse because he feared ridicule.

One oncology nurse supervisor remarked that "among side effects, hair loss is the one that patients are the most disturbed about. That's what you present to the public; it's the first thing others see."

Most people do eventually adjust, and a few actually manage to derive pleasure from or get a few laughs out of their nearly hairless state:

I don't know . . . I had never thought I was vain about my hair. It never really mattered. I had sailed through the surgery and the diagnosis so well, relatively speaking. There I was, traveling through Europe and I had cancer, and I was going through chemotherapy, and I was on top of the world . . . and suddenly, that happened to me—and prehistoric feelings of maleness were coming out. It was devastating, it really was.

Because the drugs took my hair—my scalp hair and mustache too—I became anonymous for two years. All those boring people I didn't have to talk to—I'd just walk right by them in the street. Nobody recognized me. I didn't even recognize me. I'd had my beard for ten years, and a face can change a lot in that time.

You know what? It was a trip being bald. I used to run the pulsating shower over my head!

I remember being in a yoga class where the teacher came over to me in order to correct my head position. As she touched my head and my wig shifted, she drew back in surprise and said, "Oh, your hair!" I looked up and with a devilish grin said, "It isn't mine!"

Although hair loss is one of the most well-known side effects of chemo, it is important for you to know that not all drugs cause hair loss. And those which are known for this side effect do not always cause it in every individual or to the same extent.

Fifteen percent of chemo patients do not lose their hair. Perhaps you will be one of the lucky ones. And, except in very rare cases, losing your hair from chemotherapy is a temporary state. It almost always grows back after you stop chemotherapy—and sometimes before that if your hair becomes resistant to the drugs.

WHAT YOU CAN DO

Although losing your hair is traumatic, embarrassing, and terribly inconvenient, there are psychological and practical ways to prepare yourself and to cope with its possibility or actuality. There are ways you can make the possibility or reality of losing your hair less traumatic psychologically, and make your hair look better if it becomes thinner from chemotherapy. But first, you probably want to know if there is anything you can possibly do to prevent, delay, or minimize your hair loss.

Can You Prevent or Slow Hair Loss?

Because hair loss is one of the more distressing side effects, numerous attempts have been made to prevent it. Some patients have been able to prevent some scalp hair loss through the use of tourniquets or ice-filled caps. They place these devices on their heads during chemotherapy treatments in an effort to reduce the flow of blood there and thus expose the hair follicles in the scalp to lower concentrations of the drugs. Techniques vary, but generally if they use a tourniquet they wear it during and immediately after the injection and leave it on for up to twenty to forty-five minutes afterward. If they use ice, they put it on five minutes before and leave it on for about fifteen minutes after the injection.

This practice is not the answer to all chemotherapy patients' prayers, however. While it has met with some success, the effectiveness varies greatly and total prevention of hair loss is not yet possible. The ice and tourniquets are uncomfortable. People report headaches, chills, and dizziness from them. When drugs are given by slow infusion or when oral chemotherapy is taken several times a day, the devices have to be left on too long to be safe or comfortable.

Many physicians do not endorse the use of the tourniquets or caps except under certain conditions. They feel this practice should be avoided in people for whom chemotherapy offers a chance for a cure, because there is the danger of creating a sanctuary for tumor cells circulating in the scalp. This is the case in adjuvant chemotherapy and in some metastatic diseases that can be cured as well as with leukemias and lymphomas, where the chemotherapeutic intent is to kill every single malignant cell.

Dr. William Grace, an oncologist in New York's St. Vincent's Hospital, says, "The problem with chemo caps is the propensity to develop scalp relapses in people who are being treated for a cure. This is not theoretical—I've seen it and it has been confirmed several times in the literature. I had a patient whose disease went into remission everywhere but the scalp line—where it grew."

Patients are usually responsible for bringing their own tourniquets or caps and for obtaining and maintaining ice—no mean task when the wait for your treatment can stretch to hours. Donna Park says the patient has to get a written order from the physician and that the policy varies from physician to physician at Memorial: "Because of the controversy, the decision is left up to the patient and the physician. If the patients want ice caps, they have to bring in their own. We'll put them in the refrigerator, but if something has to remain frozen, patients come in with ice chests."

Over the years, I've seen and heard about products that you rub into your scalp that supposedly prevent or slow hair loss. As far as I know, these have proven to be about as effective as over-the-counter preparations that claim to slow hair loss due to male pattern baldness. The latest product directed at hair loss due to chemo is known as "Compound 4" (etoposide) and is in development by GlaxoSmithKline. In tests with mice, half the animals given etoposide had no hair loss and another 20 percent lost only some hair where the product was applied; one-third of mice who got cyclophosphamide and Adriamycin kept their hair where Compound 4 was applied. All the mice lost all their hair where the product was not applied. Compound 4 is not absorbed into the body and therefore does not interfere with the effectiveness of chemo anywhere else in the body. As of this writing, no human trials were in the works yet, so it will be several years before Compound 4 appears on the market, and probably with a different name.

Be Prepared

The first step in coping with this side effect is to get an idea of what you will be dealing with. Be sure to talk over your concerns with your doctor. Ask how likely it is that the drugs you will be taking will cause hair loss, how much you can expect to lose, and when. Although in most cases it is impossible to be very specific or sure, in others the track record is clear. The incidence of scalp hair loss varies from individual to individual and depends in part on the drug dosage. Nevertheless, some drugs have a higher potential to cause this than others have. Drugs that most commonly cause alopecia are cyclophosphamide (Cytoxan), doxorubicin (Adriamycin), and vincristine (Oncovin); moderately common are actinomycin D (Cosmegen), the bleomycins, daunorubicin, and methotrexate. At any rate, for many patients, the experience of losing their hair is harder if the doctor downplays the possibility, extent, or importance. A wig stylist for the Kenneth Beauty Salon in New York, commented:

People who are unprepared take the bad road. I get asked a lot of questions about what I've seen or what they should expect because most of the doctors don't give their patients enough information. Some do care and understand that this is one of the major problems that people face when they go through chemotherapy. Some doctors are right up front—they tell patients they might lose their hair—either because that's the way they are or because with some types of therapies they can be more sure than with others.

Donna Park says:

It's fine for doctors to say that chemotherapy causes hair loss. But you really need to get down to the nitty-gritty. Which drugs do; which drugs don't; which ones do to a certain degree. For instance, 90 percent of the patients who receive Adriamycin do lose their hair. But you're not going to wake up the morning after your first treatment and find all your hair on your pillow. One patient I know had overheard other women talking about wigs. She became very frightened and asked, "Where am I going to find a wig tonight?" I had to tell her that she wouldn't wake up bald the next morning but that she should start looking for a wig.

When my hair fell out, I was devastated. I can't deny that vanity played its part, but a good deal of the blame lies in my not being well enough prepared. My oncologist did warn me that it all might fall out but said it was possible that only some of it might. He observed that since I had a lot of hair to begin with, I could afford to lose some. He mentioned that a lot of people on chemo get wigs, but I said, "Not me! Even if some hair falls out, I'm not so vain that I can't live with hair that looks a little thin." I thought I'd wait and see if I needed one. I don't know if he was soft-pedaling hair loss in order to be kind and not to scare me off or if it just didn't sink in that I might become totally bald and what this would mean to me. As a result, I was totally unprepared—in psychological and practical terms—when it did fall out, all of it.

As a general rule, hair begins to fall out within three or four treatments. It may begin sooner and peak one or two months afterward. In some people, it falls out very gradually or the loss is so slight it is hardly noticeable. In others, it falls out in huge clumps or all at once. Some people wear caps or scarves to bed to catch the shedding hair. People can become completely bald except for a slight "peach fuzz" effect. If the hair doesn't all fall out but becomes thinner, it can continue to grow, but with a change in texture and appearance.

Often hair growth doesn't stop completely, and some hair remains. Chemotherapy can sometimes just shrink the hair bulb, or root, which constricts the hair shaft as it grows. The hair—chemo hair—becomes thinner, sparser, weaker, with a brittle, finer texture, and takes on a dull appearance. Those with thick, strong, bouncy, curly hair find themselves with limp, straight hair. These people usually do not wear wigs and are still "presentable" but can be far from happy with their appearance:

My hair didn't fall out completely, but it was a mess. It was very thin and fine; it was always shiny, and now it was drab. I looked like a nun who had just come out of the convent. I'd turn my head, and hair would fall out—there was hair over everything. I went to my hairdresser and he asked me, "What have you done?" I burst into tears and told him I hadn't done anything, that I was on chemo. We tried henna, everything, to thicken and liven it up, but nothing worked.

I never got a wig, though I played with the idea because my hair had gotten very thin; it was straight, with no life, and it just lay there. I'd show pictures of myself to people I had just met, who didn't know me before the chemo, and say, "This isn't me—this picture is the real me." I wore a lot of hats—I love them—I had different hats for different outfits.

My hair had been falling out a little bit. I lathered up my head, began to massage my scalp, and with a sinking feeling I could almost feel the whole thing shift . . . with the water and the lather. . . . I got almost physically sick. I know I at least came close to tears; I don't think I actually cried. But I was paralyzed. I couldn't do anything. I just felt disgusting with all this hair all over the place. My wife came in and had to finish rinsing me off and cleaning out the tub while I got out and tried to not throw up. It was really devastating.

I lost a lot of my hair—but not all of it. I'd say I've lost half of it. I don't need a wig; I've always had a lot of hair. Now it just looks sparse—people come up to me and say it looks gorgeous—I used to have too much hair. I wear it very close-cropped, and I trim it every three weeks. The texture has changed—I used to have very curly hair, and now it's straight. And it breaks. It still looks good, but it's not me.

The onset of my hair loss was much more difficult to deal with than it had to be because, as I said earlier, I was so ill-prepared; my being away from home when it happened made it even more of a nightmare. I had had three treatments, and I didn't feel too bad at all. No hair had fallen out, so I figured I was home free and would be spared the worst of the side effects. Full of relief and nonchalance, I went on a trip. In a glorious example of "perfect" timing, my hair began to shed slightly on the plane. Four days later I was barely presentable: You could see right through to my scalp. There I was stuck, away from home with no scarf, no wig, in unfamiliar surroundings with nowhere to hide. I finally found a few horrendous scarves to wear, which at least left me looking human. I cried a lot during that week; I never felt so down at any other time because finally toxicity had built up. Not only had my hair fallen out, I was beginning to feel physically ill because of the nausea and tiredness that had hit at the same time. Eventually I bought a wig that looked fine, but I still felt a sense of revulsion every time I saw myself without it. Losing my hair was the most dramatic, tangible side effect I experienced. Everything else was vague and invisible or purely medical. Then I not only felt sick, I looked sick.

I have come to believe that no one is fully prepared for hair loss because it requires you to know yourself so well that you can predict how you will react. So, in retrospect, I think what surprised me most about my hair falling out was the way I felt about this event. Before the hair loss, I didn't think I was so vain that it would bother me. But it did fall out, and it did upset me—and then the fact that it bothered me upset me even further!

If your oncologist seems unable to help you cope, speaking with a counselor such as a nurse or social worker or with a patient who has had or is having chemotherapy may help you prepare yourself psychologically for hair loss. All the sources for emotional support discussed in Chapter 12 will also help you adjust to both possible and actual loss of hair.

Some people try to hold on to their hair once it starts falling out. Often they stop shampooing it or combing it because they have heard that this

walk around with a head of thinning hair, or suffer the expense, discomfort, and inconvenience of wearing a hairpiece. Bald is just their "new look." However, many others do cling to whatever is left and are deeply affected by hair loss.

There are differences between the way men and women react to losing their body hair as well. Peggy Knight, president of Peggy Knight International, finds that in her experience, women have a hard time accepting the loss of scalp hair but men are more disturbed when they lose their body hair. Again, this reflects what we perceive as normal—in the United States it's common for women to remove body hair, but for men, only some types of athletes can remove body hair without threatening their perceived masculinity or sex appeal.

BUY A WIG OR HAIRPIECE

Most experienced professionals recommend that you begin to look for a wig, and possibly buy one, *before* beginning chemotherapy and before your hair has started to fall out. Although many patients may not need or want a wig, many others will, and the peace of mind in knowing that an attractive hairpiece is handy is an important factor in how well people cope with hair loss. Donna Park says the advantage of looking for a wig early is so that "when you start to feel uncomfortable—either from the other side effects or because the hair loss is noticeable—you're not pressured to go out and buy something that you really can't afford or one that isn't right for you. You need time to shop around to find something that's right." Or some other kind of head covering should be on hand—turbans, scarves, hats, and caps are preferred by some instead of wigs or are used until they obtain a wig.

Having a wig in which you feel comfortable is an important factor in the difficult process of coping with hair loss. People say that keeping their spirits up is an important part of the treatment; then they feel "hopeful, relieved, not like outcasts."

"At least now I can leave the house without a hat or feeling that I'm going to scare the kiddies in the neighborhood," said one new wig owner. "You don't know what a feeling of comfort and confidence this is to me," said another. The better you look, the better you'll adjust to baldness. If you have a lousy wig on, you'll feel terrible. If you see someone wearing a bad wig in the doctor's office, you'll probably be turned off by that—don't be that person.

As to style, "There are really two types of people," another expert says. "Those who want to look as much as possible like they did before, and those who go in the opposite direction." If you want to look like your old self, in most cases it's best to buy a wig before your hair falls out. That way the wig specialist can see your natural hair color and hairstyle and then match it closely. Most people still have at least some of their hair when they come to a salon for a wig. If you don't, the stylist will ask you to bring in a photograph or describe how you looked pre-chemo. Some will take an instant photo of you or ask that you allow them to snip a sample of your hair for accurate color selection. (If you wait until your hair has fallen out, try to save some of your hair to bring in.) Although wigs will fit differently after your hair has begun to fall out, a good professional will be able to compensate for this as well as for hair regrowth.

You can get a wig through hairdressers, beauty salons, barbers, and wig specialty shops; directly from wig suppliers; through the mail; and in department stores. They may be made of real or synthetic hair, prestyled, ready-made (the equivalent of "off the rack"), handmade, or custom-made. The kind of wig or hairpiece you get and where you buy it depend on your individual taste, how important it is for you to duplicate your own hair, how much money you can spend, where you live, what's available, and how much time you have.

For me, buying a wig was a relatively simple matter in which luck played a big part. I just looked up "Wigs" in the Yellow Pages and made a few phone calls: I knew I didn't want to spend much. I went to a wig supplier—and that meant less than glamorous conditions. I looked at the samples, picked out a couple, hid in the bathroom to try them on, and that was that. I was lucky—I paid less than $100 for the one I ended up with. It was a mass of natural-looking curls very close to my own hair color but very different from my usual style. So I didn't have to worry about a phony-looking part or hairline or explaining everything to people I knew only slightly. It was the right style, and perfect strangers would walk up to me on the street and ask where I got my perm. I'd send them to my hairdresser, of course.

You will do best, though, if you allow yourself as much time as possible for the selection, ordering, and preparation of your hairpiece. You can begin by asking your oncologist, nurse, or social worker to recommend a source for a good wig—they have probably seen many different hairpieces and are in a good position to judge. Or you can ask a fellow patient who is wearing one that you like.

If possible, you should buy the wig in person. Only then can you be assured of getting the best fit and the most flattering style. Some recommend bringing a friend along. And to feel most comfortable and look most natural, you should have your wig fitted and styled professionally. If you get the names of several sources, you can shop around and compare. Most of the preliminary scouting can be done over the phone—find out about the types of wigs available, the price range, the waiting time, the personality of the wig stylist, and the degree of privacy. Ask what their payment policy is. If you order a wig in advance, will they refund your money if your hair doesn't fall out and you don't need the wig, after all? What if you are not happy with the wig? Will they restyle it or offer you another at no or minimal extra cost?

If you delay buying a wig until after your hair has begun to fall out, the stylist's personality and the degree of privacy offered are even more important. As one patient said, "When you lose your hair, your spirits fall and you are ashamed to be seen. A regular salon is inappropriate for a chemo patient who is not buying a wig for fun and pleasure and who doesn't want to explain or show hair loss to a stranger."

More than enough has been said or written about the psychotherapeutic overtones in the client-hairdresser relationship. Suffice it to say that this aspect can assume even more importance when the client is a cancer patient who has lost his or her hair. The sensitive ones can see the pain inside you and be patient and understanding during a time when you might be difficult to please or get along with.

Synthetic hair is less expensive than human hair in terms of both initial cost and upkeep. Synthetic wigs are easy to maintain since they do not require "setting" and don't frizz, droop, or lose their set. They come in dozens of shades that can be blended to look and feel quite natural. Even if you decide that you want a custom-made or human hair wig, you might want to buy a cheaper, ready-made synthetic one before your hair falls out. If you do lose your hair, at least you have something to tide you over until your better wig is ready.

Still, human hair wigs generally look and feel more natural. However, they are more expensive and require more care than do synthetic wigs. It's very important that a wig be easy to handle. That's why some people do not recommend human hair wigs—they're too expensive, too delicate, and require too much care. Especially if you aren't feeling well most of the time, you don't want to be bothered with taking care of a wig.

Both human and synthetic hair wigs have a mesh or lace base that varies in degree of give, comfort, appearance and practicality. Make sure your wig is comfortable, and that the base is not made of a very large mesh—this is okay for someone who still has some hair, but in a totally bald person, the bare scalp will show through. Machine-sewn ready-made synthetic wigs are made for people with hair. "Most not only allow scalp to show through the base when the wind blows, but they are scratchy and uncomfortable on a totally bare scalp," says Peggy Knight.

Handmade and custom-made wigs look better, are more comfortable and lighter on the head, and are less hot in the summer. They are much more expensive and there's a longer wait (up to six weeks) for them to be ready. Nevertheless, people do order them and some come from all over the country and the world to have their wigs made at major salons in big cities. Real hair wigs can be made from your own hair, provided that it is cut off early—once it falls out, it is too tangled to use.

With the proper care, a good wig can last for up to a year of moderate wear. It helps prolong the life and appearance of a wig if you buy two wigs. You might want one that resembles your own hair and another that's very different, just for fun. People often have a good one that's comfortable and always looks good and a cheaper one that they can wear when their good wig is being serviced, or for every day, or for times like emptying the garbage. Usually two wigs will last you for one year."

Some people become so devastated and self-conscious about their appearance that they remove their wigs only for sleeping and showering. However, even the new lightweight wigs can be pretty uncomfortable, especially after weeks of daily wear. Many people, though shy at first, eventually loosen up, give way to comfort, and do not wear their hairpieces at all times. Most children and spouses quickly adjust to the appearance of the chemotherapy patient, and of course do not love them any less because they are temporarily bald. Families understand that at a time when you are not feeling well, every little bit of understanding helps. It is a show of trust and security to let those close to you see you as you really are. As one woman said to me, "I run around a lot without my hairpiece because it's so hot and uncomfortable. My kids are used to it; they don't care—I'm still Mom."

I liked the way my wig looked, but sometimes I hated the way it felt. As is the case with my shoes, it was a relief to be rid of the wig and I couldn't wait to take it off the minute I got home. I was very self-conscious about it, though my husband, God bless him, tried to convince me he actually preferred me bald. I felt so naked, so vulnerable, so ugly. We tried to make jokes about this and he gave me the nickname Baldielocks. At times he'd make me feel better about it by cradling my head in his hands and gently stroking my peach fuzz. Still, I often wore a scarf or knitted cap instead of the wig, although this was partly because my head got surprisingly cold without the protection of my usual mane of long blond hair.

Some women look to turbans, hats, scarves, and head wraps as alternates to a full wig, especially when accessorized with a striking pair of earrings. Turbans come in many colors and are stretchy, soft, and comfortable. A turban stays on easily and stands up to wear and tear, so it is especially useful on days when you feel really sick or during a treatment cycle if you are a hospital inpatient. You can soften the somewhat severe look of a turban with a small wiglet attached to the front so that some hair peeks out from underneath. This combination is more comfortable than a wig; it is less expensive and more practical and still gives the illusion of hair. For practical ideas and techniques for head coverings and scarves, see the book *Beauty and Cancer* by Diane Doan Noyes and Peggy Mellody. In addition, contact the Look Good . . . Feel Better program, which provides education, through group or individual sessions, free program materials, including videos and pamphlets, and free makeup kits for patients in group workshop. Call 800-ACS-2345 or www.lookgoodfeelbetter.org.

Hairpieces needed as a result of medical treatment are a tax-deductible expense, and some insurance policies cover them. Wigs can be obtained free—or their cost defrayed—through the social service departments of some hospitals and clinics, the American Cancer Society, and other agencies, organizations, and foundations. You can also obtain a wig through public assistance programs.

Help for Facial and Body Hair

Although most patients find the loss of scalp hair the most distressing, some find the loss of facial or body hair just as disturbing, if not more. Donna Park remarks that some patients say that losing the hair on their heads was more acceptable than losing the hair on other parts of their bodies. And people don't realize that they can lose their pubic hair. One woman remarked that she felt like "a plucked chicken." I found it weird but not unpleasant to be as hairless as a nine-year-old again, and not to have to shave my legs or underarms for months was a definite plus.

There is not much you can do about replacing or disguising the loss of facial or body hair. You can wear eyebrow and eyelash makeup or eyeglasses with large frames and tinted lenses. If your hairstyle can cover your brow line, you can leave it a little bit longer than usual. False eyebrows, eyelashes, mustaches, and beards do exist, but people rarely use them.

When Your Hair Grows Back

Hair lost during chemotherapy almost always grows back. Regrowth often begins even before the treatment is over, as the hair grows resistant to the chemicals. When your hair initially grows back, it may look different: People with straight hair commonly grow curly hair—to the surprise of many patients. It may at first, however, be finer, or silkier or of a different color or texture. This chemo hair is a transient stage; the hair eventually becomes thicker—in many cases thicker than before the therapy—and usually eventually returns either completely back to normal or nearly so.

I spoke with this patient six months after he had completed his chemotherapy and was due for a second haircut; he said of his hair: "It feels a little softer and is curly. My barber says it feels like infant's hair. If I just step out of the shower and don't comb it, it's a mass of Byronic curls. In fact, I'm thinking of going as Byron to a costume party next month. It's definitely less gray than it was, but my beard is more gray."

Once the hair starts growing back, when and how to "come out" can be an agonizing decision; it can be a difficult transitional period. Some people are ecstatic when their hair regrows, and they discard their wigs at the earliest possible moment. I was elated when my hair began to grow back three months after it had fallen out—I felt the stubble or, as my oncologist called it, the "five o'clock shadow." I kept rubbing my head in glee and disbelief. Nevertheless, I had to wait another three months until I felt comfortable in public without a wig, my hair was so thin and fine. Still, it was only a half inch long when I began to seriously entertain thoughts of appearing au naturel. I did it in stages. First I took out the garbage, just to see how it felt to be outdoors. It felt okay! Then I carried a letter to the mailbox across the street. No one stared; no one ran away screaming! Then, getting braver by the minute, I went to the grocery store and made actual contact with people. Still no reaction. That was it from then on. I hadn't trusted my friends who said: "Do it, do it," or Michael, who said, "Well, it is awfully short." I had to test it out myself.

Others are reluctant to give up their wigs because they prefer the way they look over their real hair. A social worker told me about a patient who began shaving her head when her hair started to grow back because it was uncomfortable under a wig, which she wanted to continue to wear. Apparently, about half of us can't wait to throw out our wigs and stomp on them when our hair has grown back. The other half has learned to like our wigs, especially if they're expensive ones. We get compliments when we wear our wigs and use them when we are having a bad hair day.

Some patients who have been coloring their hair blond before the chemotherapy have a problem when their hair grows back gray mixed with brown and sticks out from under their blond wigs. Check with your doctor, and if it's okay, you can lighten up just around the hairline so it can be combed in with the wig. Some people use water-soluble rinses to cover hair that is growing in gray because of the dangers associated with stronger dyes, which may also be too harsh for the new growth.

Some people can't wait to run out and get perms to make their new hair look better. This, as is true with hair coloring, is usually not advisable unless the hair is strong and has a good texture—check with your doctor. What is advisable is a haircut as soon as there is hair to cut. Says one hair stylist: "Once hair starts growing in and looking straggly I like to have my clients come in and I'll trim it—clean it up. That makes people feel comfortable about themselves. They can look better with their own hair, and pretty soon they'll be wearing their wigs only for special occasions."

Heart Problems

Heart damage (cardiotoxicity) is the principal dose-limiting side effect of two widely used anticancer antibiotics: daunorubicin and doxorubicin (Adriamycin). The onset of the symptoms (swelling of the body, shortness of breath, dizziness, loss of appetite, and fluttering of the heartbeat) may not occur until long after you have begun getting chemo and usually as long as two weeks to six months after you have completed therapy. When cardiotoxicity occurs, the drugs' effects are usually cumulative; this can lead to chronic congestive heart failure, which may continue to progress and eventually prove fatal. Unfortunately, I have personally known at least one person whose cancer was in remission, but whose life was limited by a chemo-damaged heart and who ultimately died of heart failure.

In the acute form of cardiotoxicity, which occurs less often, you notice the effects on the heart during or shortly after the drug is administered. These immediate effects usually reverse quickly without serious complications, and your doctor will usually not consider them to be a reason to stop the drug.

Taxol is another drug that may cause heart problems; 3 percent of women who get this drug experience slow heartbeat (*bradycardia*) or irregular heart beat (*arrhythmia*). Herceptin, the new monoclonal antibody that binds to Her-2/neu, a growth-regulating protein, also may cause heart damage. Heart failure occurs in 7 percent of women who get Herceptin (currently approved for metastatic breast cancer) and in 28 percent of women who get it along with other chemotherapy drugs. That's why it is not recommended for women with prior heart problems such as high blood pressure or high cholesterol. Prednisone, a steroid hormone given along with chemo, may also damage your heart.

WHAT YOU CAN DO

At one time, 75 percent of those who experienced cardiotoxicity died, but it seems that doctors are recognizing this adverse effect earlier and treating it more successfully. The best course is prevention, and studies are under way to improve early diagnosis even more and perhaps prevent cardiotoxicity's occurrence through blocking chemicals. Two University of Florida researchers reported in 2001 that a class of enzyme called *capsases* appears to trigger cell death. If we can hinder the capsases that trigger heart cell death but preserve the ones responsible for cancer cell death, we can protect the heart.

- Vitamin E has been found to protect the heart from Adriamycin in animals and may prove to do the same in humans. There have also been promising results with other antioxidants such as vitamin C and with the nutrient coenzyme Q_{10}, which appear to protect the heart. So you may want to talk to your physician about taking these supplements.
- Your doctor may treat cumulative congestive heart failure with digitalis and diuretics.
- In some cases your doctor may give you a drug called Novantrone instead of Adriamycin; it can be just as effective but can be given for longer periods without endangering the heart.
- Your doctor may give you heart-toxic drugs by slow infusion, which, for example, reduces the heart toxicity of Adriamycin by 50 to 75 percent.

Infections

Because the drugs lower your white blood cell count and white blood cells are our infection-fighters, we are at higher risk for all manner of infection while on chemo. Infections are definitely unwanted additional problems, but fortunately, colds and flu are the most common infections that you need to worry about while on chemotherapy. They often do not progress beyond the nuisance stage:

I did get a lot more colds than I usually got. My oncologist gave me a flu shot and ordered me to stay home from work because he was afraid I might get it during the "High Holy Days" of the flu. He still insists I get a flu shot every year, even though my white blood count has never dropped as low as before and is fine now.

If anybody came in this house and sneezed, I picked the infection up. One weekend I caught a cold from my daughter. The next Monday I was due for a treatment, which my doctor wouldn't let me out of. So that day, there I was lying in bed with the shivers, I couldn't breathe, my chest and nose were killing me, and I was throwing up. I was a sight.

However, in some patients, the danger of infection can go beyond these minor respiratory diseases, making infections the major causes of illness and death in cancer patients. Almost any organ or part of the body can become infected, including most often the mouth, skin, lungs, urinary tract, rectum, and reproductive organs. These infections may be bacterial, viral, fungal, or protozoal; they may be common ones, but a higher than normal proportion are exotic types. Some patients have an episode of shingles from the varicella-zoster virus that causes chickenpox. The virus stays dormant in their bodies until the chemo activates it.

Most infections are minor and can be treated successfully with antibiotics or other medication. If you get a severe infection, you may require more aggressive therapy, which includes white blood cell transfusions. You may also get these transfusions as a precaution, before infection sets in, when your white blood count dips too dangerously low. In addition, new biological substances called CSF (colony-stimulating factor) are sometimes used to "rescue" a patient with dangerously low white blood cell counts to prevent infection. The two most popular ones are called G-CSF

SYMPTOMS OF INFECTION

There are certain general signs of infection that you should watch out for and immediately report to the oncologist or nurse. They are:

- Temperature of 100° F. or higher.
- Chills, shivering.
- Loose bowels for longer than two days.
- Burning sensation during urination.
- Coughing, sore throat, chest pain, or shortness of breath.
- Unusual discharge or blood from the urinary tract, lungs, rectum, vagina, and so on.

In addition, patients should pay attention to the visible, accessible parts of the body that are most prone to infection. Since the immune system is impaired, the usual, normal signs of infection—redness, pus, and swelling—are not present or may not be apparent because they are actually signs of the body trying to fight the infection. In cases of severe immunosuppression or suspected infection, the oncologist may request tests of the urine, sputum, and feces and of nose, ear, and throat secretions.

and GM-CSF, and they stimulate your bone marrow to produce white blood cells faster. (But these have unpleasant side effects including fever, chills, malaise, and bone pain. Infections of the exotic type and infections that are particularly acute can occur in people with the leukemias, because in these kinds of cancer the chemotherapy is intended to and does greatly reduce the number of white blood cells. Dr. William Grace says:

People on chemotherapy are going to run a risk of infection. Patients must know the signs of infection, that if they get an infection they can die, and that they should inform the doctor right away if they suspect they might have an infection. Some patients "don't want to bother the doctor." They have to learn to bother us. If they have a fever on Monday but don't call the doctor until Wednesday, it may be fatal or it may take them weeks in the hospital to recover from the infection. We now have very good oral antibiotics and can often keep patients out of the hospital if mild infections are detected early."

WHAT YOU CAN DO

When your white blood cells dip, there's plenty you can do to reduce your risk of infection.

General Prevention

- Keep well nourished—eat a higher-calorie, high-protein diet. Vitamin/mineral supplements may be a good idea, especially vitamin C, which many oncologists are prescribing for their patients.
- Be sure to drink two or three quarts of fluid every day to keep your mucous membranes moist. Some oncologists are concerned about microbial content of water. These oncologists recommend that you consider boiling your water before drinking it, avoiding distilled water, drinking bottled water or filtered water.
- Check with your doctor about what foods to eat during your therapy. For example, Dr. Philip Pizzo, chief of pediatric oncology at the National Cancer Institute, suggests that chemo patients check with their doctors about the advisability of eliminating fresh raw fruits and vegetables at certain points in their therapy, such as when the white blood cell count is particularly low or during a course of antibiotics. These foods may be potential sources of harmful organisms that can migrate from the gastrointestinal tract to other parts of the body and cause serious infection. "Normally these bacteria go in one end and pass uneventfully out the other," he explains, "but in chemo patients this may not be so." Recently, there has been additional concern about salmonella in poultry and eggs, so prepare these items carefully and cook them well.

- Observe good rules of hygiene. Bathe or shower daily if possible; wash your hands before meals and sexual activity and before and after visits to the bathroom. Keep your hands away from your face, and your fingers out of your mouth, nose, and eyes.
- Avoid crowds and particularly people or children with infectious diseases. Avoid exposure to people with herpes, chickenpox, and measles even if you had these infections in the past.
- Avoid exposure to bird and animal excreta. Infectious bacteria and other parasites may be harbored in their excrement. Let someone else clean up the mess.
- Stop smoking and avoid smoky rooms. Take deep breaths of clean air occasionally.
- Get some exercise daily (aerobic exercise may help stabilize your immune system) but don't become overly fatigued. Get enough sound sleep and/or rest as needed.
- Avoid bar soaps—they are excellent mediums for the growth of organisms. Use soap from liquid dispensers.
- Keep your skin in good condition—dry thoroughly after washing and moisturize it if it's dry.
- Guard against burns, scrapes, punctures, and cuts; take proper care of them if they do occur. Wear protective gear when gardening, washing, and cooking. Be cautious while shaving—switching to an electric shaver is recommended.
- Maintain cleanliness and proper lubrication during sexual activity. Avoid excessive friction; prevent rectal contamination.

Sometimes antibiotics are used prophylactically. Dr. Grace remarks:

We identify the people who seem to be at high-risk for infection—either due to their disease or their therapy—and treat them during their low white blood [cell] counts with preventive antibiotics that are known to reduce the risk of infections. These are most commonly used in patients with leukemia, but there's no reason not to use them in high-risk patients with other cancers.

Special Precautions for Women

The vaginal infections that plague women can be especially bothersome during chemotherapy, when lowered resistance joins forces with an altered hormonal/vaginal chemistry and less than optimum eating habits. There are several ways you can help protect yourself from these infections:

- When you take antibiotics for a bacterial infection anywhere in your body, good bacteria are killed along with the bad ones, and in their absence fungus (or yeast) can take hold and flourish. To prevent this, many doctors recommend taking yogurt with live cultures orally or as a douche to restore healthy bacteria in the body. Liquid acidophilus, available in health-food stores, is a more concentrated source of friendly bacteria and may be used instead of yogurt. Using an antifungal (or yeast) vaginal medication may also be advised while you are taking antibiotics.
- Chemicals irritate and inflame delicate tissues and upset the chemical balance of the vagina. Avoid feminine hygiene sprays, commercial douches, and deodorized tampons and napkins.
- Do not use an IUD for birth control; ask your doctor about safer alternatives. Change tampons frequently during menstruation and substitute napkins as often as possible, especially overnight.
- Watching your diet may help you cut down on vaginal infections. Though this has not yet been scientifically proved, many nutritionally oriented health professionals recommend cutting down on sugars and other refined carbohydrates because an overabundance of sugars in the vaginal tract can trigger yeast infections. Fungus-related foods that contain mold or yeast (cheese, beer, wine, vinegar, and breads) should be avoided.
- Your clothes can contribute to a higher incidence of infections. Wear cotton panties or ones with a cotton crotch. Avoid tight pants and prolonged wearing of synthetic exercise clothes or wet bathing suits.
- Maintain scrupulous cleanliness in the genital area. Make sure to wipe from front to back after bowel movements to prevent fecal matter from entering the vagina.

Infertility and Early Menopause

For many of us, chemotherapy's impact on our reproductive system is a discreet, though important, issue closely related to our ability to express ourselves sexually and to our feelings about ourselves as complete human beings. Some chemotherapy drugs, primarily the alkylating agents such as chlorambucil and Cytoxan, are well known for their ability to reduce sperm counts or sperm vitality in men. These drugs plus two others—busulfan and vinblastine—are also known to suppress ovarian function and menstruation in women. No one really knows exactly how chemotherapy injures eggs and triggers early menopause. We do know that chemo causes eggs to self-destruct, a process called *apoptosis*.

These are widely used drugs and, as a result, many people who undergo chemotherapy run the risk of becoming infertile or subfertile (less likely to get pregnant or impregnate because of damaged eggs or sperm) during therapy. This condition may be temporary and disappear after treatment is over. But it can take a long time to reverse itself, and it sometimes never does so or does so incompletely. In addition, if you are a young woman, you run the additional risk of undergoing menopause early in life, along with the usual symptoms of hormone imbalance such as hot flashes, mood swings, and insomnia. If you were already menopausal when you were diagnosed, and were taking hormone replacement therapy, your doctor may advise you to stop taking the hormones, at least during chemotherapy, and your menopause symptoms may come back.

A man whose wife was undergoing chemo said:

> *I don't like it at all. My wife's reaction isn't good, either. My wife is going to a psychiatrist. I go out a few nights a week—not for a one-night stand but to get attention and affection and to boost my ego a little. I'm a very sensual, romantic guy at heart, and that part of me is not being expressed while my wife isn't interested. The old affection isn't there now that we can't have children together. Sure we have sex, but it isn't like it used to be. The little things—like stroking—are left out.*

The total amount of these drugs and the length of time you take them play key roles in whether early menopause and fertility problems occur and whether they can be reversed. Permanent infertility is most common in patients who receive high-dose long-term chemotherapy, such as for Hodgkin's disease, and less common in low-dose short-term chemo plans such as adjuvant treatment for breast cancer. Another variable is your age. The younger you are, the more resistant you are likely to be and the better your chances are for reversing infertility or menopause caused by chemo. For example, in women undergoing adjuvant chemo for breast cancer, the cutoff age seems to be about thirty. Women under thirty tend to resume menstruation, and women over thirty tend not to.

Infertility, or the possibility of it, is more of an issue for some patients and their spouses than for others. Age, former plans, and whether they already have children affect its importance. For men, cytotoxic agents kill the rapidly producing sperm and damage the testes. This reduction in the production of sperm is not of itself directly responsible for reducing either the desire or the ability to have sex from a physiological point of view. Theoretically, unless "feminizing" hormone therapy is also being given, a man's testosterone levels are not affected and he can still achieve and maintain an erection and ejaculation. An infertile man can still enjoy sex, and so can his partner. However, in reality, some men do find that their libidos are lessened during chemotherapy. It is uncertain whether this is due to physical or emotional factors. Men taking anti-androgen therapy such as Casodex (bicalutamide) or Arimidex (anastrazole) also may experience hot flashes.

The possibility of being sterile was not a major problem for me, since I had no overwhelming desire to have children. But it does seem odd—extending your own life in exchange for a potential child. At the time it didn't bother me—except that I do like to have options, whether I intend to exercise them or not, and this may have removed one of them. Now that I'm older, and having my own child is out of the question, I sometimes feel a pang of regret. But who knows? I probably never would have had a child anyway.

Although there are measures you can take in order to have children, these alternatives may leave much to be desired, especially for young single adults who want children and for couples whose families are not yet complete. Anxiety and regret over this loss can spill into many aspects of their lives. Sometimes professional counseling helps people adapt.

Women have more to deal with than "mere" infertility. A woman's reproductive system, with its delicately balanced menstrual cycle, is much more complex than a man's. A woman is born with her total supply of ova, or eggs; unlike a man's sperm, they are not manufactured constantly in the body—they mature, one at a time per cycle, during ovulation. A woman on chemotherapy undergoes estrogen withdrawal and possibly other hormonal changes. These changes prevent the egg from maturing and cause menstrual irregularities, and women can undergo real, verifiable physical and emotional changes. Aside from the discomfort and embarrassment of hot flashes, women experience profuse sweating, vaginal infections, dry or sore vagina, uncomfortable intercourse, dizziness, difficulty breathing, mood swings, and a greater than usual uncertainty about the possibility of pregnancy. If you are getting anticancer hormonal therapy simultaneously with or subsequent to chemotherapy, these problems are compounded: you may experience signs of masculinization, such as excess facial and body hair and a deepened voice.

These effects may be almost immediate or take several months to become evident; other changes in the vagina, cervix, skin, and bones can occur eventually if the menopause becomes permanent. All these sex- and hormone-related side effects can reduce your quality of sex and your quality of life during and after chemotherapy. Even if your periods do not stop completely, you may miss the rhythm of a physical phenomenon that has occurred so regularly up to now.

Although a woman may be thrust into artificial menopause, often at a very young age, doctors often don't warn women about this eventuality. They often fail to realize, believe, or accept the amount of distress this can cause. Here are two women's experiences:

I had lost my period completely about six months after beginning the chemo; it got irregular, and very light, and then stopped. I'm on tamoxifen now, and that's made things worse. When I get a hot flash, my body temperature goes sky-high and my face gets beet red.

Sometimes my emotions will set it off. The sweat pours down, and I feel like I can't breathe—like I'm having an anxiety attack. Then there's the erratic behavior. . . . I hope this is temporary, as my doctor says. I'm a young woman yet.

When I went into chemical menopause, my doctor told me it was my imagination. Right! There in the middle of winter I was sitting in church, fanning myself like crazy, turning bright red. My periods never came back, even though my doctor said there was enough estrogen so they might. I have no symptoms now; I'm not uncomfortable with it.

Another related issue is pregnancy. Conception is inadvisable during chemotherapy. Anticancer drugs have the potential to cause birth defects (*teratogenesis*) and mutations in offspring that are exposed to the drugs while in the womb and as sperm or eggs even before conception. However, there is no firm proof that the danger occurs with every drug, and so, this problem is hard to assess. In the past, doctors were particularly concerned when a woman had cancer of a reproductive organ such as the breast, which is sensitive to the levels of hormones in the body. Since pregnancy changes these levels, it was theorized that a pregnancy could stimulate the growth of cancer and precipitate a recurrence. However, recent studies show that pregnancy does not significantly raise the rate of recurrence.

There are patients who have produced apparently healthy offspring while on chemotherapy, but it's possible that even in seemingly healthy babies chromosomal damage may be latent and may not show up until some future generation. Most of the danger appears to be in the first trimester of pregnancy, and the overall risk in later trimesters appears to be the same as under normal conditions. Nevertheless, many physicians feel that the risk is high enough to recommend that their patients use contraception during chemotherapy. Dr. Grace says, "Chemotherapy is not a form of birth control. It is difficult to get pregnant while on chemo but not impossible."

If you are pregnant at the time of diagnosis, you most likely will not be given chemotherapy unless your life is in immediate danger from the disease, and chemotherapy has a chance to produce a cure or remission. Your doctor may advise you to end your pregnancy, but again, the decision is not clear-cut. You should discuss the possible risks with your doctor. If you are a sexually active woman and you miss a period before or during chemo, you should have a pregnancy test as soon as possible. If you have a baby, breast-feeding may be hazardous to your child during chemo.

WHAT YOU CAN DO

Infertility

If you are still of childbearing age, you should talk over family planning and contraception with your physician, nurse, or social worker. (The pill and IUD are usually not recommended for chemotherapy patients.) You should do this *before* you begin chemotherapy.

- If you are a male and you may want children (or more children), you should visit a sperm bank before beginning chemo, while you still have viable sperm. Should the chemotherapy leave you permanently sterile, you may still be able to father children via artificial, or *in vitro*, insemination.

- Women about to undergo chemotherapy unfortunately do not have an equivalent option at this time and are usually counseled about the possibility of adoption. A 2001 study published in the *Journal of the American Medical Association,* however, offers women hope for conceiving where before there was none. Infertility experts have restored ovarian endocrine function in two women who were at risk of early menopause from chemotherapy and radiation. They removed their ovaries, transplanted some of the tissue into their forearms during treatment, and replanted their ovaries after cancer treatment. In another study, published in 2000 in *Nature Medicine,* scientists were able to protect mice ovaries and eggs from radiation and the chemo drug doxorubicin. They were able to do this by injecting a protective chemical into the sac surrounding the ovary. Other studies show that fertilized eggs have a better chance of surviving freezing and thawing than do unfertilized eggs. But if you do not have a partner, you will need a sperm donor to produce the embryos. Some women opt to have their unfertilized eggs frozen anyway, on the chance that future technology will be able to unthaw them and keep them viable.

Early Menopause

Health professionals sometimes dismiss the symptoms of early menopause as "psychosomatic" or tell patients to grin and bear it. Don't let them! A study published in 2000 in *Cancer Nursing* compared menopause symptoms experienced by 200 women receiving adjuvant chemotherapy for breast cancer with those of 200 women experiencing a natural menopause. They found that the women on chemo reported a higher incidence of menopause symptoms, and that specific symptoms were more severe. Hot flashes ranked first, and tiredness came in as the second most-often cited symptom. This study also pointed out that nurses have an intimate supportive role in cancer treatment and so you might have better results if you speak to an oncology nurse about this, rather than to your physician.

Menopause occurs when your ovaries stop producing the sex hormones estrogen and progesterone. Many doctors simply put women without cancer on hormone replacement therapy (HRT). If you have been diagnosed with certain types of cancer, and are suffering from menopause symptoms, they may also offer it to you, or agree that you can continue taking it if you were taking it at time of diagnosis. However, HRT has been linked with a greater risk of endometrial cancer, breast cancer, heart attack, stroke, gallbladder disease, and liver disease. This makes HRT risky for any woman. In addition, most doctors are reluctant to recommend it to their patients who currently have, or who have a history or diagnosis of, cancer that is hormone-dependent. The thinking is if our bodies' natural hormones feed the cancer, so would synthetic hormones. If any cancer cells exist in your body, the hormones might be encouraged to grow. In a 2001 presentation before the North American Menopause Society, researcher Dr. Bruce Ettinger presented a retrospective look at studies that have addressed this issue. His conclusion is that taking HRT is a gamble, but many studies have not revealed a risk, or have been inconclusive. He thinks it might be safe for a woman with a history of breast cancer but who has been disease-free for at least a year or two. However, he also said, "There is no data to support the use of estrogen earlier on, and unfortunately that is when women are asking for it."

There are alternatives, including natural therapies to ease menopause symptoms, as well as nonhormonal medications.

- If vaginal dryness is the main problem, ask your doctor about prescribing a testosterone-containing cream. Or you may find that lubricants such as K-Y Jelly, Replens, and Astroglide provide what chemo has taken away.
- Refer to one or more of the many books, tapes, articles, Web sites, and organizations devoted to helping women go through menopause naturally. Natural approaches include dietary changes and nutritional supplements; relaxation therapies such as deep breathing, yoga, and meditation; herbs, homeopathy; acupuncture; and exercise.
- Your diet may influence hormone levels. Foods containing phytoestrogens—natural chemicals found in foods that act like estrogens, but in a weaker way. Scientists believe that they bind to receptor sites on cells and this prevents the stronger estrogens from binding and causing harm. Foods rich in phytoestrogens are soy, cashews, peanuts, oats, corn, wheat, apples, and almonds. Several herbs, such as black cohosh and chaste tree berry, also seem to balance hormones. However, no one is sure whether phytoestrogens have a beneficial or harmful effect in women with estrogen-sensitive tumors, so many experts advise these women to be moderate in their consumption of these foods and avoid taking phytoestrogens in herbal or supplement form.
- To reduce the risk of hot flashes, avoid foods that are known to increase them: coffee, black tea, chocolate, colas, and anything with caffeine; alcohol; and spicy foods. It's also helpful to dress in layers and carry a fan with you.
- For nonhormonal medical solutions for hot flashes, ask your doctor about clonidine, a drug used normally to treat high blood pressure. Studies show that this drug, used either orally or in patch form, eased hot flashes in women taking tamoxifen. Three antidepressants, Prozac

(fluoxetine), Paxil (paroxetine), and Effexor (venlafaxine), have been shown to ease the frequency and severity of hot flashes in breast cancer patients on chemotherapy. In one study, Effexor reduced hot flashes by more than 60 percent. It also helped men with hot flashes who were undergoing anti-androgen therapy for prostate cancer. Side effects included dry mouth, nausea, and constipation. In the Paxil study, 40 percent of the women reported an improvement in sex drive.

- If you are on chemo a long time and are concerned about bone loss, have a bone density test. If your bones are in trouble, your doctor may prescribe a bisphosphonate such as Fosamax (aldendronate), which has been shown to slow bone loss.
- For sleeplessness, you can try over-the-counter sleep medications, or natural therapies (see also SLEEP DISTURBANCES).
- It may help you deal with the physical and emotional changes brought about by early menopause if you contact women's support groups whose members have gone through menopause themselves.
- Remember, it's important to remain sexually active—it is a common misconception that sexual desire diminishes after menopause. But this may be in part a self-fulfilling prophecy (use it or lose it).

A comprehensive approach seems to work best, and you may need to use several types of treatments. Gail Greendale, M.D., of the University of California Los Angeles School of Medicine, developed a program for breast cancer survivors that included symptom assessment, education about treatment and sexual health, psychological counseling, clonidine, Replens, and instruction in pelvic exercises. After four months, women who followed the program reported a substantial reduction in vaginal dryness, hot flashes and incontinence, and their sexual function improved as well, compared with breast cancer survivors who were not on the program.

Kidney Problems
See BLADDER AND KIDNEY PROBLEMS.

Liver Problems

Many of the drugs used in cancer chemotherapy produce some degree of liver impairment (*hepatotoxicity*); most are difficult to measure and unnoticeable because of your liver's ability to withstand a tremendous amount of abuse. And abuse is what it gets during chemotherapy because the liver works overtime to detoxify harmful substances before they are excreted from the body.

Although any drug can stress the liver, some are more stressful than others. Methotrexate and 6-mercaptopurine are the two drugs usually associated with cirrhosis and fibrosis (scarring) of the liver, especially during long-term use. Other drugs, such as L-asparaginase, carmustine, Cytoxan, dacarbazine, doxorubicin (Adriamycin), mithramycin, streptozocin, and thioguanine, have also been implicated in liver dysfunction. Combination chemotherapy, preexisting liver dysfunction, and alcohol intake can compound these drugs' effects on the liver, which may become evident within one or two months after treatment or as late as two years afterward. Symptoms include jaundice, nausea, fatigue, and pain on the right side of the body.

WHAT YOU CAN DO

- Reduce the toxic burden on your liver as much as possible by avoiding other harmful substances such as cigarette smoke, air pollution, dry cleaning fumes, fatty foods, foods and beverages with lots of chemicals and unnecessary drugs.
- Do some form of moderate exercise regularly to keep your elimination process efficient.
- There is some evidence that the herb known as milk thistle (Silymarin) helps the liver detoxify, but most practitioners recommend that you do not take this during the active part of your treatment. Rather, use as part of a comprehensive detox program under a knowledgeable practitioner's care.

Lung Problems

Lung damage (pulmonary toxicity) is a relatively rare side effect, although many drugs have the potential to cause it. Busulfan, carmustine, chlorambucil, Cytoxan, the bleomycins, and methotrexate have been known to cause lung damage in a small percentage of patients. A dry cough, shortness of breath, high pulse, and a low-grade fever characterize the damage, which is a kind of scarring (fibrosis). Pulmonary damage may be reversible with time if you stop the drug early and you take corticosteroids. However, some people do suffer irreversible damage, and as a result, they are chronically short of breath and must change their lifestyles accordingly.

Pulmonary toxicity may occur after the first treatment; this is usually due to a hypersensitivity to the drug and is helped by corticosteroids. However, sometimes the damage doesn't become evident until long after chemotherapy, even years after the therapy has ended.

Because this reaction is so rare and the early symptoms are subtle or unreported, lung damage may be undetected until quite late. Dr. William Grace, an oncologist at St. Vincent's Hospital in New York, says:

Early diagnosis is the key. If it goes too far, there may be no coming back. If a patient has symptoms and an X-ray shows nothing, you go on to test for pulmonary functions. I think that what you often see is a busy oncologist who keeps giving the drug because toxicity is not detected soon enough. Subclinical or early forms of toxicity are often not recognized.

WHAT YOU CAN DO

- To prevent or minimize the possibility of lung damage, reduce the amount of tobacco (or anything else) you smoke; quitting is even better. Also avoid air pollution as much as possible.
- Take deep breaths several times a day; this will expand your lung tissue and may prevent fibrosis.

- Eat a diet rich in antioxidant nutrients such as vitamins C and E and beta-carotene; you may wish to also take antioxidant supplements under a professional's supervision.

Milk Intolerance

Some people are born without the ability to digest milk, while others have no problem. As a chemotherapy patient, however, you may develop this inability because the drugs destroy the cells in the intestine that produce the enzyme (lactase) that digests milk sugar (lactose). Without lactase, you can't digest the milk sugar, and watery, fermentative diarrhea, flatulence, and cramping result. Since you may be relying heavily on dairy products and adding milk-based nutritional supplements to stave off weight loss and malnutrition, this might be an important symptom to diagnose and treat, even if you've never had a problem with milk before.

Though there are various laboratory tests to definitively diagnose lactase deficiency, they are not often done because of the time and expense involved. Therefore, you need to pay attention to the following clues: gas, indigestion, diarrhea, or vague abdominal pain thirty to sixty minutes after drinking milk or eating a milk product.

WHAT YOU CAN DO

- If you suspect a lactase deficiency, consult your doctor. He or she may recommend that you begin a lactose-free or lactose-reduced diet in addition to adopting the measures suggested in the section on diarrhea.
- Cut down on or avoid completely foods high in lactose: milk, cream, ice cream, most cheeses, and custard or pudding desserts. You may be able to tolerate milk and milk products in which the lactose has been totally or partially broken down: acidophilus milk, lactose-free cottage cheese, buttermilk, yogurt, fermented cheese such as cheddar, and sour cream. In addition, there is a product (Lact-Aid) that can be added to milk, or taken orally, or sprinkled on dairy food to

predigest the lactose. This has also been added to many dairy foods for your convenience.

- Read labels carefully and watch out for other foods that have milk or lactose in their ingredients. Some of these include instant coffee, imitation dairy coffee creamers, cocoa and chocolate drinks, breads, party dips, commercial instant potatoes, cakes, cookies, pies, cordials and sherries, sherbet, creamed soups, and chewing gum.

- Lactose is also a common ingredient in many oral medications and vitamin and mineral supplements, so if you are very sensitive to lactose, check these labels carefully also; you may need to find a substitute.

- If milk and milk products usually are prominent in your diet as a source of protein, look for foods made with soybean milk, or soymilk. You can now buy these alternative milks plain or in many flavors, in containers just like those with cow's milk. You may also start eating tofu or other soy products such as hot dogs, luncheon meats, cheeses, yogurts, and various forms of "ice cream" desserts.

Mouth, Gum, and Throat Problems

Chemotherapy drugs—particularly the antimetabolites and antibiotics— often produce sores in the mouth (*stomatitis*), sores in the throat and in the food pipe (*esophagitis*), and sore, bleeding gums. Some researchers estimate that all cancer patients who receive chemotherapy or radiotherapy for head and neck cancer are affected. About 40 percent of other chemotherapy patients are affected, and 70 percent of patients undergoing bone marrow transplants will experience this and most likely in severe form. These side effects are caused when chemo destroys fast-growing surface cells in these areas. As a result, minute raw or bleeding ulcerated patches or spots appear. You may also develop a bacterial or fungal infection or spontaneous bleeding from your gums. You may experience dry mouth, difficulty chewing and swallowing, an unpleasant taste or odor in your mouth, and alterations in the taste of foods. Esophagitis causes mild to severe chest pain that can resemble heartburn.

These side effects can be very painful and distressing and can lead to other complications, such as loss of weight and malnutrition; gum trouble can lead to a loss of teeth. The soreness usually peaks one week after a treatment and clears up in a few days as the body repairs itself.

WHAT YOU CAN DO

There is relatively little that standard treatment has to offer specifically to prevent these side effects from occurring. But there are ways to alleviate them, minimize them, live with them, and prevent complications. If your symptoms are severe, your doctor may need to reduce the doses of the drugs that cause them.

Preventive Dentistry and Oral Hygiene

Starting chemotherapy with a clean, healthy mouth and maintaining good oral hygiene will go a long way toward minimizing and preventing later mouth problems and infections. Many oncologists—though not all—advise preventive dentistry for patients they feel might be at high-risk for oral problems as a result of chemotherapy. Here's what one dentist said on the subject, in an article published in *Family Physician:*

> Oral care is very important in patients receiving chemotherapy, but it is often overlooked in the urgency of a patient's cancer treatment. Ideally, dental evaluation and preventive care should become a part of the workup preceding chemotherapy. These measures reduce potential complications that may be difficult to control later.

• Always inform your dentist, preferably before you do it, that you are undergoing chemotherapy. Although many patients can safely undergo procedures such as simple fillings and tooth cleaning while on chemotherapy, it is never certain how any one patient will react, so it is best to take care of cavities and rough edges on your teeth before treatment begins. It's also advisable to get a thorough cleaning because the inevitable minor bleeding that occurs during cleaning could become serious and because accumulated tartar can harbor bacteria that might infect mouth sores later on.

• If you have gum problems or teeth that are so decayed that they might be abscessed, it is wise to make an appointment with a dentist and schedule as much work as possible before the treatment begins. You generally should not have serious procedures such as periodontal surgery and tooth extraction while you are on chemotherapy, and chemo may aggravate the conditions that make these procedures necessary.

• Sometimes chemotherapy can be delayed a few weeks for this purpose if the likelihood of oral complications from the treatment is great. Your oncologist may be able to recommend a dentist who specializes in the rapid and sometimes radical procedures that are necessary.

• If you wear full or partial dentures, have the fit checked before beginning chemo and if necessary have them refitted to avoid irritation and possible infection. You shouldn't wear poorly fitting dentures at all but you may wear well-fitting ones after the worst of the side effects of each treatment have subsided. Orthodontic devices (braces) usually are too irritating and need to be removed during chemotherapy.

• Floss daily and clean your mouth after each meal and at bedtime; use a soft-bristled brush and a minimal amount of toothpaste. Rinse afterward with warm saline water (one tablespoon of salt or one to two tablespoons of baking soda, which is milder, in one quart of water). This solution raises the pH of the mouth and helps prevent the growth of acid-loving microorganisms such as *Candida*, which causes yeast infection. Patients are usually advised not to use a commercial mouthwash unless it is alcohol-free, so check the label.

• If your blood count is low and stomatitis is severe, avoid dental floss and water picks. Clean your teeth gently with a soft-bristled brush or cotton swab or with special sponge-tipped swabs (Toothettes) impregnated with a mild toothpaste. After each cleaning, use the following healing, bacteria-fighting rinse, which can also be used by itself to clean your teeth if brushing or swabbing is too painful. To make it, mix one part hydrogen peroxide with five parts saline water;

add a few drops of alcohol-free mouthwash if desired. Prepare it fresh each time you use it; salt water can be made and kept ahead of time, but the peroxide will lose its effectiveness unless added immediately before using. Swish a mouthful around your mouth for a minute (it will bubble and foam) before spitting it out. Repeat once or twice. You may need to experiment using various proportions and combinations of water, soda, and hydrogen peroxide until you find a rinsing solution you can use frequently without it burning.

Medication and Other Measures

• Some doctors paint individual mouth ulcers with an antacid such as milk of magnesia. To do this yourself, use a cotton-tipped swab. Allow the antacid to stand until the liquid rises to the top, pour off the liquid, and dip the swab in the thick white residue. Apply it to the ulcer. This relieves pain and promotes healing. Also, if you simply swish antacid around your mouth it will also stick to ulcerations and protect them.

• If the pain is severe, your oncologist may prescribe topical anesthetics such as Xylocaine to kill the pain. These come in spray, lozenge, and liquid forms. If you use such a preparation, be aware of extremely hot foods—you may burn your mouth without realizing it and create further damage.

Dr. William Grace prescribes viscous lidocaine, a kind of jelly, for his patients with mouth or throat ulcers:

This is a kind of Solarcaine for your mouth and is quite good for keeping people's nutritional status up. You may have to swish and swallow a few times to get total anesthesia, and it works only for about twenty minutes to a half hour, but you can get a lot of food down in a half hour. The food doesn't taste like much because lidocaine also numbs the taste buds, but some people learn how to keep it off their tongues so that taste perception is maintained. The other thing with stomatitis is that people have a hard time coping with the pain, but painkillers can be given to relieve that.

- If an infection is present, your oncologist will prescribe medication: an antibiotic for a bacterial infection or an antifungal for a yeast or fungus infection. Local medication is usually "swished and swallowed"—if the mouth is infected, it is assumed that the esophagus is also.
- If your lips become dry and cracked, it will be difficult for you to open your mouth wide enough to clean or medicate it. Keep your lips moist with a soothing cream, drink plenty of liquids.
- If you have a history of herpes (cold sores/fever blisters) on the lips, be sure to tell your oncologist, who may prescribe an ointment to use to help prevent sores from forming while you are on chemotherapy.
- If your mouth is very dry, your doctor may prescribe an artificial saliva.

Eating Tips

- Since malnutrition slows the healing process, and deficiencies in zinc, folic acid, riboflavin, and vitamins B_{12} and C can increase the severity of these symptoms, make sure you try to eat well. A deficiency in the B vitamins may also cause cracks in the corners of your mouth. If you have trouble eating because of these side effects, discuss with your doctor the advisability of taking a nutritional supplement.
- A preliminary study shows that a dietary supplement called glutamine, an amino acid, may significantly reduce mouth pain. When patients were given a "swish and swallow" form of glutamine on treatment days and for at least fourteen days after, they had four and a half fewer days of pain compared with patients who used a placebo solution.
- Avoid irritating foods: tart, acidy foods such as citrus fruits and juices, tomatoes, carbonated beverages; hot, spicy foods; and foods that are very dry, coarse, crunchy, or salty and require a lot of chewing and/or saliva to digest, such as chips and pretzels, raw vegetables, nuts, and whole grains.
- Avoid tobacco, alcohol, and extremes in temperature—these can injure delicate tissues.
- Emphasize nonirritating foods such as fruit nectar, creamed soups, soft cheese, eggs, milk shakes, cooked cereals, eggnog, pudding, ap-

plesauce, mashed potatoes, and macaroni and cheese. Yogurt may be particularly soothing.

- Try overcooking and pureeing foods such as vegetables and meats to make them easier to eat. Try using junior baby foods. Adding plenty of liquids such as sauces and gravies to foods or using moist heat in cooking (stewing and steaming) will make food easier to chew and swallow. Have casseroles and soups.

- Drink plenty of fluids. If you are eating less, make nutritious high-calorie, high-protein drinks. Liquid supplements may be needed to help keep up your nutrient intake. Sipping tepid tea may soothe your mouth and throat.

- Some people find cold foods such as ice cream, ice cubes, frozen yogurt, Popsicles, and sherbet soothing, but others find these things painful.

- If you have esophagitis, milk and milk products such as sour cream, yogurt, and cottage cheese tend to coat the throat and protect the cells. You can eat these every two to four hours.

Nail Problems

Discolored and disfigured nails are a rare complication of chemotherapy. Your nails can become brittle, cracked, and ridged; they may tear, flake, and break off painfully near the quick. The main culprits seem to be bleomycin, busulfan, cyclophosphamide (Cytoxan), doxorubicin, and 5-fluorouracil.

WHAT YOU CAN DO

- Minimize the dangers and damage to your nails by wearing rubber gloves and protective gloves when performing chores; using rich hand creams may also help if you massage the cream around the nail beds.

- Remedies for hardening and strengthening brittle nails have not been proved, but they are generally harmless and, unless you experience a reaction to the ingredients, may help.

- Give yourself gentle manicures and pedicures because you may be more susceptible to infection and bleeding than usual, so don't cut or yank cuticles.
- If your nails are very damaged, thin, and weak, avoid harsh chemicals such as nail polish and nail polish remover. Otherwise, nail polish may help support and protect your nails, especially if you use the kind with nylon fibers. Use as many coats as necessary to form a thick enough shield.

Nausea and Vomiting

Most chemotherapy drugs cause some degree of nausea and vomiting after injection or administration. Some drugs, however, are notorious for their ability to cause these reactions in a high percentage of patients. Researchers have found that a high potential for nausea and vomiting exists in cisplatin, cyclophosphamide, daunorubicin, doxorubicin, dacarbazine, mechlorethamine, and streptozocin; a moderate potential exists in carboplatin, cytarabine, carmustine, methyl-CCNU, etoposide, ifosfamide, methotrexate (high dose), the mitomycins, lomustine, and procarbazine. The other commonly used drugs have low potential to induce vomiting. We don't know why some drugs in particular cause more vomiting than others—as a group they neither have any other attribute in common nor differ significantly from other chemotherapy drugs that do not cause vomiting.

The intensity, onset, and duration of nausea and vomiting that you may experience from a drug is an individual matter—it depends on your unique biochemical makeup, how well nourished you are, the dose of the drug you are getting and the rate your doctor administers it, and the other drugs you are getting. Psychological factors have also been implicated, especially in the case of anticipatory vomiting. This type of reaction occurs even before the drug is actually given. If you experience nausea and vomiting, they may begin within a few hours after a treatment but are short-lived, or they may last for twelve to twenty-four hours, or you may suffer from a constant, low-level nausea that persists throughout the course of treatment but does not lead to vomiting.

Usually the onset of nausea and vomiting is delayed a few hours—from three to four, possibly up to twelve after administration. In some drugs it is swifter—as soon as a few minutes after injection. If you experience a constant low-level nausea, you may find this sensation heightens soon after a treatment. Though reactions can vary somewhat from treatment to treatment, your reaction (unless treated) to the same drug is usually fairly consistent. If you are a violent vomiter, you will not suddenly begin to experience persistent nonproductive nausea or vice versa. Two people describe their usual reactions:

About four or five hours after my treatment the puke attack would begin. It went like this: The first one usually wasn't so bad because I'd have something in my stomach to throw up. Then I would throw up every twenty minutes for the next hour. Gradually they would get closer and closer together—every fifteen minutes, every ten minutes, every five minutes—by which time it was the dry heaves, pure bile. Then it would gradually slow down to every ten minutes, fifteen, twenty. Then would come the final one—I'd always know it was the final one. I'd put one hand on my forehead, one on my stomach, and breathe a big sigh of relief. Then I'd go to bed and sleep.

I never threw up, I was just nauseous the five days that I was on the chemo. I'd work all day in the hospital without eating; I couldn't—I didn't want to vomit. Because once I started, I was afraid I wouldn't ever stop. The nausea was even worse when other patients got sick themselves. That was awful.

My own particular reaction was the constant low-level nausea. Though it rarely went away and would heighten at certain periods during my therapy, it was never bad enough to make me throw up—but I seldom throw up anyway and am able to count on the fingers of one hand the number of times in my entire life I've been sick to my stomach.

Because nausea and vomiting are so unpleasant, they may be the side effects you fear the most. Vomiting can also become one of the most serious from a medical point of view. Deleterious results of prolonged, regular chemotherapy-induced nausea and vomiting include intolerance of the treatment, a generalized weakness, serious weight loss, loss of substances vital to the body such as water and nutrients that lead to malnutrition, dehydration, and an electrolyte imbalance that brings on irritability, lethargy, convulsions, and respiratory and heart problems. Though this is extremely rare, vomiting is sometimes so violent and prolonged that ribs and vertebrae have been fractured and the delicate tissue in the digestive tract has been torn.

Nausea and vomiting, therefore, jeopardize the successful treatment of cancer and reduce the quality of life. A survey of fifty-six oncology centers revealed that up to 10 percent of patients who potentially could have been helped by chemotherapy refused it because of actual or anticipated nausea and vomiting. Dr. Richard Gralla, formerly of Memorial Sloan-Kettering, says, "If the quality of life is terrible, it makes it that much more difficult to come back for the chemo even though they know it's a good thing to take. Even if you make up your mind to go through with it, it still makes your life miserable."

THE CAUSES OF NAUSEA AND VOMITING

Though some drugs may irritate the digestive tract directly, we think this effect is only a possible contributing cause of the nausea and vomiting associated with cancer chemotherapy. Rather, the drugs are capable of somehow triggering the parts of the brain that control nausea and vomiting. It may be the drugs themselves that do this, or it may be that the drugs cause a neurotransmitter in the brain to trigger the vomiting.

Nausea is a very common protective mechanism found in many species of animals. When you eat or drink something (the most likely ways for substances to enter the body), it gets into the bloodstream. There are certain receptors in the brain that are constantly sampling the blood. When harmful substances reach a certain level in the blood, it causes nausea. "When you take foreign substances in, there are very few ways you can get rid of them," explains Dr. Gralla. "One of them is by vomiting. Unfortunately, the body doesn't know that you didn't take chemotherapy by mouth but by injection."

Many other factors and conditions can produce nausea and vomiting in cancer patients, such as tumor pressure on the GI tract, metastases in the central nervous system, other drugs you are taking, pain, and chemical abnormalities caused by the cancer or the treatment. It is important to determine whether there are any contributing underlying causes of nausea and vomiting because this can influence the measures used to alleviate them.

WHAT YOU CAN DO

Both you and your doctor have many tools and techniques available to reduce the awfulness of nausea and vomiting—and to prevent them in the first place.

Using Drugs to Control Nausea and Vomiting

Drugs that cause vomiting are called *emetics;* the drugs used to control nausea and vomiting are called *anti-emetics* ("emesis" is the medical term for vomit). Until recently, the inability to deliver safe, effective, consistently reliable anti-emetics that are inexpensive and easy for outpatients to take has without a doubt been one of the more embarrassing and frustrating failings in the history of the cancer support system. Those most widely used in the past not only have been disappointingly ineffective but also have rather undesirable side effects of their own—sedation being the most notable. It has been difficult to find drugs that suppress vomiting, partly because the portion of the brain that controls this function lies so close to the area that controls the heart and lungs. Anything that would interfere with vomiting could affect the functioning of these vital organs as well.

Dr. William Grace, an oncologist at St. Vincent's Hospital in New York, feels that much of the problem lies in the way the available drugs are—and are not—used. Some doctors are not well informed and don't sit down and take the time to "fine-tune" their patients' therapies or to explain to them how to take their antinausea medication. "The common perception is that the disease makes you sick, the drugs make you sick, they're all going to be sick people," he says. "But that's not true. A lot of these things can really be done well. A lot of people are getting quite sick because there's not enough attention being paid to detail, to giving chemo-therapy well."

Fortunately, there have been a couple of breakthroughs in recent years, and as a result, chances are improving that you can get through this particular side effect much more comfortably. This improvement is due to three relatively new drugs—metoclopramide (Reglan), ondansetron (Zofran), and granisetron (Kytril)—and the increasingly popular practice of combining different drugs to greater effect.

Reglan belongs to a group of drugs called dopamine antagonists. Meto-clopramide had for years been used in relatively low oral doses with little effect. But when it was used in high doses intravenously in experiments by Dr. Gralla and others, it was shown to be highly effective against the side effects of cisplatin, a drug that results in severe nausea and vomiting that had proved unresponsive to the other antiemetics.

Zofran is effective in 85 percent of the people who take it and for most people it works well even against chemo regimens most notorious for caus-ing severe vomiting. Another advantage is that it doesn't cause the drowsi-ness that most other antiemetics do. Kytril, an even newer drug, is usually given along with another drug, Decadron, to enhance its effects. It is given intravenously prior to chemotherapy and may be given again afterward if needed.

Other, older drugs that your doctor may recommend include Com-pazine (prochlorperazine), which may be taken orally, and Trilafon (per-phenazine) and Torecan (thiethylperazine), both of which may be taken orally and administered intramuscularly or intravenously. These may still be beneficial if your chemotherapy drugs have a low or moderate potential for causing nausea and vomiting. Sometimes other drugs are effective in patients who do not respond to these oral medications. This group of drugs includes Haldol (haloperidol), administered orally or intramuscularly, and Inapsine or Innovar (droperidol), administered intravenously.

Corticosteroids, as a class of drugs, have been found to have anti-emetic properties, although it is uncertain why. Corticosteroids such as dexamethasone (Decadron) and methylprednisolone in high doses have been found to give good results.

Valium and Dalmane are sedative/hypnotics and are also used to re-

duce nausea in patients. Many oncologists are prescribing Ativan, an antinausea medication that also acts as an antidepressant and sleeping pill.
One intriguing side effect of this drug, and one that many patients consider a big plus, is that it can also cause amnesia. As a result, it helps dim
the memory of any vomiting they experienced that antiemetic drugs failed
to control. As Memorial Sloan-Kettering's Dr. Fahey has found, "A lot of
patients do better if they are mildly sedated with antianxiety drugs begun
before treatment and continued through it, right along with the chemo.
With some therapies, you're really better off if you're in kind of a fog, if
you just 'lose' that day."

Marijuana, a member of this class of drugs, also has been shown to be
an effective anti-emetic for some chemotherapy patients. In spite of its il-
legal status as a recreational drug, its therapeutic use for cancer patients
has gained broader acceptance and gotten a lot of publicity. As a result,
you may be able to get legal "joints" from your oncologist or capsules or
suppositories containing THC, the active ingredient in marijuana. The
synthetic form of the active marijuana ingredient is called dronabinol
(Marinol) and is available by prescription.

Though it does work for some people, and it may work better than other
anti-emetic drugs, marijuana is no panacea. Its side effects can vary con-
siderably, and they depend on many factors, including the strength of the
drug and the patient's expectations and prior experiences. The side effects
that might benefit cancer patients include the well-known "high" or sense
of well-being, its relaxing and tranquilizing effects, an increase in appetite,
and a lessening of pain. Marijuana, however, may also cause undesirable
side effects such as paranoia, disorientation, an inability to concentrate,
acceleration of the heartbeat, dry mouth, and red eyes. Be sure to check
with your physician before taking marijuana; you may have a physical
condition or be taking other drugs that are incompatible with marijuana
and that might have an adverse effect.

These unpleasant side effects are particularly unacceptable in older
patients, and many who have been given THC once have refused to take it
again. Research is being conducted to develop synthetic THC that will
have fewer side effects than the natural THC found in marijuana.

Patients find that marijuana works best if they begin using it *before* a treatment and continue to use it regularly afterward until the time comes when they would usually stop vomiting. Three to five puffs begin to have effect in a few minutes and last for about two hours. When taken by mouth, in brownies or cookies, or as a capsule, the effect begins in forty-five minutes to two hours and lasts two to six hours. Marijuana is also available as rectal suppositories—when used this way, the effect begins in thirty minutes and lasts up to six hours.

For more information see *Marijuana Medical Handbook: A Guide to Therapeutic Use* by Ed Rosenthal or look for "medical marijuana" on the Internet, using your favorite search engine.

Antinausea drugs are far from perfect. Not all work as effectively as we'd like; some work better against some emetics than others. Some of the drugs need to be taken hours before chemo is given (some recommend twenty-four hours) and then repeated at two-, three-, or four-hour intervals until the nausea is scheduled to subside. Oral anti-emetics have the advantage of being self-administered by the patient, but they may be unreliable and only partially effective against many emetics or, for some drugs, unavailable in this form. Intramuscular or intravenous administration, the most effective mode for some high-dose anti-emetics such as metoclopramide or corticosteroids, on the other hand, must be done by a trained professional, is time-consuming, and so is limited to hospital inpatients for the most part. In addition, there is the cost: Oral anti-emetics may cost as little as one dollar for twenty-four hours worth of treatment, whereas twenty-four hours of a new intravenous anti-emetic given in the hospital can cost more than $100—in addition to the other costs of chemotherapy, including the anticancer drugs themselves. None of the anti-emetics are without side effects, with sedation being the most prevalent. Marijuana, although it falls somewhere in the medium-price bracket as an anti-emetic, in many instances is purchased illegally and so poses its own additional unique disadvantages.

My oncologist gave me a prescription for Compazine when I started the chemo. But my reaction was a slight constant nausea, which heightened in waves without any warning. So I felt I never really needed the Compazine too badly—besides, I would have had to take it every day. I ended up never using it and throwing the pills away. I thought I was putting enough chemicals in my body as it was and decided to grin and bear it. I was one of the more fortunate ones in that I didn't have the severe reaction that necessitates the use of imperfect anti-emetics that these patients experienced:

> *I spent the year pretty much stoned. I smoked marijuana every time I went for a treatment; I also took Compazine at the same time. I don't know whether there was any effect or not, but I was afraid to try a treatment without that stuff. I had such a terrible time with it, what would I do if it were even worse without it? I didn't want to know.*

> *You wouldn't believe the drugs they gave me for the nausea. They tried everything on the market. First they tried Compazine. They tried it in different dosages, but that didn't work. They tried it in suppositories, but that didn't work either. Then they tried another drug. That didn't work. Finally they tried a new drug that came in a patch you put behind your ear; I'd start putting that on the night before they gave me the treatment. That didn't work either. They suggested I try marijuana. At first I didn't mind the idea of getting high for medical purposes. But then I thought, "I've already had one kind of cancer. Now I'm going to start smoking something that might give me lung cancer just so I won't feel the side effects of cancer therapy? What am I, crazy?"*

> *One of the amusingly frustrating aspects of my treatment had to do with marijuana. I felt I was cheated—I had heard about using grass to control nausea, and never having smoked controlled substances before, I was looking forward to this opportunity to try it. But they just gave me something through the IV along with the chemo that knocked me out.*

The problems with anti-emetics are far from completely solved, but there are ways of getting around them and ways to enhance the drugs' effectiveness.

- *Timing:* Dr. Grace says, "You always start antinausea medication before you give the chemo. You've got to put the drug on the emesis center to change the emesis threshold. Once people start to be sick, forget it. It's very hard to stop it. The physician must use anti-emetics prophylactically—he must have the pills around, or write the prescription, and explain to the patients how to take it. This is a very labor-intensive field, and doctors must take the time to be compassionate." Dr. Ronald Bash also recommends that his patients begin taking an anti-emetic several hours before a treatment. He favors prescribing them in suppository form because many patients tolerate them better than oral medication. In addition, anti-emetics should be continued for a day or a day and a half after the treatment, because nausea can persist this long.

Sedation, a common side effect of anti-emetic drugs, can limit your mental and physical activities. This disadvantage, too, may be sidestepped by judicious use of timing and may even become an advantage. Patients find it often helps if they can sleep through the hours in which the worst nausea and vomiting are likely to occur. The sedative effects of the anti-emetics can help them to do this. In fact, tranquilizers, sedatives, and antihistamines have all been prescribed for their anti-emetic effects.

Dr. Gabriel Hortobagyi, a breast cancer specialist at MD Anderson Cancer Center, recalls how sedation used to be a problem with younger patients: "They were out of commission for hours. They couldn't drive, take care of their kids, or see a movie." But with ondansetron, the only side effect seems to be a headache, which isn't even experienced by every patient.

Those who are receiving chemotherapy as inpatients are often given an intravenous anti-emetic right through the same IV that the chemo goes through. They then spend a whole day and/or night sleeping. Outpatient treatments and anti-emetics can also be scheduled so the patients sleep through the worst of it. If you are home, try to have someone check on you periodically because it is possible to vomit in your sleep, inhale it, and suffocate. Elevating the head of the bed with either pillows or a prop under the mattress will help prevent this from occurring.

In addition, oral chemotherapy can all be taken at once, in the evening, instead of throughout the day. If it is taken along with an anti-emetic and a sedative, patients sleep through any nausea. Though there is a theoretical possibility that a higher concentration of the drug in the urinary tract could increase the risk of toxicity (cystitis), Dr. Grace doesn't see this effect in his practice: "If patients drink a lot of water at night, they wake up to urinate. The difference is infinitesimal; patients just don't have urinary problems."

• *Type and Dosage:* You may need to experiment with drugs and their amounts in order to hit on the right anti-emetic therapy for you. When one anti-emetic doesn't work, you should switch to one of another class, or increase the dosage, or combine drugs of different classes. Chemotherapy appears to stimulate several sites in the nausea-vomiting mechanism, and no single agent blocks all these sites. So, just as combinations of cancer chemotherapy drugs are usually more effective against cancer, combinations of anti-emetics work better than single agents do. This approach can also be helpful if an effective anti-emetic begins to lose its power. If patients get "breakthrough nausea"—a little more nausea with each cycle because of the accumulative toxicity—"the patient," says Dr. Grace, "might have to escalate the war. You increase the dose or add another anti-emetic."

Using Psychology to Control Vomiting

Nausea and vomiting can have a strong psychological component. The atmosphere and spirit in which chemotherapy is given perhaps can play a role in how nauseated a patient gets, as can the patient's expectations. Dr. William Grace feels strongly about this:

You can't have cancer patients come in and expect to get sick. From day one we tell them that with the proper anti-emetics the probabilities are very remote. Also, people who get chemotherapy should get

it in a private room which is warm and well ventilated so that any-
body who is sick in another room is neither heard nor seen by the pa-
tient. In some facilities, you sit in a room and everybody watches
everybody else getting sick. You get a visual reinforcement that the
stuff going in your arm is going to make you sick; there is also au-
ditory and olfactory reinforcement. People like to talk to each other
before and after, but getting chemo, itself is, I think, a very private
thing. I don't think they like to get chemo together, especially if
something bad is happening.

In addition, you can develop conditioned aversions to specific foods
and begin to refuse certain foods because you have "learned" to associate
them with the treatment and vomiting. This situation is very much like the
conditioned response that Pavlov elicited from his dogs, which learned to
salivate at the sound of a bell because they associated it with being fed.
Refusal of food becomes a conditioned response not related directly to the
presence or absence of nausea; as a result, you can avoid certain foods or
all foods throughout the therapy, not just during the time after therapy.

Another example of conditioning as a result of chemotherapy is called
anticipatory nausea and vomiting. This occurs in about 25 percent of those
taking chemotherapy and when it occurs, you feel the side effect before
the drugs could possibly have taken effect, often before they are even administered. You may wake up nauseated on the day of treatment, or begin
to feel symptoms on the way to your doctor, or just as the needle is being
inserted. Sometimes just seeing the physician, whether on a treatment day
or not, passing the hospital, or being in the same neighborhood as the
clinic can trigger nausea and vomiting. A patient remembers, "If I even
smelled rubbing alcohol, I would start retching from the association." Anticipatory nausea and vomiting can make posttreatment nausea and vomiting even worse. Your oncologist may give you anti-anxiety medication or
sedatives such as Ativan and Decadron before the treatment to help relieve your anxiety and block anticipatory nausea. In addition, you may use
relaxation therapies to reverse this reaction. Matthew Loscalzo, who treats
patients for this and other problems related to cancer and chemotherapy at
Johns Hopkins, says:

Anticipatory nausea and vomiting is a conditioned aversion. Usu-
ally by the third or fourth session, upon waking that day the patient
may vomit, just at the thought of going in to the hospital. One thing
I do with patients is to let them know that this is at first a physio-
logical response to the drugs. The body becomes nauseated, and the
patient learns to associate the entire environment of the hospital
with the side effect. People tend to learn very quickly when they are
under stress, or are emotionally depleted, or when their anxiety level
is high.

It is not simply a psychological process—there is nothing psy-
chologically wrong with you. You simply have to relearn something.
It's in part a physiological process like learning to play the piano.
After a while, your fingers play the piano and you don't have to
think about it. It's the same with this.

Relaxation techniques are also being used to reduce the postchemother-
apy nausea and vomiting that result after a chemotherapy treatment has
been given, though with not quite such dramatic results. Loscalzo continues:

With postvomiting and nausea there's a good reason for people to be
ill. Their bodies have been subjected to chemotherapy. It's very dif-
ferent from the conditioned aversion experienced before a chemo
treatment. It can, however, also be exaggerated. We can help these
people with their anxiety, but only up to a point. They are still going
to feel ill—that is normal. But we can help them to reduce some of
the distress that they're feeling because they can control their anxiety.

This patient underwent relaxation and hypnosis to relieve her anticipatory nausea and vomiting:

I was getting sick even before I had the treatment. One of the nurses
mentioned that a doctor was using hypnosis for chemo patients and
it seemed to work well. In the beginning I had five sessions a week
with the hypnotherapist. This was disturbing because he was in the
same building as my chemotherapist, and the second time I went I

got sick because of the association. My hypnotherapist assured me it would never happen again—and it didn't. I stopped having the anticipatory nausea and vomiting.

He also tried to help me control the nausea after the chemo, but that he couldn't do completely. What did happen was that I was able to recover from the chemo faster. The nausea went away faster, and I could eat sooner. He just suggested it to me while I was in the trance. He told me what was going to happen, what I should expect to eat. Within twenty-four hours I could handle light food.

M. L. Frohling has used these techniques at Denver Presbyterian Hospital and illustrates another example of how these techniques are used to control side effects:

There was one patient who had to be hospitalized for severe nausea and diarrhea. She was getting chemotherapy after surgery as a precaution. She didn't believe there was any cancer left in her body, and she perceived the chemo as coming in and killing off only healthy cells. Through visual imagery I was able to help her realign her belief system to be more oriented toward regaining her health instead of thinking the chemo was destructive. Once her conflict was resolved, she had her third round of chemo without a bit of nausea.

Using Other Nondrug Measures to Reduce Nausea and Vomiting

Cancer professionals have devised many hints to help their patients reduce nausea and vomiting. You might want to try them if your nausea and vomiting are mild, or you don't want to take anti-emetics, or you want to do something on your own to help reduce this side effect instead of or in addition to taking anti-emetics.

• Methods of consuming foods and beverages that have worked under other nausea-inducing conditions such as illness, stress, or pregnancy may work in this case. For example, nausea in the morning may respond to remedies recommended for morning sickness—eating melba toast, dry toast, or crackers upon awakening and before getting up.

- It is important to avoid dehydration—drink plenty of water and other liquids, especially before and as soon after a treatment as possible. Carbonated beverages such as ginger ale, 7 Up, and Coca-Cola can help curb nausea. Clear liquids such as fruit juices, clear soups, Popsicles, and gelatin desserts are usually tolerated.
- Bland, light foods—mashed potatoes, applesauce, sherbet, toast, yogurt, and cottage cheese—stay down more easily.
- Avoid sweet, salty, greasy, and hot or spicy foods with strong odors.
- Eat foods cold or at room temperature to avoid releasing strong odors that can sometimes trigger nausea.
- Sometimes sour or tart foods—pickles, lemons, sour hard candy—or rinsing the mouth out with lemon juice and water can help curb nausea.
- Always sip liquids and eat foods slowly. Avoid drinking during meals. Eat in a still, relaxed, quiet environment.
- Experiment with the amount and timing of your meals. For some patients, avoiding any food or drink for one or two hours before and after a treatment helps. Sometimes eating a large meal three to four hours before the treatment and eating lightly the rest of the day does the trick. If neither of these helps, try eating several small, light meals during the day.
- If the smell of food nauseates you, let others do the cooking and avoid the cooking area. Stick with foods that do not have strong odors.
- Ask to have the timing of your treatment changed—some patients report a decrease in nausea when the treatment is given early, others when it is given late in the day. The method of administration can sometimes make a difference: The slower drip (infusion) method can cut down on nausea.
- Oral chemotherapy that makes you nauseous can be taken along with food or milk and/or an antacid. This sometimes reduces nausea, but check with your physician to make sure there is no incompatibility between drugs.

- Distract yourself. Watch TV, go to the movies, or socialize to take your mind off nausea.
- Many patients report that exercise reduces nausea. This worked well for me, and swimming worked best of all. However, activity after meals can increase your discomfort and perhaps even trigger vomiting.
- Use relaxation techniques such as meditation, hypnosis, and visualization. Studies have shown that these therapies do help reduce nausea and vomiting in many patients (see Chapter 11) and are especially effective in anticipatory nausea and vomiting.
- Try acupressure or acupuncture, which some people have found to be successful in controlling nausea and vomiting. You might also try a device originally designed to stop motion sickness, seasickness, and morning sickness. The device (made by Marine Logic in West Palm Beach, Florida, and available in diving shops and pharmacies for around $15) is a pair of wristbands that exert gentle pressure on the p-6 acupuncture point. The manufacturer claims a success rate of 70 percent with morning sickness, and while results from physicians using the product for chemotherapy are not complete as of this writing, they show great promise—and no side effects.

Many patients find that one or a combination of these methods helps them handle nausea and vomiting. Often they come up with tricks of their own—some of them bizarre—to help them get through it:

I tried to do something to occupy my mind, to talk myself out of feeling sick. I convinced myself that having a Coke and a doughnut before a treatment helped.

I craved fruit juices. And I ate salty pretzels before a treatment— somehow they were not too unpleasant when I vomited, and they stayed pretty much the same on the way up as on the way down.

Chicken soup and toast were the only things I tried. But after a while I didn't try anything. I'd wait until I came home from work, have a brandy, and get knocked out. I'd go to sleep immediately, and I guess that's why I thought it was the only thing I could tolerate.

I smoked cigarettes while I was on chemo, though I don't anymore. They were my crutch. You'd think that they would have made me sicker, but every time I felt a wave of nausea, I'd light up and it went away. Maybe it was the deep breathing rather than the cigarette.

Nervous System Problems

There are several chemotherapy drugs that are known for their effects on the nervous system. As a result of taking vincristine or vinblastine, or taxol, you may experience peripheral neuropathy (nerve damage in the hands and feet), the symptoms of which include a tingling or numbness in the fingertips and/or toes. You may feel clumsy and have trouble opening jars or tying your shoelaces. In addition to peripheral neuropathy, there may be damage to the nerves that control the action of the intestines, which results in constipation, sluggish bowels, or a colic-like pain. Sometimes the facial nerve is affected and there is a deep aching pain in the jaw or throat. A loss of deep tendon reflexes or increased motor weakness causes foot or wrist drop, difficulty walking or rising from a chair, clumsiness, or a loss of coordination. In addition, the impotence of which some men complain is possibly a result of nerve damage.

Vincristine was part of my chemo protocol, and I did experience some tingling and numbness in my fingers and toes. It came on so gradually that I barely noticed it. It was winter, so I thought maybe the cold had something to do with it. I never would have said anything if my oncologist hadn't eventually asked me about it. I got quite constipated for a while, but we don't know whether that was from the drugs or from my different diet and decrease in exercise. I noticed one foot would sort of lag behind when I walked, but I thought I was just tired.

In addition to these fairly concrete, measurable signs of neurotoxicity, there is a constellation of others that are vague and much harder to put a finger on. They can result in a mental fuzziness or cloudiness, a feeling of being doped up, off balance, and not "with it." Some people on chemo, myself included, just feel slower, duller, and clumsier both mentally and physically. Though it is difficult to distinguish the emotional and physical contributors from the direct pharmacological culprits, certain drugs are associated with these effects.

Vincristine and vinblastine, for example, can cause muscle weakness; vincristine also can cause muscle cramps. Both drugs have been known to cause mental depression. L-asparaginase may affect the nervous system by causing mental depression, hallucinations, confusion, lethargy, and nervousness. Procarbazine's effects include depression, tiredness, agitation, dizziness, hallucinations, confusion, weakness, and unsteadiness. Floxuridine can cause depression and lethargy; mitotane, depression, drowsiness, and tremors; thiotepa, dizziness; 5-fluorouracil can also cause clumsiness and a little bit of slowness. Dr. Grace says, "Since neurological damage is not a well-known effect, it is often not recognized or looked for. Some people say they become complete klutzes—they just fall down. People also can't do serial sevens—subtracting seven from one hundred, then seven from that result, then seven from that, and so on. They can't balance their checkbooks, or themselves."

Three patients relate their neurological side effects:

I lost my balance a few times, and I actually fell. My legs got so wobbly, like butter. My doctor called it "sea legs"—he said that many patients get it. It's been nearly two years since my last treatment, and I still feel like my legs haven't gotten their strength back. I still feel like they could buckle under me any time. I'm a forty-four-year-old person! Sometimes I walk like an old person—with little tiny steps. My doctor says they should get stronger; he's heard of this.

While on chemo, I lost my equilibrium. I tripped and broke my leg two months after chemo began; that healed well. Several months after that I lost my balance and broke my shoulder and arm. And then I fell in my kitchen—I fractured my ribs and tore a muscle in my arm. Then I punctured my eardrum with a Q-Tip because I again lost my balance and felt uncoordinated. I lost my hearing in that ear. People said they used to cry when they saw me.

I used to flounder for words, have trouble finishing sentences. I also found I was forgetting things—I'm not talking about forgetting keys—I would forget entire conversations.

Thus far, we know more about short-term and long-term neurological effects in children who have had chemo than we do about adults. But adult patients do notice difficulties that doctors have trouble explaining or pinning down. Peter Silverfarb, a prominent researcher in this area, reports that almost all commonly used chemotherapeutic drugs affect cognitive abilities (memory, attention, concentration), and that if you look for subtle and mild symptoms, they will be found in many chemo patients. But thus far there is very little concrete proof.

Part of the problem lies in differentiating cognitive impairment caused by the drugs from the signs of mental depression. They may exist simultaneously and make each other worse, and both may be due to chemicals. Another problem is the generally held belief that the blood-brain barrier protects the brain from harmful chemicals circulating in the blood.

Although the research documenting this type of neurological damage is still inconclusive, patients like my friend who complained, "I'm slow, I'm confused, I'm stupid, I don't feel like me at all. Am I going crazy?" need to be reassured that they are not crazy, that what they are going through is probably related to the chemicals in their system, and that they are not imagining it.

With cisplatin, another side effect on the nervous system occurs. This takes the form of ototoxicity, where there is a hearing loss and/or tinnitus (ringing in the ears). When there is a loss of hearing, it's usually only in the high frequencies. Ototoxicity occurs in approximately 30 percent of the patients who receive cisplatin. It may also occur in patients receiving mechlorethamine. A testicular cancer patient who experienced both hearing loss and tinnitus says:

I had a dramatic hearing loss for a while, which worried me because so much of my job entails telephone contact. I've gotten some hearing back, but telephone conversations are still very difficult. The doctors aren't sure whether it will ever come back, and they say if not, maybe a hearing aid will help later on.

I sit at my desk in the dead of winter, in a high-rise building in the middle of the city; there is construction going on outside, and I could swear there's a nest full of blue jays fighting right outside my window. Every once in a while in the evening I'll be sitting listening to records or reading the paper and I'll turn to my wife, just to be sure about this, and ask her, "There is not a nest of birds fighting outside the window, is there?" She'll say, "No—it's back again, isn't it?"

Neurotoxicity is, for the most part, temporary and reversible. (Those who undergo therapy with vincristine or vinblastine in high doses or over a long period of time are at a higher risk to develop neurotoxicity that is less reversible.) Its symptoms may peak a few days after a treatment and then gradually subside. They usually disappear completely after treatment has been concluded. But this may take up to two years, and in some patients, they may never go away completely.

WHAT YOU CAN DO

Neurotoxicity can be dangerous. You should tell your doctor immediately if any of the above symptoms occur. Although tingling toes may seem like "nothing," they could indicate more serious nerve damage that should be caught early.

- If you experience constipation, you may need to use stool softeners, laxatives, enemas, and an increase in dietary fiber to counteract sluggish bowels.
- You can minimize ototoxicity from cisplatin by using forced diuresis—massive doses of fluid given intravenously before and after the

drug—and by giving the drug very slowly. Hearing tests can be administered regularly to prevent severe, irreversible hearing loss.

• Exercise may reduce the risk of other forms of neurotoxicity because when you exercise, you're using the nervous system. "I don't know of any hard data," says Dr. Grace, "but I will tell you this: I see less neurotoxicity in active people. Those who are most inactive have more problems with clumsiness and confusion. Practice makes perfect—you get more coordinated by being physically active. I do tell them, though, to avoid sports that require skills or are dangerous. I recommend vigorous walking, for instance, and advise them to stay off bikes and be careful when walking down stairs." Other than that, he says, "There is not much you can do for neurotoxicity other than reduce the drugs. The doctor has to be very careful in addressing this toxicity."

Numbness or Tingling of Hands and Feet

See NERVOUS SYSTEM PROBLEMS.

Pain

Most people associate cancer with pain, sometimes great pain. Yet the amount of pain and the way you respond to it vary tremendously from person to person. It depends on the type of cancer and its location, the stage of the disease, the type of treatment, your past experience with pain, and your cultural background and psychology.

Pain is rarely caused by chemotherapy; one of the goals of chemotherapy is to reduce pain by shrinking the tumor. (One exception is the pain you feel if a chemo drug leaks out of your vein, causing *extravasation.*) Other side effects, both physical and emotional, can make pain seem worse and vice versa. "Prolonged pain destroys the quality of life. It can erode the will to live," writes Dr. Ronald Melzack, who has been studying pain for decades. "Severe, persistent pain can impair sleep and appetite, thereby producing fatigue and reducing the availability of nutrients to organs."

It is estimated that 60 to 90 percent of cancer patients have enough pain that they require pain medication. Fortunately, pain can be controlled today, if it is properly recognized and treated. There are all manner of drug and nondrug therapies for pain relief. Still, one-fourth of cancer patients suffer needlessly because of misinformation or a reluctance to use narcotics the way they should be used.

Gabriel Hortobagyi, a breast cancer specialist at the MD Anderson Cancer Center, says, "The common mistake made by physicians and patients alike is to be too conservative about pain control. Pain is an extremely destructive symptom. With the tools we have available today, there is very little reason why a person should not be able to have virtually complete control of pain their whole lives."

Diane Blum, director of Cancer Care, Inc., a social services and psychosocial support agency, describes part of the problem: "People with pain don't want to ask for medication. People believe pain is inevitable or that it builds character. They say they are going to concentrate on the chemo or nutrition—they're not going to bother their doctor about pain. It's sad because it takes so much energy to cope with pain, and you need that energy to cope with the disease."

Another issue is fear of addiction. Dr. Hortobagyi says that people have got to realize that "people who have real pain do not become addicted to narcotics. They need to have as much as it takes for them to have pain control." A related and serious stumbling block is that many of us were raised to believe that taking narcotics is "wrong." But Hortobagyi argues, "They are applying this principle to their own situation, and it's totally out of context. In their situation, narcotics is the drug of choice, and there's nothing wrong with taking it."

WHAT YOU CAN DO

Dr. Hortobagyi feels that both patient and doctor need to be savvy about pain control: "People wait until their pain gets real bad before they ask for or take pain medication. It's much easier to control pain when you start, when there is very little pain. You can control it well and get virtually uninterrupted pain relief." As a patient, you need to talk to your doctor about any pain you are experiencing. Cancer Care advises patients to:

- Keep a record of what makes pain better or worse and what triggers the pain or relief
- Describe the pain. Is it shooting, sharp, dull, burning, aching, numbing, tingling?
- Rate your pain on a scale of zero to ten.
- Rate the effectiveness of medication the same way.

Take Pain Medication

Pain medications (analgesics) range from mild pain relievers, such as aspirin and Tylenol, to stronger ones, such as Darvon, to weak narcotics, such as codeine and Percodan, to strong narcotics, such as morphine, Demerol, and Dilaudid. Some drugs that are not painkillers per se (coanalgesics) can reinforce the effect of painkilling drugs. Tricyclic antidepressants are especially effective for pain arising from malfunctioning nerves, such as shingles. Cortisone-type drugs are also sometimes prescribed. Combining drugs of different types, such as Tylenol and codeine, makes them more effective. Treatment should be carefully individualized as to drug, dosage, and timing so that you don't feel pain but the trade-off in terms of side effects from pain medication is acceptable to you.

For severe, persistent pain, morphine is the drug of choice. Enlightened practitioners know that when morphine is given or taken at fixed intervals around the clock, pain is much better controlled, smaller doses are required, and so side effects are fewer than when it is dispensed "as needed," that is, when pain has returned. This preventive approach is easier to achieve, and patients have more control over their medication now that morphine no longer needs to be injected. Morphine is available in oral forms including slow-release capsules, in skin patches that last for three days, and in suppositories. Portable pumps can also deliver a slow, steady infusion of injectable morphine within or outside the hospital.

These advances reduce but do not eliminate entirely the side effects of

narcotics, including sedation, confusion, and disorientation. Another notorious effect is constipation, which, Diane Blum insists, "needs to be
talked about up front." This type of constipation usually cannot be prevented by the usual dietary measures or by stool softeners or mild laxatives. You will probably need stronger laxatives on a regular basis to
counteract this universal side effect of narcotics.

Nondrug Measures against Pain

In addition, there are nondrug measures that are effective for some people.
These measures are generally used to enhance the effects of medication so
doses can be lowered. They include acupuncture, biofeedback, relaxation
techniques, hypnosis, and visualization and are best begun when the pain
is still mild or moderate.

Sexuality Changes

Many patients are eager to know about how chemotherapy affects people's
sex lives. As Grace Christ, formerly of New York's Memorial Sloan-Kettering
says, "Sexuality is a product of many things. Chemotherapies do impact on
sexuality—but we're not sure as to how." Some patients report an increase
in sexual activity; others say there is no difference. Many, however, do report a decrease to varying degrees:

*I would say there's moderate sex on chemo. We weren't exactly
swinging from the chandeliers . . . but I did feel like "doing it." I
did feel somewhat asexual because of the combination of a lost
breast and the lost hair. Frankly, I couldn't imagine how anybody
would want me.*

*Sex? There is no sex on chemo. My husband and I always had a
really nice sexual relationship, and suddenly I had no interest whatsoever. It wasn't because of the mastectomy; it had nothing to do
with my feeling less desirable. I was just indifferent. He and I sat*

down and talked about it, and he really understood. Fortunately, we learned to live with it; we knew it was temporary.

Obviously chemotherapy side effects such as bone-deep fatigue, infection, nausea, weight fluctuations, hair loss, depression, low self-esteem, and fear of losing a partner can lower our libidos and inhibit us sexually. Chemotherapy may also affect hormone levels and otherwise throw our reproductive systems off course, as when young women are thrown into premature menopause. (See INFERTILITY AND EARLY MENOPAUSE.) While anyone with any type of cancer may be affected, those with reproductive cancers would most likely suffer more. For example, a study published in the *Journal of Consulting Clinical Psychology* found that 30 percent of the women with gynecological cancer experienced a decline in the frequency of intercourse, and suffered from a "severe," "distressing," and "pronounced" lessening of sexual excitement.

As with other side effects, there are no hard and fast rules. Science has taught us that the brain is the most potent sexual organ there is: The mind is the true source of our sexuality. Our mental attitude can be a surprisingly powerful force both in overcoming any obstacles chemo has placed in our path and in adapting to those it cannot override. Though sexual intercourse may be put on the back burner, you may find that sexual expression is not. Sex during chemotherapy may not be quite the same as before, but it can still be enjoyable and satisfying for both you and your partner.

WHAT YOU CAN DO

If sexuality is important to you (and to many people it is not, at least at this time) and you find yours is being adversely affected, you can find help through many channels. Having honest, open discussions with your partner is an excellent place to start and may be all you need to set things on a better course. In addition, you might seek out medical solutions to physical side effects that affect sexuality, look for outside psychological support, or brush up on your sex education and learn about alternatives to previous sexual habits and preferences. In a 2001 study from the College of Nursing and Health Professions at the University of North Carolina, researchers studied women who had been treated for breast cancer. The women had either a mastectomy or lumpectomy, and most had adjuvant chemotherapy as well. They found that the women experienced a sense of loss: loss of a part of the body, loss of regular menstruation and youth, loss of sexual sensations, and loss of womanhood. As a result, the women experienced an "altered sexual self." The women who adjusted the best were those who sought information about the sexual side effects of cancer, and those who had strong intimate relationships.

Remember, it is natural to have some concerns and questions about sexuality in relation to cancer treatment, although health professionals rarely discuss this issue openly with patients and volunteer very little information without prompting. If you do speak up, you may even find that they avoid answering your questions, but don't allow this to convince you that your fears and thoughts are imaginary or foolish. A study done in England, in 2001, revealed that only 25 percent of clinicians and 20 percent of nurses discussed psychosexual issues with their patients. (Although most all of them thought that medical staff should do so.) Don't give up if sexual satisfaction and expression rank high on your list of needs and their absence or diminishment poses a threat to your quality of life.

Between You and Your Partner

The keys to enjoyable sexual activity for anyone are the ability to communicate openly, relax, and be flexible. This is no less true for people who are having chemotherapy. The quality of your relationship, your sexual skills, and the affection between you and your partner that existed previously also help determine your level of sexual enjoyment during chemo.

If chemo does impose changes on the way you're feeling emotionally and physically, let your partner know about your new needs and limitations. For example, you may be ready to resume sexual activity but your partner may not realize it, or sex may be the furthest thing from your mind but not your partner's. You might want to be sociable or affectionate at this time, but not sexual.

Psychological and emotional factors may cause us to withdraw from the whole experience as a way of protecting ourselves from possible failure or rejection. Whether we try to express our sexuality or we withdraw depends also, to a large extent, on our sexual partners, be they permanent (a spouse or steady lover) or randomly available. Although rejection is a real possibility—partners may find chemo patients unattractive, or fear catching the disease, or be afraid of hurting them, or be reluctant to bother them "after all they've been through"—these anxieties are often not grounded in reality.

Often, whatever differences happen because of chemo are fortunately short-lived. If you had a good relationship and enjoyed sexual activity before your illness, chances are that these things will reassert themselves eventually of their own accord. Sometimes the increased closeness that a serious illness can bring between two people not only will change their sexual relationship, but will ultimately change it for the better.

There's more to sex, love, and affection than intercourse and/or orgasms. Even when you are too ill or tired or when surgery is too recent for you to indulge in the athletics of the whole sexual gamut, you and your partner can express yourselves sexually—and have a very good time doing it. As adults, we have come to think of kissing, cuddling, and caressing as preludes, but they are quite nice all by themselves.

In my household, sex wasn't exactly a thing of the past, but it sure wasn't what it used to be. We often found ourselves content with the less vigorous forms of affection and appreciation. That was what I needed most at the time, not more excitement! The simple fact of having a warm, caring body next to mine was immensely reassuring, comforting, therapeutic, and meaningful. Gentle, heartfelt, loving stroking and hugging were good for my body and soul; they helped heal me emotionally and increased my sense of physical well-being, too.

And just as you can have intercourse without orgasm, so you can have orgasms without intercourse. As Kinsey and Masters & Johnson have shown in their studies, the parameters of healthy sexual behavior are broader than we thought; patience and a willingness to experiment may open up whole new vistas of sexual pleasure. Many chemotherapy patients turn to self-stimulation and find it a reasonable solution to needs that might otherwise go completely unfulfilled at this time.

It's difficult for anyone to start new relationships but this leap of faith and trust can pose a special challenge for people on chemotherapy. You may feel reluctant and awkward about bringing up the subject of your cancer and its therapy at first. But once the discussion has begun, communicating your feelings can help strip away superficialities and cultivate a closeness that might not otherwise have occurred or might have taken forever to develop. On the upside, as a person with cancer, you have the ultimate satisfaction of knowing that you are loved for yourself, not just for the way you look or for your ability to become a parent. (Chemotherapy can cause infertility, as discussed in INFERTILITY AND EARLY MENOPAUSE.)

Getting Outside Help

Sometimes the chemo-related sexual changes are such that they can't be dealt with between partners. At times, referral to a sex clinic or therapist may be in order. But often just talking things over with a sympathetic person can be a help. A nurse, a social worker, other patients, support groups, or your gynecologist or urologist will help you find some answers. A sensitive oncologist may be able to answer your needs for sex counseling or information; he or she may also be able to suggest material for home reading (or viewing). However, many patients find it difficult to bring up the subject with their oncologists, who rarely bring it up themselves.

Lari Wenzel, a medical psychologist, says:

> I think the problem is much greater than people will admit. The problem starts when the physician doesn't ask, and most patients aren't going to bring it up. It's not a routine part of your physical exam. And unless you have a very close relationship with the doctor and you are very assertive, it's just a problem that's not acknowledged the way it should be.

Both patient and doctor may feel awkward and uncomfortable discussing intimate sexual details. Physicians often are not equipped or eager to do sex counseling, or they don't realize that sexuality can be a concern at this time. Dr. William Grace, an oncologist at St. Vincent's Hospital in New York, says: "A lot of people just resign themselves and say, 'Well, I'm not going to be sexually active at this time.' A lot of people don't want to talk about it; it's very hush-hush. I'd say only about 10 percent of my patients bring it up, and when they do, it's usually with a nurse, who then tells me."

Lari Wenzel emphasizes that "as cancer care becomes more sophisticated, it's incumbent on all health professionals to recognize multiple needs in their patients—not just the medical needs." To that end, she feels strongly that "any cancer treatment program should have the built-in opportunity to acknowledge the possibility of sexual problems. This could be part of an overall emotional assessment—a brief questionnaire or interview that asks whether they are suffering from depression or anxiety. How is this interfering with their functioning at home, on the job, or with their sexual functioning?"

Although sexuality may get brought up during a support group, Mary Hughes, a psychiatric clinical nurse specialist, thinks that individual therapy is a more comfortable setting. Timing also enters into it in terms of being ready to look at long-term living. "In groups, you're still focusing on survival," she says.

According to Wenzel, preliminary research shows that in many cases psychosocial intervention can help. In a study of women with gynecologic cancer, a substantial proportion of those who received counseling said they had returned to their predisease frequency of intercourse compared with the women who received no counseling.

Fortunately, many problems have simple solutions. "A lot of patients' sexual problems are related to the physical side effects of chemotherapy," continues Dr. Grace, and here the oncologist's medical skills can surely help. "They may have painful intercourse due to vaginal dryness. If there is an infection present—infections like *trichomona* and *candida* have an increased risk at this time—we treat that." If you suffer from fatigue, nausea, constipation, or diarrhea, you can take medications and measures that reduce them, too.

Skin Changes

Chemotherapy can affect your skin in many ways. Most effects are minor and disappear between treatments or after the course of therapy is over. Your skin may become dry, itchy, flaky, oily, or sensitive to skin creams, lotions, soaps, or other products. The reason for this is that since the skin cells multiply rapidly, the skin sheds more than usual and becomes thin. Your sweat glands may also be affected and shut down, which can also leave your skin drier than usual. A breast cancer patient recalls:

> *I was concerned that my skin was going to get old fast from the chemo. I didn't get wrinkles or creases, but my skin did get very dry. I looked like I had dandruff all over my body—not just my head. When I peeled off my stockings I'd shake them out and flakes of skin would fall. It was disgusting! I used a lot of Nivea. And when my scalp got dry I used mineral oil on it, and baby oil, but that just made my thin hair look limper and thinner.*

Your skin may be prone to more bacterial and fungal infections than usual because of its increased sensitivity and your lowered resistance to disease in general. Some drugs cause changes in skin color, and these changes may be triggered or worsened by exposure to sunlight. The areas usually affected by the drug-sun combination are the backs of the hands, bodily creases, nails and nail beds, the face, and the elbows. Rarely, the skin over the whole body can be affected. Drugs that increase sunburn are actinomycin D, beomycin, dacarbazine, doxorubicin (Adriamycin), 5-fluorouracil (5-FU), methotrexate, and vinblastine (Velban).

Some drugs can cause a local irritation or red rash around the injection site. This is not serious and should disappear within an hour or two after the treatment. Some drugs may also cause the veins to darken. This is not serious either, and the vein is not damaged; the darkness should disappear within a week or two. Patients may also experience mild discomfort during an injection, both from the needle and from the drugs themselves. This should not be confused with *extravasation,* a potentially serious complication that occurs at the site of the injection when some of the drug escapes into the surrounding tissue rather than entering into the vein where it belongs. This is a slight, though real, danger with intravenous therapy.

WHAT YOU CAN DO

For Minor Skin Changes

- You may need to alter your usual routine and change skin-care products. Men may need to start using moisturizer and be gentle when shaving.
- If your skin is dry and sensitive, protect it from harsh, cold, dry weather and too much water.
- Avoid long hot baths because they tend to dry skin even further. Quick showers and sponge baths with super-fatted nondrying soaps are better.
- Apply emollient and moistening creams and lotions daily; apply immediately after washing while your skin is still damp so they help seal in moisture.
- If the air in your home is dry, raise the humidity with a humidifier (make sure it is mold and microbe-free).
- If your scalp becomes itchy and flaky, try using a dandruff shampoo. You might try rubbing oil into your scalp, although as mentioned above, this can make thinning hair look worse.
- If you wear a wig or head scarf or hat, it can increase perspiration, dandruff, and itching and can irritate a sensitive, newly bared scalp. Cleanse frequently with a mild shampoo and keep your head uncovered whenever possible.
- Treat yourself to a professional (or do-it-yourself) facial—they can be marvelously relaxing and restorative inside and out.
- If you have been wearing minimal makeup, you may find that the natural look doesn't work for you anymore. Treat yourself to a makeup consultation to get advice about evening out skin tone and giving your face a lift with color. Department stores will do this for free, or you may want to see a professional makeup consultant pri-

vately. Try to find someone who has experience with cancer patients; your oncology clinic may be able to give you a referral, or ask the American Cancer Society about their free program for people with cancer called Look Good . . . Feel Better.

- Treat local infections with local medication; refer to "Infections" for information about protecting the immune system and avoiding infections.

- Many patients are advised to avoid the sun, although others are permitted to sunbathe in moderation. Use common sense and enjoy the outdoors. Check with your doctor to see if your drugs can cause photosensitivity (increased sensitivity to sunlight); if they do, wear protective clothing, hats, and a sun block while in the sun.

For Extravasation and Other Serious Problems

There are varying degrees of extravasation, which depend on the amount of drug that escapes and the nature of the drug itself. Most but not all drugs cause problems if they leak into the surrounding tissue. Methotrexate, for example, is harmless—in fact, it can be injected into the muscle. But your doctor should always take extra precautions with a drug such as Adriamycin, which is perhaps the most caustic anticancer drug. Dangerous drugs that can cause *necrosis* (tissue death) should not be the first or the last substance to enter the vein; they should be safely sandwiched between either harmless drugs or a saline solution. After the treatment is over and the needle is withdrawn, rather than applying pressure with the arm in the usual lowered bent elbow position, some doctors have their patients raise their arms up over their heads as they apply pressure to the injection site. This collapses the vein nicely and prevents any remains of the drugs from backing up out of the vein and causing problems.

The sooner extravasation is caught, the better. Always tell the doctor or nurse about any pain or burning sensation during the injection so they can check whether the reaction is normal or if something is amiss. Try to keep movement to a minimum during treatment and complain like hell if you are being treated by a clumsy technician.

Even though my oncologist was very careful, I had a minor brush with extravasation myself. I usually avoided looking at the injection site during a treatment, but I couldn't help but take a peek the time I felt more pain than usual. I saw a mound of purple swelling in the crook of my arm, but I wasn't really worried—yet. My oncologist told me the mound was blood mixed with vincristine. I made some jokes about whether this was how people got those special effects in the movies; he patched me up and continued the injection in another vein. The pain became so bad, I hardly slept that night, and when I called him, he prescribed a very strong cortisone cream. In a few hours, it felt much better and the swelling went way down. I put ice on it all week, and when the time for my next shot rolled around two weeks later, it was almost completely healed.

Another danger with intravenous chemotherapy is "blown" veins. Preferred veins, those used again and again during blood tests and chemotherapy, get a real workout. Eventually, they may say "enough" by shutting down in protest, becoming hard, and no longer allowing the blood to flow through. This is not particularly dangerous since other blood vessels will learn to take over, but it may make treatment gradually more and more difficult as more and more "good veins" get used up. These problems are becoming rarer with the increased use of indwelling catheters and ports, which protect the veins from chemotherapy drugs.

Occasionally, phlebitis may occur. This is a painful inflammation of the vein that is somewhat common in patients taking drugs they are sensitive to. Treatment for phlebitis includes the application of heat and oral painkillers. This condition takes several weeks to subside.

Sleep Disturbances

Nighttime is often a difficult time for a chemo patient, and for many reasons. Some drugs may directly cause nervousness or agitation. The corticosteroids, such as prednisone, are notorious for their stimulating effects, which may be advantageous during the day but disastrous at night. Many people have trouble falling asleep while taking these drugs, but they are unaware that there may be pharmacological reasons and blame their sleeplessness on everything else. Another drug, procarbazine, can cause insomnia and nightmares.

Pain and discomfort seem to grow and fears and problems loom larger in the still of the night, when daytime activities are not around to distract you. Surgical pain, emotional stress, and sleeplessness can feed on one another in a vicious cycle. It may be even more difficult to sleep if you are being treated in the hospital and sleeping in a strange bed, with nurses and staff buzzing around, your roommate groaning or snoring, and machines whirring or clanking.

WHAT YOU CAN DO

The most common medications to help you sleep can also cause drowsiness, fatigue, and gastrointestinal symptoms as well as interact with anticancer medications—the last thing a chemo patient needs on top of chemo side effects. A study from Queen's University in Canada, which involved cancer patients suffering from insomnia lasting more than six months, found that nondrug methods such as these improved their sleep quality.

- Discuss any sleeping problems with your nurse or doctor so he or she can begin to help you do something about them. If you are taking a corticosteroid like prednisone, your oncologist might suggest that you take the drug early in the day in order to give the stimulating effects time to wear off before bedtime.
- Take measures to relieve any emotional anxieties that are coming between you and a good night's sleep. See Chapters 7, 11, and 12 for information about relaxation techniques and coping with emotional effects of cancer and chemotherapy.
- Establishing a ritual usually helps lull people to sleep. Reading, listening to soft music, watching TV, taking a hot bath or shower, having a soothing massage, doing some deep breathing or stretching or relaxation exercises, and even drinking the proverbial glass of warm milk are several conservative, nondrug methods you can use to help you get to sleep.
- Drinking fewer caffeinated beverages such as colas, coffee, and tea also may help.

- There are many natural remedies for anxiety and sleep problems, including the herb valerian and homeopathic remedies such as Calmes Forte that you may find helpful.

You may have not needed these techniques in the past, but that's no reason not to explore them now and to use them for as long as you need them. Nor should you hesitate to ask for or use some kind of sleeping pill to get you through a particularly tough time. Sometimes a single good night's sleep can make all the difference in your outlook and general well-being. Sleep is especially important for the chemo patient because it enables you to better face the next day's challenges.

Sore Mouth

See MOUTH, GUM, AND THROAT PROBLEMS.

Sore Throat

See MOUTH, GUM, AND THROAT PROBLEMS, and INFECTIONS.

Taste Changes (Taste Blindness)

Many chemotherapy patients experience a loss of taste or a change in the way foods taste, which occurs because the lining of the tongue and the chemical receptors that detect taste are altered. Patients often find that food tastes "different" or "bad." High-protein foods such as meat—beef and pork in particular—usually lose their appeal; it is thought that this low tolerance for meat stems from a lower threshold for bitterness because chemical imbalances in the body react to amino acids in the food. Patients have said, "I found myself gagging on certain foods, like steak," or "I didn't like meat at all—I'd cook it for my family, but I wouldn't eat it myself."

Sweets can also seem less seductive than usual. Some researchers have found that patients have an elevated threshold for sweets up to a certain point. Once that point is reached, though, additional sweetness becomes intolerable. Many patients find in general that "nothing tastes right," and their appetites suffer. One patient remembers:

> *I didn't like anything sweet. My appetite wasn't normal; I usually just had one serving of what we were having, no seconds. I cooked still, that didn't bother me. Just the sweet stuff—cake, candy. I still baked for my husband, and it didn't bother me to see him have it; I just didn't want any for myself.*

WHAT YOU CAN DO

There are few ways of getting around these chemo-induced alterations in taste. You may find that this condition is aggravated by a bad, metallic taste that certain drugs leave in your mouth. But here are some suggestions that may help:

- Sometimes hypnosis and visualization help. (See Chapter 11.)
- Incorporate other, nonbitter high-protein foods if you find you have an aversion toward meat. Fish and poultry are usually still palatable, for instance, and dried beans, cheese and other milk products, eggs, and the complementary proteins found in beans, whole grains, and nuts can be made into many appetizing dishes.
- Protein supplements may be helpful. Those derived from soybean supply complete protein, and there is no danger of lactose intolerance. Protein supplements are available in liquid and powder form and usually supply 28 grams of protein per two tablespoons—the same amount you get from a three-ounce steak.
- Add extra seasonings and spices to foods if you can tolerate them.
- Acidic foods such as oranges and grapefruits tend to stimulate the taste buds, so include some with your meals.
- As when dealing with loss of appetite, attractively served, well-prepared food served in a comfortable setting can be helpful in restoring (or ignoring) the way food tastes.

- A zinc deficiency can alter your ability to taste food; ask your physician about taking a zinc supplement.

Weakness

See FATIGUE AND WEAKNESS.

Weight Gain/Water Retention/Bloating

The popular picture of the chemotherapy patient is someone who is sick, vomiting, not eating, and losing weight to the point of emaciation. Many patients do lose weight, but many others, particularly women on adjuvant chemotherapy for breast cancer, instead find themselves tipping scales in the opposite direction. This can be aggravated by or partially caused by an increase in appetite, water retention, and abdominal bloating. Even though I lost weight on chemo, I developed a little potbelly during the time I was on prednisone; this bloating disappeared when I stopped taking the drug. Many women, however, find it a real problem to lose weight they gained while on chemo that is not due to water retention. Donna Park says this weight gain can be devastating:

> *The women are often gaining tremendous amounts of weight, so they have an altered body image not only because of the mastectomy but because of the weight they gain. They put on fifteen, twenty, thirty pounds—it depends on how careful the patient is. We're not sure if it's only because of the prednisone. One of the theories we have is that patients are eating constantly to relieve their continuous nausea. Another theory is that they're feeling, "Well, I don't know what next year will bring, so I'm going to eat to make myself feel better." Or it might be because they are engaged in less activity, so they burn fewer calories.*

A bloated feeling and appearance can have many causes other than glucocorticoids such as prednisone. Some anticancer drugs can set off processes that render the stomach and intestines less capable of digesting food. Or the digestive process may slow down because of nervousness, tension, lack of exercise, or constipation. Eating gas-producing foods or swallowing air as you eat can contribute. As a result, the lower abdomen bloats, and you look and feel too full too quickly.

Marylin Dodd, in *Managing the Side Effects of Chemotherapy and Radiation,* says that chemo drugs can change the way your body metabolizes fats contained in food, resulting in an increase in appetite and in fat deposits in the body. A non-chemo-related book, *Fight Fat After Forty* by Pamela Peeke, documents the propensity for stress itself to increase body fat, particularly around your abdomen—and cancer patients have plenty of stress. In any event, something seems to be throwing a monkey wrench into the way food is being metabolized, which leads to weight gain that is mostly fat rather than muscle.

One contributor to overweight is the binges that go on between treatments when the patient feels well. For example, "I'd lose weight for the five days I was on chemo, but the moment I stopped, I ate like a pig. I hate pizza normally, but I'd bring home a big pizza and just gorge myself. Ice cream, anything. Just to get rid of the memory of the nausea."

As Ms. Park mentioned, constant nausea may drive you to a constant nibbling in an effort to mask the unpleasantness; a bad taste in your mouth, a common side effect of many drugs, can do the same.

Whatever the reasons, weight gain is a particularly common and frustrating side effect for women on chemo for breast cancer. The weight just keeps coming, especially when they are on chemo for a long time. They hate the weight gain, partly because of the change in appearance, self-image, and self-esteem, but some also worry about the possible connection between obesity and the progression or development of breast cancer. To be sure, these are legitimate concerns, but if you are in this situation, you may be able to take heart from the somewhat positive observations of several cancer patients and physicians. They have noticed that some patients seem to tolerate chemo better if they eat to the degree that they become somewhat overweight. I have personally known two women who deliberately ate more and gained weight during chemo, and they are informally called "our miracles"—both were on chemotherapy for over three years with minimal side effects and far outlived their prognoses. No one really knows why this should be so. Perhaps they were getting more protective micronutrients (such as vitamins and minerals) along with the calories, or perhaps fat itself has some as yet unknown protective effect. Certain fats, called essential fatty acids, do appear to have a protective effect. What we do know is that there may be some undiscovered process at work and that this information may help some patients find weight gain a bit easier to take.

It's always preferable to prevent a weight gain than to have to lose it afterward. Chemo may permanently alter your metabolism, as this patient discovered:

> *One thing I was very down about was the way I ate—I put on thirty-five pounds while I was on chemo. I changed my eating habits and had a huge breakfast, lunch, and dinner. This was not me—but when I ate, I felt stronger. Now I'm fighting to take it off—even though I went back to my old eating habits, I've only managed to lose about twelve pounds.*

WHAT YOU CAN DO

Prednisone and dexamethasone are corticosteroids given as part of several chemotherapy plans. Their side effects include an increase in appetite and salt and water retention. Nutritionists usually recommend a diet low in salt and refined carbohydrates and high in protein and potassium to help keep weight gain and water retention to a minimum. Here are some other tips to help keep the scale's numbers down.

Food and Cooking

- Do not add salt to foods during cooking, and leave the saltshaker off the table when you eat.
- Watch out for hidden salt in prepared and convenience foods. Avoid anchovies, bouillon, soups, canned fish, bacon, cold cuts, corned beef, frankfurters, sausages, potato chips, corn chips, pretzels, salted

nuts, soy sauce, catsup, and hard cheeses. Look for salt-reduced versions of these products.

- Look for cookbooks with salt-reduced recipes and tips that help you lower your salt intake without sacrificing too much flavor. Use herbs, spices, and lemon juice to perk up recipes.
- If the problem persists or is severe, your doctor may prescribe a diuretic (a pill that rids the body of excess water). Some foods are natural diuretics: citrus juices, parsley, some herbs, and water itself. Exercise (swimming in particular) seems to act as a diuretic, too. If you take a diuretic, eat foods high in potassium—bananas, apricots, cantaloupe, orange juice, and potatoes—which diuretics deplete from the body or take a potassium supplement.
- Eat small, frequent meals and avoid hard-to-digest fatty or high-protein foods. Eat slowly and eliminate foods such as onions and cabbage that cause gas. Hydrochloric acid tablets or other digestive aids taken with meals may help reduce the bloated feeling and appearance.
- Since lactose intolerance can cause bloating, try avoiding dairy products to see if that makes a difference. (See MILK INTOLERANCE.)

Behavioral Changes

- To reduce edema in the ankles and legs, avoid standing in one place for long periods of time and elevate your feet as much as possible. You may find special support hose or pressure stockings helpful.
- If you find yourself nibbling all day, perhaps low-calorie food items such as raw vegetables, fresh fruit, hard candy, fruit juices, ginger ale, and no-calorie herbal teas will serve this urge as well as more fattening foods do.
- Adjust your chemo regimen. According to Dr. Grace, some of his patients find that if they take their oral chemotherapy spaced out over the day instead of all at once, the slight nausea they get helps keep their appetite down. Some patients also take Dexatrim while on chemo—this not only curbs the appetite but counteracts some of the fatigue caused by the therapy. He suggests that if patients take a corticosteroid such as prednisone, they take it on alternate days instead

of every day. "They don't get anywhere near the amount of bloating they usually get, even though they take the same total amount."

- If you are eating to "make yourself feel better" because of anxiety about your prognosis or condition, talk with your oncologist or use the psychological/relaxation therapies described in Chapter 11.

- Exercise more. Exercise is highly beneficial to chemotherapy patients (see Chapter 9), but you may not be getting as much as usual. Activity helps burn off calories, curb your appetite, improve your mood, and reduce nausea that you may be trying to alleviate with a steady stream of food. Exercise also takes up the time that you might otherwise fill by eating, as does any distraction. Only four things made me forget about the nausea: food, sleep, exercise, and the movies.

CHAPTER SEVEN

The Emotional Impact
of Chemotherapy

Because you are a cancer chemotherapy patient, your emotional balance receives a terrific one-two punch: one, the diagnosis of a disease that is highly symbolic and threatens your very life; two, undergoing a long-lasting toxic treatment that threatens the quality of your life but whose effectiveness is uncertain. In addition to your own personal reactions to your new situation, you need to cope with the reactions of others to your disease and its treatment. You will need to adjust to new environments and new people; you must find ways of dealing with big and little stresses and responsibilities. Don't be surprised if the emotional stress of cancer chemotherapy is far more devastating than the stress of the physical side effects.

Just as no two patients will have the same physical response to chemotherapy, so too will people's emotional reactions and resulting behavior be as individual as fingerprints. Unlike the physical side effects, which are concrete, measurable, and observable by others, the emotional consequences of cancer and chemotherapy are not tangible, easily measurable, seen, or felt by anyone else. This does not mean, however, that they are not real or that they have to be endured. As Karen Ritchie, chief of psychiatry at MD Anderson Cancer Center, says, "To call the nonphysical problems a lower priority is a mistake. They should be treated, just as nausea is treated."

The emotional reactions of cancer patients vary:

I can't really describe how I felt. I think I just didn't want to believe it. I just felt so deserted that day.

I had adjusted pretty well to the mastectomy—I was glad I still had my eyes, my arms, my legs—you know, I didn't really miss having a breast, and the rehabilitation wouldn't be too involved. But the chemo really blew my mind. I had a fatalistic attitude at first.

I was an ultramarathon runner and found myself barely able to do a ten-minute mile. When my doctor told me the final diagnosis, I had an out-of-body experience. I felt like I was viewing the situation as if it were someone else being told. After about ten minutes, I came back to earth and started talking to people about my options. Soon after that I started poring through the medical literature. I went straight to the acceptance stage; I became galvanized into action.

A lot of people look at you and say, "God, I'm so sorry." And deep down inside they're thinking, "Thank God it isn't me." I would, too—I'll be honest about it. If there were some way I could have given it to someone else, I would have.

Making Sense of It All

Dr. Judith Bukberg, a psychiatrist who specializes in treating cancer patients, says:

I think there's too much stoicism in the world. People seem to have the idea that because this is real—because something real and bad is happening to them—that all kinds of emotional reactions are to be tolerated. That's ridiculous. Sure, you have a reason to be depressed, but that doesn't mean you can't do something about it.

People also don't want to upset other people—either their families, friends, or doctors—and so they put on a great face to the world, and meanwhile God knows what's going on inside of them.

People want to protect each other, but it isn't always helpful in the long run—either to themselves or their relationships.

That cancer patients do suffer a lot of stress and emotional turmoil was shown in a study done by the Psychosocial Collaborative Oncology Group. The investigators found that 47 percent of the patients who were interviewed and tested showed serious emotional turmoil, mostly depression or anxiety, in trying to adjust to their illness.

The emotional effects of cancer and its treatment—how it influences your behavior, work, social interaction, and overall quality of life—are called *psychosocial effects.* The study of the psychosocial impact of cancer and chemotherapy is still young. Its importance has only recently been recognized. Nevertheless, some basic patterns have emerged as to what emotions patients are likely to feel, when they are most likely to feel them, and what can be done to help patients cope with their emotions. By becoming familiar with the way others have seen things, you may develop a framework that makes some sense out of your own experience. By becoming acquainted with various probabilities and possibilities, you can begin to get a handle on your emotions and thus be in a better position to cope. You will be aware of the availability of others who can help.

Emotional Stages of Cancer

One concept of the impact of cancer—and chemotherapy—involves thinking in terms of the emotional stages that many people go through when faced with death or any stressful, unpleasant situation. You will probably recognize this pattern in yourself or in your family:

- *Denial.* "No not me! It's all a mistake. I don't believe it; this can't be happening. I don't want to think about it."
- *Anger.* "Why me? What did I do to deserve this? Why not somebody else?"
- *Bargaining or guilt.* "I promise I'll do anything to be cured—I'll

change my life, my personality, I'll be 'good.'" "I'll stop cheating on my income tax." "I'll be more considerate of other people's feelings."

- *Depression.* "I feel so low and discouraged. Nothing matters, nothing will help, what's the use?"
- *Acceptance.* "Okay, this is the way it is. Now let's get the show on the road and do something about it."

The five-stage cycle begins around the time of diagnosis; it continues into the therapy and persists long afterward. With each subsequent stressful event such as surgery, the beginning of chemotherapy, the failure of chemotherapy, the cycle repeats. Some people may need to skip stages or remain in one stage longer than others. Denial, for instance (which can masquerade as healthy optimism and vice versa), was once thought best gotten over quickly. Now mental health experts think it may be an appropriate, helpful stage that should not be rushed. Richard S. Lazarus writes in Paul Ahmed's book, *Living and Dying with Cancer* that denial or self-deception is "often a valuable initial form of coping, occurring at a time when the person is confused and weakened and therefore unable to act constructively and realistically." Denial is a way to buy time, to recover from the shock so we can digest the news and gradually come to deal with the threat. When our reasoning powers return, we will be able to act rationally. Some people just need more time.

In the hospital after my surgery, people were amazed by my good spirits. An army of friends practically never went home, and the jokes were flying fast and furiously. "The *Pearl Mesta* of the cancer ward" is what they called me, but I realize now it was good old denial doing its job and helping me survive.

Living with surgical scars, pain, and loss of functioning, going for chemotherapy treatments and suffering the side effects—all can be more distressing because they remind us of our situations and so make denial harder. Every time I went to the oncologist for treatment, I was reminded that I had cancer. It wasn't only the side effects I knew the drugs would bring that made me not want to go. It was that gut-wrenching kick to my psyche: I'm going here because I have cancer and may die.

Confronting the Basic Emotional Issues

Another approach to making sense out of emotional turmoil centers on feelings of alienation, mutilation, mortality, and vulnerability. Most cancer patients at some point are confronted by these basic issues, from which spring a host of emotional reactions.

ALIENATION

You may be afraid of being abandoned, of being unacceptable, and of becoming isolated. You may feel alone in the world, unconnected, apart, and unable to relate to other human beings. These feelings may originate within yourself or be based on real situations and the very real reactions of others. Although cancer has come out of the closet, and even celebrities and politicians are talking about it to the media, cancer is still a disease with many negative connotations. Many of these feelings are unfounded or exaggerated, but this does not diminish their impact. You may feel sorry for yourself and shut out the rest of the world. You may think of your diagnosis as a punishment for past wrongdoings or negative personality traits, or as an automatic death sentence. You may start to withdraw and break off contact with loved ones as a preparation for what you may see as an imminent final separation. (You may indeed be *physically* alone and apart because of time spent in hospitals, or undergoing treatment, or being away from work or being sick and unable to socialize.) People may withdraw emotionally from you for various reasons, including fear that you are going to die. Or they may feel guilty, angry, or resentful.

Sometimes feelings emerge because you and the people around you fall prey to the nonsensical myths and superstitions that surround cancer. For example, some people still believe that cancer is something of which to be ashamed, that it is a form of punishment for being "a bad person," or that it is contagious. For example:

> *We call it "the big C." Amazing how you put cute little nicknames on everything. Cancer is a very difficult word to say. And when you tell people you have it, they can't look you in the face.*

While I was on chemo, I would not permit anyone to kiss me or to come too close to me. I just felt—and they also helped me feel—like a leper. I would never permit anyone to eat from my food, even my husband. Except when we went out to a restaurant once a week with other people, he would offer me food, and I would take it from his fork. I would subject him to something that I thought was contagious because I wanted them to see that he was not afraid.

FEELING MUTILATED

Many aspects of cancer and its treatments are disfiguring and invasive; you may feel mutilated as a result of surgery, for example, and mourn the loss of a part of your body, your attractiveness, and your ability to function. You may not feel "whole" and may experience changes in body image. Chemotherapy changes the way you feel, but it also can change the way you look. You may lose or gain a large amount of weight, lose your hair, or feel you just don't look like yourself. These changes can leave you with a sinking feeling, but can be even more devastating when they are visible to others. If you are being treated for cancer of a reproductive organ, you might be feeling that you are less than a woman or not quite a man. I, for example, would avoid looking in the mirror, though at the same time, I was strangely attracted to do it—fascinated—like rubbernecking at an accident. I couldn't believe the scar, the bald head, the lack of eyelashes and eyebrows, the circles under the eyes, the pallor. I'd feel where my breast had been—gone. Touch where my hair had been—gone. Who was this person? I felt like such a phony. I had to wear a wig and a prosthesis just to feel "normal," to be accepted.

FEELING ONE'S MORTALITY

When you are diagnosed with cancer, you become more aware of the inevitability of death—your own, whether from cancer or another cause. Death is no longer the abstract philosophical concept it is for most other people—it is a reality. Mortality is an unavoidable issue regardless of the prognosis and goal of the therapy—be it cure, remission, or palliation. The younger you are when cancer strikes, the more unfair this loss of innocence and eternal life seems to be. Most days, I'd chug along just fine, even though it was in the back of my mind. But every once in a while it would get to me: *This disease could kill me.* I'd flip out and scream and cry from fear and remorse. I'd imagine my own death and rage against the unfairness of it all—I wonder what the neighbors thought. I was only thirty-one years old. I didn't want to die!

FEELINGS OF VULNERABILITY

Many cancer patients become distressed by the loss of control over their lives and their health. They hate feeling dependent, helpless—at the mercy of their disease and other people. They feel a loss of self-esteem and self-confidence, which is worsened by the fatigue, debility, weakness, and consequent inability to perform their usual functions. Feelings of worthlessness may surface. The uncertainty of treatment, the duration of the disease, and the steady stream of side effects create an atmosphere of unending sickness. For some people, the fact that the cancer itself is defined as a disease of uncontrolled growth reinforces feelings of the loss of control. For example, these two cancer patients said,

Every time another side effect appeared, it was another blow. I kept feeling worse and worse; I worried what could go wrong next and where it would all end.

I'm not afraid of pain or of death. I'm afraid of being disabled . . . of being stuck in bed, not even able to wash myself.

Every patient will not necessarily go through the full spectrum of possible emotions; nor will he or she feel them all at once. At various times some feelings will recede and others will come into the foreground. Studies of cancer patients have found that people (except for those with lung cancer) are usually most vulnerable psychologically three to four months after diagnosis.

As a result of her experience in social work, Grace Christ finds it useful to think in terms of a series of potential crisis points. Chemotherapy patients and their families are under the most stress during these times and must perform adaptive tasks at each of them if and when they occur: (1) the time of diagnosis, (2) the beginning of treatment, (3) negative physical reactions to treatment (side effects), (4) failure of conventional treatment, (5) the end of a treatment protocol, (6) the recurrence or metastasis of the disease, (7) the beginning of investigational treatment, (8) the end of active treatment, and (9) terminal illness.

How You Cope

Chances are that if you cope well generally, you will manage to cope with chemo, too. People who cope best tend to be flexible and have the ability to shift their perspectives and see situations in new ways that allow problems to be solved. Other useful characteristics include independence but a willingness to lean on others when necessary, cooperativeness without complete passivity, and a positive attitude. People who cope poorly are often already in emotional turmoil from personal problems and disrupted family background, have a pessimistic attitude, expect no help from others, have poor self-esteem, and rely on tension-reducing devices rather than on activity to change the source of tension.

Dr. Judith Bukberg points out that what is especially stressful for one person may be less so for another and that how—and how well—you cope with cancer and chemotherapy depends on three basic factors: how much stress you are actually under, how you perceive the stress, and your own unique coping style, abilities, and support system. Age, sex, personality, intelligence, values and beliefs, the type and extent of the cancer and treatment, what they mean to you, and the quality of your relationships with others will enter into the coping process.

HOW MUCH STRESS ARE YOU UNDER?

Some therapies are indeed more stressful than others. You may be experiencing a great deal of toxic effects and thus more emotional stress. Your life may be quite disrupted by physical symptoms or the location and timing of the treatment. Some cancers are more malignant than others, and some prognoses are worse. You may have other stresses outside of the treatment or caused by the treatment (such as financial problems or family troubles) that are already straining your ability to cope.

HOW DO YOU PERCEIVE STRESS?

You can perceive a situation such as chemotherapy treatment to be a threat, a source of pain, a challenge, or an attempt to help. Some people are much more able to contain anxiety, or they just don't get anxious easily. Others become fearful and nervous very readily. Also, your past medical history can influence the way you feel about medical treatment; if you've already had a bad experience with a certain procedure, you will be more anxious about it than will someone who hasn't. "People who come from loving, trusting families," says Dr. Bukberg, "have more trust in health professionals and are more able to put their lives in their hands."

HOW DO YOU HANDLE STRESS?

Dr. Bukberg defines coping as "something that an individual does—either as an automatic response or as a thought-out, planned response to a stress—that is designed to decrease the amount of emotional upheaval and/or in some way to affect the environment to reduce the stress." Each person has certain coping mechanisms—a certain way to deal with things—as a part of his or her personality. People have tendencies to respond one way or another, based on what else has happened to them in the past and what has worked under previous conditions. Broadly speaking, people cope actively or passively. As Dr. Bukberg observes, referring to a concept introduced by Dr. Lipowski, some people tend to avoid all kinds of stress—they deny or minimize a problem. They may disregard the facts, the true meaning of a piece of information, or their emotional states. At the other end of the spectrum, some people become "hypervigilant." They are anxiety-prone, intellectualizing, and somewhat obsessive—they loathe ambiguity and uncertainty, and they want to know as much as they can and become totally involved in their treatments.

Some people rely on their religious convictions. Others become stoical or rationalize their cancer by saying there are people who are worse off. Some merely defer thinking about it until they are strong enough to cope. Some, accepting every blow, attempt to treat their problems lightly and try to shrug everything off with jokes. Others are problem solvers. There are many, many ways of coping, and usually a person will need to combine several of these ways to get the best effect.

All these mechanisms do help us relieve stress. But they may not work as well as they have in different circumstances in the past. They may work temporarily or partially but not enough to reduce our fears, anxieties, or depression to a bearable level. If your usual ways of coping are not working now or are not working as well as you'd like them to, perhaps this is the time to expand your coping repertoire.

For any given stressful situation, there are usually several options, some or all of which you may not be aware of. Here, for example, is a stressful situation experienced by many chemo patients: You are not happy with your oncologist—he is abrupt and cool, he doesn't treat you like a human being or ever tell you anything. This is making you anxious, and you are tired of feeling like a pincushion with a checkbook instead of a patient. Your usual passive, accepting, or minimizing attitude is no longer working. What do you do? Dr. Bukberg says:

> *There are three options. You can do something behaviorally such as talking to your doctor about it or changing to another doctor. Or you could do something cognitive, which would be to try to understand, for example, that he may be upset at having to cause discomfort to people or at having so many people to see that he can't get more involved—in some way redefine the situation so it is more manageable to you. Or you could do something that is directly tension-reducing such as relaxation techniques or hypnosis, where you are primarily reducing the tension that is aroused by the situation.*

No coping mechanism is intrinsically "good" or "bad," "right" or "wrong." A mechanism may, however, not be *useful* in a particular situation. When your usual style of coping is not working well enough—when it does not solve a problem or at least bring stress down to a tolerable level—it is time for a change. Change doesn't mean admitting that you were "wrong." Your favorite sneakers may serve you well in weather when you can wear them; they may be comfortable and familiar. But come a snowstorm—they do not work well. Learning how to cope better may take practice. It may take work. It may be painful and slow in spite of your immediate need for it: Trading in your old ways of thinking and acting for new patterns is not easy. But coping can be learned just like any other skill.

In addition, the changes that chemotherapy puts you through may not seem pleasant at the time, but many people find it is ultimately a positive experience and feel it changes them for the better. Patients say it can be a tremendous personal growth experience. Dealing with their troubles in a time of crisis makes them more mature, more tolerant, more understanding of others, and they feel more—not less—in command of their lives. Their relationships with others can improve, too, as loved ones grow along with and become closer to the patient.

Expand Your Coping Repertoire

There are five basic, interrelated areas for you to explore if you want to expand your coping repertoire—relaxation, attitude, communication, education, and support services. Chapters 11 and 12 will also give you some ideas for supporting your mind, body, and spirit through the tough times.

RELAX WITH MIND-BODY TECHNIQUES

Try one or more of the techniques described in Chapter 11. These may not solve your problem, but they will provide you with a mini-vacation from the reality of your stressful life. Like a good night's rest, they provide you with the psychic strength and foundation to cope with whatever the day brings. Many of these techniques have emerged from the new field called psychoneuroimmunology (PNI), which is beginning to show us just how large a role patients can play in their recovery. Mind-body techniques unquestionably have improved many people's quality of life and perhaps even affected the outcome of their illness.

WORK ON YOUR ATTITUDE

We hear it all the time: Accentuate the positive, eliminate the negative. The power of positive thinking. Look at the bright side. How, you might ask, can I remain cheerful and optimistic when I've got cancer and am going through a debilitating therapy? Obviously, this is an unenviable situation for which no one would wish. But there *are* two sides to everything. Is the glass half empty or half full? Of course it is both, but which reality you choose to emphasize makes a big difference in how well you tolerate chemo.

Many patients and many health-care workers have found that a positive attitude—toward chemotherapy, their chemotherapists, and life in general—helps people cope better. Those who are highly motivated and do not let chemo get them down, who strive to assume as normal a life as possible, who remain actively involved and live their lives to the fullest, who work and play and cultivate hope instead of passivity, inactivity, and despair—these are the people who do best during their time on chemotherapy. This patient's good attitude helped her cope well:

> *I told my mom, "It's cancer," and we both started crying. We cried*
> *for about five minutes and then I said, "Okay, that's enough." I then*
> *went on an errand. That's how you have to handle it. You cannot let*
> *it monopolize your life. I've seen too many who died because they*
> *gave up. And you can't give up.*

Rena Blumberg wrote of her experiences during an intensive course of chemotherapy for metastasized breast cancer during which she remained energetic and able to "celebrate" each day. She calls her book *Headstrong*, a word meaning "to have your own way," but she means it in a very positive sense. She writes:

For me, "having my own way" meant I was going to survive. To live—and live fully. This took willfulness, to be sure. And at certain moments, particularly during chemo, yes, it took downright obstinacy. But more than any other attitude, I feel this "headstrong" approach to coping with cancer was the quality that allowed me to survive and to get on with the business of living and living joyously.

However, blind, unquestioning faith or a complete Pollyanna stance may be harmful. You can't always ignore the negative—doing so is unhealthy if it prevents you from taking any corrective action. But by allowing the positive to take precedence you become free and have more energy to take care of the negative.

It certainly helps if you are sure that you want the treatment and remember that the purpose of chemotherapy is a longer, better life. As Dr. Michael Van Scoy-Mosher, an oncologist at Cedars-Sinai Medical Center in Los Angeles, says, "Patients need to realize that chemotherapy is not the enemy—the cancer is."

The Wellness Community, which provides psychosocial support to people with cancer, believes that attitude is a crucial component of a comprehensive treatment plan. They have coined the term "Patient-Active" to describe a person who is part of the team fighting for his or her recovery.

In his book *From Victim to Victor,* Harold Benjamin, the founder of the Wellness Community, suggests that you consider eleven ways to become Patient-Active. Briefly, these include making plans for the future, not allowing people to abandon you, not becoming a recluse, pursuing happiness, being with other cancer patients, becoming a partner with your physician, keeping up hope, maintaining intimacy and affection, and maintaining as much control over your life as possible.

COMMUNICATE

The value of telling others about your hopes, fears, needs, and wants is a recurrent theme in discussions with patients and health-care workers and in the literature on coping with cancer. Just talking about your feelings and admitting you have them can be therapeutic even if you don't find the exact words to describe them. An open, communicative relationship with your doctor or nurse can be a real advantage and play a central part in how well you do with chemo. But a lack of communication with friends and family is one of the most common and troublesome scenarios of cancer patients. This is often the fault of both the patients and their families and friends to one degree or another and is a shame because they all can be the most valuable source of emotional support for each other. It is ironic, then, that poor communication often results from each party's concern and desire to protect the feelings of the other. Although people who are close to each other may be more sensitive to unspoken feelings, they are not clairvoyant. People cannot begin to grasp what you are going through unless you tell them. And you cannot expect people to understand and act on your wishes if you do not give them any clues.

Of course, it is difficult for some people to talk with each other under normal circumstances, and the stresses of cancer can accentuate the problem. Lari Wenzel observes:

> *There are certain patients who have difficulty addressing their emotions or fears. They may have lived their entire lives in this fashion. Having the diagnosis of cancer will not necessarily lead them toward self-disclosure. For example, men tend to verbally acknowledge their feelings less than women do, probably due to the socialization process. Generally, people who are well educated about their disease tend to be more acutely aware of their feelings and can discuss them at length.*

Dr. Bukberg says she has had people come to her for therapy because they believed their families couldn't tolerate hearing about their situations. "They really needed to sit down with somebody and talk," she says, "before they could get it together and do the talking that needed to be done with their families."

The severe stress of cancer and chemotherapy can aggravate or accentuate one's style of coping, exacerbate present problems, or bring up old ones. In couples, observes a social worker who has treated many cancer patients, this can create a problem:

Typically, a man may want to cope through action, by doing an activity. The female may want to cope by talking. If that becomes exaggerated—the male wants to distance himself more, the female wants to talk, they may find they have a problem. Sometimes this takes the form of what I call dissynchronization. An example is the forty-year-old man with acute leukemia. He and his wife would sometimes have trouble communicating and used fighting as a way of reengaging with each other. That was their style. When he went back into remission, they were both very relieved, but the rhythm and pacing of their relationship had been thrown off. They found that they were both very distant from each other, very uncomfortable, and unhappy. She was afraid to face the possibility of his death, of fighting with him and being angry with him, and of being open and valid with him because she was so afraid of what she might do to him. But also she was fearful of getting reengaged with him and going through the same pain again. But she was able to look at what she was doing and work out another mode of relating. It made marvelous changes in their relationship.

EDUCATE YOURSELF

Often mental states such as fear, anxiety, anger, confusion, and repression are due to a lack of information. Fear of the unknown and an inaccurate picture of reality are two circumstances you should guard against. The reality of your situation is tough enough to deal with—why add to it unnecessarily? A well-informed patient usually does better in many ways than an uninformed patient. You can feel you are in control and make wise decisions only if you have the facts and can compare the options. The better you understand your therapy—what its goals are, what the side effects may be, and what can be done about them—the better you will tolerate it and the less ominous it will seem. It may help to have a clear picture of your prognosis and to realize that a diagnosis of cancer is not an automatic death sentence: Heart attack victims generally have a much worse prognosis than people with cancer do.

Posing questions to your doctor or nurse is the best way to start getting whatever information you need and want. Write down your questions as you think of them so you don't forget them; take notes or bring a cassette tape recorder. Many patients find that bringing along a clear-thinking friend or relative is a great help—when you're under the kind of stress cancer imposes, it's usually difficult to retain everything you hear.

Dr. William Grace, chief of oncology at New York's St. Vincent's Hospital, notes that "things go in one ear and out the other. I insist that my patients have notepads. They write everything that I tell them. And then they write down their questions to me, while leaving enough space between them to write the answers. This is a stressful environment, and otherwise, they forget."

Remember: Physicians may sometimes seem to be magicians, but they are never mind readers. They are trained to tell you only the basics and to depend on you to cue them as to how much further detail to supply. Patients vary greatly in their need to know and in their ability to absorb information. So if you want more than you have gotten, you must come out and ask. Don't be shy or feel guilty for taking up your doctor's time. On the other hand, if you want less information—if you can do without the technical details—let the doctor know that, too. Too much information, especially when given in a small time span, can be overwhelming and thus just as harmful psychologically as too little information.

Sometimes an outside person such as a social worker can help. Patients sometimes have inner conflicts about the amount of information they want and what it means to them, as this case illustrates:

A classic problem is "The doctor isn't telling me anything." Well, that may be, but it could also be that the doctor is telling the patients more than they can process. Or maybe they haven't asked the questions.

I once saw a patient, a young man with advanced cancer who was very sick. He complained that the doctor wasn't telling him how the chemo was working, and he didn't know whether he should keep fighting. I said, "Have you asked him?" He said, "Well, no." I gave him some ideas about questions to ask the doctor, such as "What would happen if I stopped? What would happen if I stay on the drugs? Would you still take care of me?" He asked me to write them down. He ended up not asking the doctor. In fact, he already knew the answers but was struggling with the conflict inside himself.

If you want to learn more about your cancer and its treatment, you can go beyond your health-care providers and turn to booklets, medical journals, and pamphlets. If you are unable to go to bookstores and libraries, you can turn to the Internet or ask a friend or relative to do the legwork. This is one concrete way people can help you, and they are usually more than happy to do so, as was the case with this patient:

My doctor was very vague about everything—especially my prognosis and the other treatments available. And I wanted to know before he began pumping that stuff into me. My friends were very supportive and photocopied articles from medical journals for me to read while I was still in the hospital. It made me feel a lot better knowing what the whole story was.

You may have trouble deciphering some of the medical terms and concepts in the technical or scholarly publications, so perhaps your physician, oncologist, or other doctor will help explain whatever you don't understand. Other sources for information are cancer agencies and societies, and large cancer centers listed in the Resources section (Appendix B).

SUPPORT SERVICES: ASKING FOR HELP

Many chemotherapy patients and their families are very good at coping and can bounce back easily—or they become experts quickly. However, many other patients and their families can use some outside help. This does not mean that they are weak or helpless. It simply means that outside help can make them cope better during a time of extraordinary stress. Diane Blum, director of Cancer Care, Inc., says, "Ups and downs are to be expected. Cancer is a crisis, no matter how good the prognosis, no matter how mild the treatment. You can't get through it without some kind of strong emotional response."

It is logical to turn to friends, family members, and perhaps coworkers for emotional support, and we may be more comfortable expressing our innermost thoughts to those who are close to us. However, this may not always work out or be enough. We may, for one reason or another, get negative reactions. Those people may withdraw: Sometimes the very people to whom we would like to turn are having trouble coping themselves. We may, in fact, feel less comfortable baring our souls to people we know than to people who will be less judgmental and more objective and who are experienced listeners, counselors, or therapists.

Fortunately, as I discuss in Chapter 12, there are many alternative sources for emotional support, both for ourselves and for our families. We may turn to our doctors or nurses, certainly, but they are often not trained to give emotional support. Social workers, the clergy, support or self-help groups, and patient volunteers are better targets for our outpourings. Or a psychotherapist, a family therapist, or a stress management technique may be what we need.

Of the huge variety of forms of psychosocial support, one or more is bound to be right for you. You might require help for extended periods— all through chemotherapy and possibly thereafter. More commonly, though, patients and their families find that they need a "leg up" only periodically, when some new twist in the situation makes them feel too overwhelmed to cope on their own. (These "twists" may coincide with the crisis points mentioned earlier.)

Dr. Bukberg says that the appropriate help depends on what the problem is and who the person is:

A group is a very, very good place to start. If the problem is that you're feeling kind of alone and going through a rough situation, and other people obviously do not understand in the same way that another person going through it can, if you're feeling very different from other people—and these kinds of things can make you feel so awful—for a lot of people a group is probably the best thing.

Sister Rosemary Moynihan would like to see a range of options but acknowledges that "groups are good for some people. The main advantage is they help normalize the experience, lessen isolation, give people a better sense of how others deal with this, to learn different ways of coping."

Diane Blum agrees: "There's a wonderful moment in support groups when a person says, 'I didn't know other people felt that way.'" But for people who don't get to support groups, she recommends education programs: "A lot more people are willing to sit and listen . . . they get the information they need, and the acknowledgment that the way they're feeling is not unique. Often someone will come up to the staff afterward and talk about feelings that they didn't want to talk about in front of the group."

Grace Christ thinks that "talking with a patient volunteer—someone who has gone through the experience—is also valuable." And Jimmie Holland, M.D., chief of psychiatry at Memorial Sloan-Kettering, extols the virtues of working over the telephone: "I think the telephone is underused and underappreciated for its value. Here at Memorial we do a lot of work with people who live too far away or who can't come in for face-to-face contact."

Today we have another source of support: the Internet—and it is changing the nature of cancer communication. Now you can access organizations devoted to specific types of cancer, such as breast, lymphoma, leukemia, and prostate cancers by Internet as well as by phone. Most of these organizations have hotlines, where you can anonymously request information or get emotional support from trained volunteers or staff. Online you can not only access state-of-the-art information about cancer and its treatment (some of it inaccurate, unfortunately), but also a wealth of Web sites devoted to survivor stories, encouragement, chat rooms, and bulletin boards to exchange information and support electronically. You may prefer a face-to-face support group setting; you may not. Or you may want to incorporate both into your overall coping strategy.

Dr. Bukberg points out that "the behavioral approach may also be a good first step for people who are having a lot of tension, anxiety, and/or those who are having difficulty with anticipatory nausea. Progressive relaxation, hypnosis, and imaging techniques are appropriate." (See Chapter 11.) She continues:

> But if, after people have tried something like that, anxiety is still really high or depression is still really bad—if it's interfering with

their functioning, if people can't concentrate on work, if their rela-
tionships with others around them seem to be disrupted—then it's
worth taking a look and trying to see what else may be going on,
what else could help. Sometimes counseling that's meant to explore
an individual's particular situation can just help clarify things.

Occasionally psychotherapy can help, according to Dr. Bukberg. "Psychological meanings that a person may not be so much aware of also affect how they are experiencing a stress, and people sometimes find themselves reacting in surprising ways. Psychotherapy can uncover what some of these additional meanings are, and sometimes that helps." She gives the example of people whose self-esteem is very tied up in particular parts of their bodies—their breasts or their hair. "The loss of these is obviously much more devastating than it is for people who have other things in their lives that are more important for their self-esteem."

Dr. Holland is seeing a more appropriate use of medication to diminish anxiety:

Although patients are still afraid of becoming addicted, if we can
persuade them to take antianxiety medication during a crisis, they
do much better. Getting sleep at night again is especially helpful.
They have less anxiety, fear, and distress and have no trouble stop-
ping the medication when the crisis is over. You also reduce post-
and pretreatment side effects such as nausea and vomiting if they
come to a treatment feeling relaxed, rather than tense and worried.

Depression and the Blues

Depression is perhaps the most common and debilitating emotional reaction in chemotherapy patients. At some time or other almost everyone—even the staunchest optimist—feels pessimistic, down, sad, weepy, blah, and blue:

I'm a very lively person. I'm not a depressed person. But I do get de-
pressed over my illness. I wish I were healthy like everyone else.

I would be depressed many times. I kind of spaced out, just with-drew. I would cry very easily. I felt so different from the person I had been, the person I knew. I felt like an observer of life because I was so debilitated, so out of it most of the time. And I was so used to be-ing a participant.

As the patients and cancer professionals who are quoted on the next few pages show, depression is quite common. They also show that the coping techniques just discussed can help a great deal to lift you out of your depression and prevent it from becoming incapacitating or unbearable.

Depression in chemo patients can happen at any time, but it doesn't usually settle in until after some earlier reactive stages have been experienced. Many patients are well into their treatments and have been through all the terrifying (and in a sense exciting) and demanding parts before the pressing weight of depression becomes noticeable or intolerable. One oncology nurse finds that, for instance, with people on a two-year protocol, "Once they get through the first year and into the second, it's really just awful. But at any midway point patients tend to have a downward feeling—'Are we ever going to get this over with?'"

A recent study suggests that younger women (in this study, that means under 50 years old) are more likely to feel depressed in the year immediately following a diagnosis and treatment of breast cancer. Lari Wenzel, Ph.D., the lead researcher at the University of California at Irvine who conducted the 2001 study, found that 30 percent of younger women reported feelings of depression, as compared with 20 percent of the older women. Dr. Wenzel speculates the discrepancy may be due to the possibility that older women have developed more coping strategies.

In my case, the tensions and insults accumulated gradually until one final event provided the crucial jolt. I seemed to be coping just fine until the side effects really kicked in. My oncologist said that the toxicity had finally built up, and I started to feel really sick about one month into the treatment, and really down. And then my hair fell out, which made it even worse. A little while later John Lennon was killed, and that really did it. Between that and the cancer, I felt as if a part of my past had died, was gone forever, and nothing would ever be as carefree, as good, as it had been before.

Grace Christ explains that depression in chemotherapy patients is usually a "reactive" depression. "Chemo patients are depressed for a good reason," she says, in that they are feeling sad and down as reactions to a specific external event.

Lari Wenzel points out:

The conditions surrounding the treatment could promote feelings of depression. If you are feeling physically ill all the time or a good deal of the time, you are not looking your best, your life has been disrupted, and you know your life is also being threatened, which is why you are undergoing the treatment . . . it's quite easy to understand why people become depressed.

Matthew Loscalzo says:

There are many different theories on depression. Some propose it's due to a learned helplessness. We often see this in our patients at Memorial, and I think it's one of the key issues. Another theory is sensory deprivation: People who are not stimulated amply get depressed and tend to withdraw. Cancer patients are physically depleted, with chemical changes taking place because of the cancer and chemotherapy; their personal space is violated by everyone from the cleaning lady to the doctors, and by everybody else in between. They don't understand what the doctors are saying half the time. And they're not up to snuff—their thinking processes may not be too clear because of the cancer or treatment or both. Patients need to be actively involved in their own care.

In addition, there is some evidence, and some professionals believe, that the drugs themselves cause chemical changes that lead to depression. Mood changes are not unusual when the hormone-producing endocrine system gets thrown out of order. For example:

After the second treatment I got a depressed feeling after I got home; I felt very down. The next treatment I got a depressed feeling on the way home. Then I felt it as I got to my car and became weepy as I drove home. Then it was when I got to the front steps of my doctor's office. By the time of the ninth or tenth treatment I really went berserk. At the end I couldn't make it out of his office. What upset me was that I always felt I had been a together person.

I had terrible mood swings. If you looked at me, I cried. I never knew if it was the surgery or the drugs, but I was in chemical menopause at that time. And I remember my mother going through menopause and having some tremendous mood swings. She was a real bitch at times; I became a bitch at times. Even I didn't like me. I remember one day I came home from work; I was off the next day. I just locked the door and didn't answer the phone, didn't do anything. I just sat. God, I didn't like myself for a long time! I didn't put on lipstick or take care of my hair. I didn't care what I looked like. Hell, I didn't like me, so why should anyone else?

WHAT YOU CAN DO

Depression is bound to go hand in hand with not feeling well for a prolonged period of time. As one patient said, "It just wears you down." So it is likely you will be able to alleviate some aspects of depression when you take care of your physical side effects, as suggested in the previous chapter. Your support group or your oncologist may be able to guide you further or suggest more.

- Be active. Patients often find that mental or physical activity is an antidote for the blues—the fact that they don't feel like themselves does not stop them from doing whatever makes them happy. Sitting around doing nothing but feeling sorry for yourself is not only boring, but also encourages you to dwell on your problems. Time could be so much better spent on enjoyable, esteem-building distractions such as hobbies, friends, social functions, work, and support groups.
- Exercise has many advantages and has gotten many a chemo patient out of the dumps. (See Chapter 9.)

- Some people have let—or have learned how to let—others help keep them cheerful and maintain their perspective. I was at the very bottom of my depression—the pits—when a girlfriend of mine called with some horrifying news. A young man we knew—in his twenties and about to be married—was in an accident and was paralyzed from the neck down. As awful as it was, it really shook me out of my own depression. What the hell was I so upset about compared to his bad luck? At least I could walk, go to work, and do things.

Mental health professionals are careful to point out that there's a difference between what most patients call depression and a medical diagnosis of clinical depression. This distinction changes treatment options. Matthew Loscalzo explains:

Depression is to be expected in about 25 percent of patients. However, recent data show that cancer patients are no more depressed than other equally ill patients. There's no question that chemo patients get the blues and get sad. They may feel "depressed." But we have to separate out fatigue and those sad feelings in someone who is chronically ill or is receiving certain drugs from clinical depression. That's a very specific diagnosis with specific ways of measuring it. With true depression, you are depressed about yourself. But chemo patients are depressed about something outside themselves.

As Dr. Bukberg says, "There are depressed people who just don't get better." The signs include being in a depressed mood, losing interest or pleasure, sleeping too much or too little, poor appetite, constant fatigue, feelings of worthlessness or excessive or inappropriate guilt, diminished ability to think or concentrate, and recurrent thoughts of suicide. "If depression is persistent, a trial of antidepressant medication should be considered," Bukberg says. She points out that a variety of studies show that psychotherapy works for depression in some people, medication works in others, and a combination might be best of all.

PART THREE

Guide to Complementary Therapies

As a chemo patient, you are so much more than just a walking tumor—you've also got a body and a mind. How can you take care of these aspects of yourself while the chemotherapy is dealing with the cancer? Conventional medicine offers some drugs to help you get through the worst of the side effects. But these don't always do the trick, they don't have the possibility of enhancing the anticancer effects of the drugs, and they have side effects of their own. One solution is to use complementary therapies—those therapies that are outside conventional medicine—in addition to chemotherapy. The approaches in this section—nutrition, supplements, exercise, mind-body therapies, psychological support, and other therapies such as herbs—can help you cope with chemotherapy in a variety of ways.

Before chemo, they can prepare your mind and body for what's to come so you start therapy in the best possible shape mentally and physically. During chemo they can help shield your healthy tissues from the effects of the chemo without lessening their effects on the cancer cells—in fact, there's ample evidence that they can increase the chemo's effects while reducing the drugs' unwanted side effects. Finally, after chemo, they can help clear your body of the toxic residue left in your body, help repair damaged tissues, and restore your mind and spirit. Because they help strengthen your immune system and other defenses, they may also continue to support your body's innate ability to keep cancer and other diseases and conditions at bay.

If any of these therapies interest you, I encourage you to find out more about them and to look for a knowledgeable practitioner to supervise and guide you. And of course, discuss with your oncologist what you would like to do so your complementary practitioner and your oncologist can communicate and work together.

CHAPTER EIGHT

Diet and Nutrition

While good nutrition is important for everyone, diet and nutrition are the most potent tools in any program geared to helping you cope with chemotherapy. Before, during, and after chemo, the food you eat and the supplements you take can play a central role in your emotional and physical health and well-being. Before starting chemo, you can boost nutrition and build up your body's stores of vitamins and minerals. Good nutrition can prepare and strengthen your tissues and organs to withstand the onslaught of the toxic chemicals to come. After chemo, you can use food to help your body detoxify and to help give your body the building blocks it needs to restore and rebuild what chemo has broken down. Proper nutrients may help return your energy to normal and help rebalance your hormones. Some estimate that 60 percent of all women's cancers and 40 percent of all men's cancers are related to nutritional factors. Even the American Cancer Society, which generally takes a conservative stance, attributes one-third of cancer deaths to poor diet. Because diet is so universally linked with the development of cancer, eating a good diet may reduce the risk of a new cancer from occurring. It may also help prevent or slow a diagnosed cancer from growing or recurring.

We now know that a good diet is important in preventing cancer and so many other diseases and conditions. Proper nutrition is crucial for providing us with physical and mental energy. Why then does it so often get ignored by doctors when a person is facing chemotherapy? Have we suddenly turned into a different species from a planet where food doesn't matter? If anything, food matters *more* when you are on chemo. I can't do the subject justice in this one chapter, but there are many excellent books on nutrition and many of them focus on cancer in particular. If you want to know more, I recommend you take a look at them. Several books are listed in the Bibliography and Suggested Reading section (Appendix C). In the meantime, here is a summary of why you need to pay extra attention to food while on chemo, and why you may also want to augment your diet with nutritional supplements.

What Chemo Does
to Your Nutritional Status

Two things are clear: One, diet and nutrition are an important source of support when you are living under the special conditions and stresses that cancer and chemotherapy impose. And two: Every person who undergoes chemotherapy is probably malnourished to some degree which can worsen side effects, quality of life, and prognosis.

The chemicals used in cancer chemotherapy affect your mind and body and thus your diet in many ways. As described in Part Two, the drugs can cause you to lose your appetite, change your ability to taste foods, bring on nausea and vomiting, and damage the mucosal lining of your mouth, esophagus, stomach, and intestines. All this can lead to alterations in the kinds and amounts of food you eat as well as your body's ability to absorb and utilize what you do eat. Some drugs can themselves chemically deplete or destroy nutrients in the body. As a result, chemotherapy alone can cause multiple obvious and not-so-obvious nutritional deficiencies.

In addition, you are being exposed to many other factors and conditions that deplete your body's supply of nutrients and/or increase its demand for them. Physical and psychological stress such as the diagnosis of cancer itself, surgery, and radiation have well-documented deleterious effects on nutritional status. The mere fact of being hospitalized—the physical and psychological stress of the treatments and the poor diet—has been shown to cause nutritional deficiencies. You might have other deficiencies or imbalances as a result of the cancer itself or as carryovers from dietary conditions that contributed to the development of cancer in the first place.

My oncologist says:

It's well understood now that many patients who have gone through surgical operations and who are in the process of receiving toxic medications have serious nutritional deficiencies. One of the most serious forms of malnourishment that occurs anywhere on earth occurs in the modern hospital. A person is thought to be okay because he is on intravenous feeding. The fact of the matter is that the total amount of nutrition he receives over the course of twenty-four hours is about the same as a couple of Coca-Colas.

There is an appalling lack of knowledge about the changes in one's dietary needs during chemotherapy. Therefore, as the authors of *Nutrition for the Chemotherapy Patient* write, "In clinical practice, nutrition is often neglected. The assessment of nutritional status . . . is generally quite casual" and is based on a "quick glance" and a "mental estimate" of how much body fat you have. Unfortunately, you can look well developed and well nourished, but underneath the layer of fat you may have lost significant lean body mass (muscle). "Further, where there are no overt signs of vitamin deficiency . . . the physician usually assumes the vitamin status to be normal. In fact the patient's vitamin status . . . is often marginal at best."

Dr. Samuel Dreizer and colleagues at the MD Anderson Cancer Center have been treating chemo patients for over twenty years and find that the nutritional status of most of these patients ranges from the "subnormal to the extremely precarious." It's not uncommon for patients to have severe deficiencies in vitamin B_1, vitamin B_2, vitamin K, folic acid, niacin, and thiamine and the symptoms of sore, cracked lips and mouth, skin rashes, and bleeding. They have reversed these deficiencies and others with oral or intravenous supplements.

Not to mention the fact that even most "healthy" or "well-nourished" Americans do not pass nutritional tests and surveys with flying colors. If you are an average American who has been eating the Standard American Diet (SAD), you are deficient in many nutrients before you even start getting chemotherapy. In other words, you enter the race with a nutritional handicap.

Chemotherapy patients often lose weight (although some actually gain it), become deficient in many vitamins and minerals, lose energy, and generally fall into a malnourished, unhealthy state at the very time they need to remain as strong and healthy as possible to fight the cancer, repair the damage done by the disease, and withstand the side effects of therapy. If this happens to you, it not only lessens your quality of life while on chemotherapy, it could be setting you up for problems in the future, as well.

Where to Get Help

The ways in which nutrition, diet, cancer, and chemotherapy interrelate is a frustratingly complicated field of study. Much more work needs to be done. Yet evidence is accumulating, and you can put it to work for your benefit. As D. M. Hegsted, professor of nutrition at the Harvard School of Public Health, declared in "Optimal Nutrition," an article published in the May 1979 supplement of *Cancer:* "The fact that we do not know the optimal solution cannot and does not prevent us from using whatever relevant evidence is available to make the best judgment possible. If we wait until we know everything we need to know, we will wait forever." He is addressing the problem of nutritional links with the onset of cancer, but the same arguments are being made for treatment, too.

Self-education is the first step toward making that judgment. You can probably safely make simple changes in your eating habits on your own; in fact the American Cancer Society has an excellent set of "Guidelines on Diet, Nutrition, and Cancer Prevention" available on its Web site. But because the information is so complex and evolving, if you are thinking of making any drastic changes in your diet or taking large doses of vitamins, minerals, or other nutritional supplements, a qualified dietitian, nutritionist, or nutrition-oriented physician can intelligently advise you. Although you should let your oncologist know if you are concerned about nutrition, you shouldn't expect your oncologist to dispense nutritional advice— most traditional doctors are lamentably ignorant about nutrition. Some are downright hostile toward the nutritional approach to anything, perhaps because nutrition has been overhyped or perhaps because they fear patients will forgo conventional cancer treatment and focus only on nutrition.

This problem is well recognized by experts in the nutrition field, be they of a conservative or a progressive bent. However, this state of affairs is gradually improving; imagine my own surprise when my surgeon, who had always seemed very traditionally minded, started asking me whether I take vitamins B, C, and E and selenium! Lisa Logan, former nutrition support clinical dietitian at Presbyterian Denver Hospital, says:

Many oncology patients have very complex medical problems, and frequently nutrition may be the last problem addressed. The current literature, which supports early nutrition intervention to lessen complications and improve tolerance to therapy, can no longer be ignored. So I have seen a gradual improvement in the awareness of physicians I work with. Also, many hospital outpatient clinics have nutritionists that deal specifically with oncology patients. Physicians concerned with the importance of nutrition will refer their patients for more extensive nutrition assessment and intervention.

Dr. Shari Lieberman, a nutritionist in private practice, speaks from her own professional experience:

The problem with conventional doctors is not that they don't believe in nutrition but that they are uneducated in that area. They don't admit this to their patients, but they admit it to me. They tell me to do what I think is best and to let them know what I'm doing. The added need for nutrients during chemotherapy is well documented, particularly as it relates to physical and physiological stress. So doctors that argue about this are just not reading. Maybe there's a little bit of tunnel vision.

Dietitians are trained in food service science and have a minimum of an undergraduate course in nutrition. Although some hospital dietitians are doing progressive work, generally they are conservative. Nutritionists have a minimum of a master's degree in the nutritional sciences, which allows them to understand the subtleties of nutrition and the therapeutic nature of the components of food. Not all nutritionists are progressive. Ask your health-food store to make a recommendation, or someone in your support group. Then make sure to ask where they got their training and education— some people call themselves nutritionists but aren't.

Dr. Michael Schachter is a physician in private practice who combines nutrition and holistic health with mainstream medicine. He treats many cancer patients who are on chemotherapy with other physicians, and he thinks oncologists tend to resist the idea of nutritional therapy as an adjunct to chemotherapy for several reasons:

In some respects the two approaches are antagonistic—one tends to break down the body, the other tends to build it up. Or it may be related to the old expression, "If you're not up on something, you're down on it." They may think if there's some value to nutrition, then they should be doing it, too—but they're not doing it. So to protect themselves they have a very strong negative feeling about it.

The position of many oncologists is they say the nutritional approach has not been sufficiently proved. But studies relating nutritional factors to cancer may take many years to complete, and cancer patients can't wait for these to be finished before taking action to help themselves. Some chemotherapy patients feel pretty terrible, and clinically they feel a lot better when they undertake a nutritionally supportive program along with their chemotherapy.

We are happy to work with oncologists, if they are willing to work with us. Frequently oncologists do not support their patients being on a nutritional program, but patients are convinced that it will help. Consequently, patients surreptitiously undertake nutritional programs. We often get feedback from the patient that his oncologist is extremely pleased at how well he is doing, that the patient is zipping through the therapy with a minimum of side effects. I can also say that more and more oncologists, though skeptical of nutritional therapeutic approaches doing much good, are not taking as hard a line as they did previously. They say to go ahead and do it if you want to, as long as you take the chemotherapy, too.

My oncologist, who stresses the importance of individualizing all aspects of cancer treatment, sometimes suggests adding nutritional therapy to the chemotherapy regimen despite its "unproven" nature:

My approach is that there are many things we don't know in medicine. But there are substances which are of use in assisting people to be able to perform better and do better which have negligible side effects. These can be useful in improving the strength of a person who is receiving therapy for malignancy. So I have tried to bring in elements that might be of benefit in terms of improving the body's strength. I have had to look at many sources, both traditional and nontraditional. Traditional approaches tend to look at data more critically and use double-blind testing to validate the doses of substances that are required. The nontraditional ones tend to say, "Why don't we just try this and see what happens." That latter approach has also produced some interesting effects. So I am in the position at this point in time of having to take somewhat sketchy, experimental data and apply it, perhaps in advance of its complete understanding.

My basic point of view is that you keep your eyes open. You keep trying to apply as many things that may help as you can get your hands on, without being kooky. One has to be modest but listen to everything. I feel that as an internist I have to be well versed in everything that happens.

What Good Nutrition Can Do for You

Proper nutrition can help you in four important ways.

IMPROVES TOLERANCE OF THERAPY

A well-nourished body is stronger and more resilient than a poorly nour-ished one. Studies have shown that nutrition can decrease the severity and duration of side effects such as vomiting, nausea, weakness, lowered im-munity, and susceptibility to infection. Nutrition may also minimize other side effects that we do not know about yet. In general, however, people who eat well while on chemotherapy tend to feel better and stay more physically active and more mentally alert.

INCREASES THE EFFECTIVENESS OF THERAPY

When you feed yourself, you also feed your cancer cells. Studies have shown that well-fed cancer cells multiply more readily and so are more susceptible to anticancer drugs than are slow-growing, undernourished cells. In addition, a good nutritional status may allow you to withstand higher doses of drugs and so increase the effectiveness of the therapy in that way as well.

SPEEDS RECOVERY FROM TREATMENTS

Nutrients are the building blocks your body uses to rebuild the normal tis-sues that have been affected by the chemotherapy. If the proper nutrients in the proper amounts are available, you can recover much more quickly and efficiently than if you have nutritional deficiencies.

REGULATES YOUR WEIGHT

Many people lose weight on chemotherapy, but some (notably women on chemotherapy for breast cancer) gain weight. Underweight and overweight are both undesirable for you at this time: They can lead to weakness, lethargy, depression, embarrassment, and lack of self-esteem. Being careful about what you eat will help avoid both these extremes.

The Basic Healthy Diet

There is so much evidence that the typical American diet is a contributing factor to many diseases—cancer being one of them—that several government agencies (such as the Department of Agriculture, the National Cancer Institute, the Senate Select Committee of Nutrition and Human Needs, the Department of Health and Human Services, and the National Academy of Sciences) have released very similar dietary guidelines urging Americans to change their eating habits. The National Academy of Sciences surveyed the scientific literature and concluded that cancers of most major sites are influenced by dietary patterns. Based on animal studies and observation of many human populations, it has been found that we eat too much fat, too much salt, too much sugar, too much cholesterol, and too much food in general. And our health is suffering because of our indulgence.

Simply stated, a basic healthy diet consists of a variety of foods that will give you the most vitamins, minerals, and other nutrients, plus the optimum amount of protein, carbohydrates, fats, and water needed to keep your body working normally. The following daily menu fulfills these guidelines. It is rather moderate, when you consider other eating plans such as veganism (no animal products whatsoever), or macrobiotics. But it is revolutionary compared with what most Americans are eating in that it is lower in calories and emphasizes foods from plants rather than foods from animals. It encourages you to eat fresh fruits and vegetables; recommends whole grains and other relatively unprocessed foods rather than packaged convenience foods containing refined ingredients such as white flour, sugar, and chemical additives; is moderate in protein; and is low in fat. While this way of eating may be a bit of a challenge even when you are not on chemo, it is the kind of diet that I have been eating for more than twenty years. While I do a lot of my own cooking, it is becoming easier and easier to eat this way, even when you are eating out in restaurants, if you know how to order. More and more restaurants are offering healthy items on their menus, and are happy to prepare food to your specifications. In my recently published book *Dare to Lose,* which I wrote with Shari Lieberman, Ph.D., we provide guidelines for preparing food at home as well as for ordering in restaurants. This book will also give you a healthy way to lose any excess weight you may have accumulated while on chemo.

DAILY MENU

Every day's menu should include fruits and vegetables, protein, grains, healthy fats, and plenty of liquids.

Fruits and Vegetables

Eat at least five servings of fruits and vegetables daily. There is evidence that vitamin C and beta-carotene protect against the development of cancer. Colorful fruits and vegetables—oranges, grapefruit, apricots, cantaloupes, peaches, strawberries, dark leafy green vegetables, carrots, winter squash, tomatoes, green peppers, and sweet potatoes—are high in one or both of beta-carotene and vitamin C. Cruciferous vegetables (broccoli, Brussels sprouts, cabbage, and cauliflower) contain these vitamins plus certain compounds called *indoles,* which research indicates can increase the body's capacity to convert carcinogens into harmless substances. Fruits and vegetables are also high in fiber. Lower fiber consumption has been implicated in bowel and breast cancer, and the National Cancer Institute recommends that we increase our intake. Incorporate fruits and vegetables into your mealtimes and choose them for snacks as well.

Protein

Eat three servings of protein daily. Choose from low-fat plant-based protein-rich foods such as beans and legumes, tofu, nut and grain milks (soy, oat, rice, or almond); organic eggs; low-fat dairy; fish and seafood; and free-range poultry occasionally and in small portions. Minimize fatty meats and cuts of meat, such as beef and pork. Isoflavones, found in legumes (beans, peas, and lentils), appear to inhibit or block estrogen receptors and may reduce the risk of estrogen-dependent cancers, and slow down established cancers. However, recent animal studies show that taking high doses of supplements of genistein, a type of isoflavone, could cause breast cancer cells to proliferate. In addition, women in Japan eat soy foods that are prepared differently than they are in the U.S.: These tend to be fermented forms such as miso and natto, and their portions are smaller. So, at this point, nutritionists are somewhat confused about soy beans, soy products, and soy supplements. That's why Dr. Lieberman recommends that if you incorporate soy into your diet that you do not also take supplemental isoflavones and that you eat small portions of these foods, "not a whole slab of tofu."

High-protein diets are associated with an increased risk of many cancers. Pickled, smoked, and salt-cured foods in particular appear to increase the incidence of cancers of the stomach and esophagus. Japan, Iceland, and China, where these foods are consumed in great quantities, have higher incidences of these cancers. So avoid consuming a lot of hot dogs, bologna, salami and sausages, ham, bacon, and smoked fish; salt should be reduced to five grams per day.

Grains

Eat four servings of grains daily. Emphasize whole grains such as dark German health bread, oat bran, oatmeal, whole-wheat pastas, and whole grains such as brown rice, barley, and kasha (buckwheat groats). Whole grains are higher in vitamins, minerals, and fiber, which may reduce risk of several types of cancer, not to mention constipation.

Fats

From a health standpoint, it's best to choose foods that are low in fat and not to add much fat to your foods. A high-fat diet is associated with a higher risk of cancer, heart disease, and diabetes. If you do add fats, add a little organic nuts or nut butters, olive oil, or flaxseeds. These contain less harmful saturated and polyunsaturated fats and more of the beneficial type of fats known as omega-3 fatty acids. Several studies show that people who consume greater quantities of fat have a higher incidence of cancers of the breast, bowel, and prostate. Most experts now recommend that Americans reduce the current level of their fat intake by more than one-fourth so it accounts for 30 percent or less of their total calories rather than the usual 40 percent. To do this, we should resist adding butter, margarine, mayonnaise, gravies, and fatty sauces to our foods, as well as eat less beef and other fatty meats, reduce our consumption of cheese and other whole-milk, full-fat dairy products, and avoid fried foods. There are loads of vegetarian and low-fat diet books and cookbooks available that show you how to prepare foods using methods that require little or no added fat, such as baking, roasting, steaming, and broiling.

Liquids

Drink eight to twelve glasses of liquids daily. Filtered or other pure water is best, but you may also drink diluted fruit and vegetable juices, soups, and herbal teas. Try to minimize caffeine-containing beverages such as coffee and colas, as well as alcoholic beverages. Alcohol, especially when combined with cigarette smoking, has been connected with higher rates of cancer of the breast, mouth, larynx, liver, and lungs. Drinking "in moderation" is advised—probably no more than two drinks per day.

TAILORING THE DIET

With some exceptions, the basic healthy diet is the same for everyone, whether you've been diagnosed with cancer or not, whether you are about to go on chemo, are already on chemo, or have finished chemo. However, it is likely that you will need more protein and calories than usual after surgery to help you heal, and during chemotherapy to help your body replace lost healthy cells and keep up your weight, fat stores, and lean muscle mass. Even though you may not be feeling well or don't feel like eating these particular foods, it is important to eat well. On the other hand, you might need to make certain adjustments so you can get through the therapy. It may be all you can do to eat *anything* while on chemo, and you may want the cozy familiarity of your usual foods. You may not feel comfortable making big changes in your eating habits—after all, so much of your life is already changing. Don't stress. These changes can wait. But if you do feel up to it, and if you want to take further steps to safeguard your health, use these guidelines when making your food choices.

I recommend you consult with a nutritionist experienced in cancer nutrition, at least once. In addition to chemo-related tailoring, you also may need to make certain adjustments if you have other conditions such as kidney problems, diabetes, cardiovascular disease, or irritable bowl syndrome. And remember, if side effects make it difficult for you to eat according to this plan or if you have lost or are losing weight, turn to the eating-related side effects in Part Two for tips on overcoming your difficulties. If you can't eat enough while on chemo, and you are losing too much weight, you may want to add a liquid nutritional supplement. This is fine—just try to avoid the commercial drugstore and supermarket variety and buy yours from a health-food store. Many liquid supplements are full of sugar and unhealthy fats.

Added Benefits
from Nutritional Supplements

Although these eating guidelines are a step in the right direction, a growing number of experts say they do not go far enough—not for the average population and especially not for the cancer patient who is at high risk for disease already and who is being further weakened by various therapies.

They point out that first of all, since cancer chemotherapy patients are at a high risk to develop second cancers and other illnesses, they should modify their diets as much as possible to reduce this risk. They feel that the recommended dietary allowances (RDAs) of vitamins and minerals in the so-called balanced diet are hard for anyone—and impossible for the chemotherapy patient—to get every day. They also claim that the RDAs are far too low anyway for optimum health in the average person and do not even begin to answer the needs of the chemotherapy patient. They argue that supplements of vitamins and minerals should be added to the nutritional regimen because they can protect organs from the toxicity of the drugs, counteract the carcinogenic activity of the drugs and other chemicals in the food and the environment, and improve the functioning of the immune system, which plays a role in destroying cancer cells but is being weakened by the therapy.

Generally, a multivitamin/mineral supplement, which will help make up for the nutrients that your diet is lacking, can be taken safely and is advised. In *A Comprehensive Guide for Cancer Patients and Their Families,* Dr. Ernest Rosenbaum writes:

> *In some cases vitamin and mineral supplements may be needed because of the side effects of certain types of cancer or of therapy, which may result in vitamin or mineral losses or increased requirements. Vitamin and mineral supplements may also be needed by patients who are unable to eat a balanced diet, or who have loss of appetite, malabsorption or weight loss, or who drink or smoke excessively.*

The majority of chemotherapy patients fit into at least one of these categories. Remember, too, not to rely solely on supplements—real foods contain nutritional elements that supplements don't, perhaps some we don't even know exist.

But how much should you take? Few oncologists would object to your taking a one-a-day-type multivitamin that would supply you with the recommended daily allowances. But should you go higher, as I did?

My oncologist says he is "not a megavitamin person" and thinks it's important to distinguish between megadoses of vitamins and large doses of vitamins. He will sometimes prescribe "large reasonable" doses of vitamins and minerals that might be useful as adjunctives in terms of trying to build the body:

> *Data produced by the National Cancer Institute, for example, have shown that vitamin E is useful as an antioxidant, and it has many other remarkable effects and no negative ones. There's lots of evidence to suggest that zinc is useful in the management of immunodeficiency disease of many origins. There is some data to suggest that selenium is useful under some circumstances. In reasonable doses, vitamin C does tend to promote restoration of normal tissue*

strength. Vitamin A in reasonable doses has been shown to be an immunostimulant under some circumstances. B vitamins have been shown to be useful during the recovery from many conditions; B vitamins are rapidly used up during cell death and cell restoration. So, for instance, one or two milligrams of vitamin B$_1$ just isn't enough.

Dr. Schachter points out that it's important to eliminate harmful substances as well as add beneficial ones:

Patients must have appropriate quantities of each of the nutrients in order to optimally support their body defenses. At the same time, nontherapeutic toxic substances should be eliminated as much as possible. We start out by recommending the elimination of junk foods, refined carbohydrates, chemicals, and so on. We emphasize the ingestion of complex carbohydrates—whole grains, vegetables, nuts, and seeds—and that patients try to cut down on their meat and get organic beef if they can. And then we add a nutritional supplementation program—vitamins, minerals, enzymes—as a kind of insurance.

With regard to cancer, we're especially interested in trying to stimulate the body's defense system. We believe in the surveillance theory that people are developing cancer cells all the time. So we try to supplement liberally with nutrients that are thought to improve the body's defense system. We're also interested in protecting the organs against chemotherapy. One of the things that chemotherapeutic agents can do is form free radicals which damage the cell membranes and lead to carcinogenesis. By taking large (but not toxic) doses of vitamins A, C, and E and selenium, you're nourishing the organs that are being bombarded by toxic substances and protecting them from some of the damage.

Dr. Lieberman comments:

I'm not against chemotherapy per se. It's just that it's done in a very nonthinking way. It's done to people who aren't eating, who aren't

taking any supplements, who end up with multiple nutritional defi-
ciencies, which is the last thing you want to do to a cancer patient.

When people talk about eating a well-balanced, nutritional diet
and they say you can get everything you need from food, that is un-
educated. In order to get the RDAs of all the nutrients—which as far
as I'm concerned are the bare minimum—you have to eat about
2,500 calories a day. That's a lot for the average person, and for
people on chemotherapy—forget it.

The thing that I emphasize for people who are going to take
chemotherapy is that they can use nutrition to minimize the risks
and negative effects of the chemotherapy. You can take supplements
of selenium and vitamin E, which are antioxidants, and of A or beta
carotene. Studies have revealed that cancer patients typically have
low levels of these nutrients.

Nutritional therapy as described above sounds straightforward, but the
practice is not without its controversies. We don't know everything about
the way the body responds either to chemotherapy or to the various nutri-

GOALS OF NUTRITIONAL THERAPY

Progressive nutritional therapy for the chemotherapy patient seeks
to improve his or her health generally and protect specifically
against carcinogens (such as anticancer drugs). It is based on
three principles:

1. Avoid foods and nontherapeutic substances that are known
   to be or are highly suspected of being carcinogenic or that
   make the body a hospitable place for cancer to develop.
2. Include nutrients that bolster the body's own defenses.
3. Include substances that have the direct or indirect ability to
   inhibit the formation of cancer in the body.

BASIC SUPPLEMENT PROGRAM

Before, during, and after chemotherapy treatment, you may want to take a multivitamin-mineral formula containing approximately these amounts of nutrients:

Vitamin A	10,000–50,000 IU
Beta-carotene*	5,000–11,000 IU
B-complex	50 mg–150 mg
Vitamin C	5,000–10,000 mg
Vitamin D	400 IU
Vitamin E**	400 IU–800 IU
Boron	1–3 mg
Calcium	1,000 mg
Chromium	200–400 mcg
Copper	2 mg
Iodine	150 mcg
Iron	15 mg (optional)
Magnesium	500 mg
Manganese	15–30 mg
Selenium	200–400 mcg
Zinc	15–25 mg
Essential fatty acids	250–3,000 mg
Garlic	200–1,200 mg

*Make sure your beta-carotene is natural and not synthetic. This information will be listed on the label.
**Make sure your vitamin E is natural. It will be listed as D-alpha tocopherol rather than D,L-alpha tocopherol.

Adapted from *The Real Vitamin and Mineral Book*, by Dr. Shari Lieberman and Nancy Bruning. Avery/Penguin Putnam, 1997, second edition.

ents, let alone about how chemotherapy and nutrients interact in the body. What to take? How much to take? When to take them? For example, some oncologists warn that antioxidant supplements—vitamin C, vitamin E, beta-carotene, selenium, coenzyme Q_{10}, flavonoids—should not be taken for two or three days before and after a chemotherapy treatment. Some say you should give it an even wider margin. Their logic is that some anti-cancer drugs—namely bleomycin, daunorubicin, doxorubicin, mito-mycin, and mitoxantrone in particular—work by creating free radicals. Antioxidants are known to protect normal cells from free radicals, but tak-ing supplements to support this protective mechanism might also protect the cancer cells. Some recommend that you do not take folate or folic acid if you are getting methotrexate or leucovorin because they kill cancer cells by depriving them of this nutrient. You'll be relieved to hear there is no ev-idence that these or other nutrients interfere in any way with the drug's ef-fectiveness.

In fact, it is now "medically accepted" that people on methotrexate for some types of cancers take a folic acid supplement. Retinoids (vitamin A) help reduce the incidence of second cancers in people who have already had one head or neck cancer. In one study, vitamin E supplements re-duced the number of people who lost hair from doxorubicin by two-thirds. Magnesium is often prescribed to replace the magnesium depleted by some chemo drugs such as cisplatin. Potassium is depleted by 5-FU, and zinc and selenium are also depleted by chemo; these minerals are impor-tant for immune function and your sense of taste.

In our book *The Real Vitamin and Mineral Book,* Dr. Lieberman and I cite more recent research showing that many substances not only possess cancer-inhibiting effects, but they may also offer some protection against the negative effects of chemotherapy and environmental toxins and may even make the drugs more effective. For example, vitamin E may protect the heart and enhance the effectiveness of Adriamycin; selenium may act additively or synergistically with chemo and radiation; and vitamin E and coenzyme Q_{10} prevent cell damage, particularly of the heart, from Adri-amycin. In one intriguing study done at the University of Wisconsin, breast cancer patients with high blood levels of vitamin A responded twice as well to chemotherapy as did women with lower levels. Dr. Lieberman feels that "subsequent studies will no doubt reveal other natural substances with similar properties."

Once she consults with her patients' oncologists, many of them have no objection to a supplement program. But if they do, they are often willing to compromise and have their patients refrain from supplementation for two days before the chemotherapy treatment and resume supplementation two days after treatment. (See page 289 for Dr. Lieberman's recommendations for a supplement program for people who are on chemotherapy.)

Dr. Kedar Prasad, of the University of Colorado Health Sciences Center in Denver, has written extensively on the subject of using high doses of antioxidant nutrients as an adjunct to chemotherapy (and radiation). He says that scientists who debate the use of antioxidant supplements fail to make a distinction between the effect of antioxidants produced by the body (endogenous antioxidants such as glutathione and the enzyme superoxide dismutase) and those introduced to the body in the diet or supplements (exogenous antioxidants such as vitamins A, C, E and carotenoids). Endogenous antioxidants protect both normal cells and cancer cells against damage by chemotherapy; but exogenous antioxidants protect only normal cells and actually enhance the destructive effects of chemotherapy on cancer cells. Furthermore, he says, these exogenous antioxidants "also initiate changes in expression of those genes that are involved in regulation of growth, differentiation and apoptosis (death) only in cancer cells." For more information about antioxidants and cancer therapy, see Dr. Ralph Moss's book, *Antioxidants Against Cancer* or Burton Goldberg's *An Alternative Medicine Definitive Guide to Cancer.* For a more technical book that could persuade your doctor, see *Natural Compounds in Cancer Therapy* by John Boik.

In his book *Beating Cancer with Nutrition,* Patrick Quillin explains it this way: Antioxidants have been shown to dramatically improve the tumor kill from pro-oxidative chemo and radiation while protecting the host tissue from damage. Essentially, the proper selection of nutrients taken before and during chemo and radiation can help make the medical therapy more of a selective toxin against the cancer. Cancer cells are primarily anaerobic (meaning "without oxygen") cells. Cancer cells do not absorb nor use antioxidants, with the exception of vitamin C, the same way that healthy aerobic cells do. Vitamin C (ascorbic acid) is nearly identical in chemical structure to glucose, which is the flavored fuel for cancer cells. With this background, it should not be surprising that researchers at Sloan-Kettering found that radioactively labeled ascorbic acid was preferentially absorbed by implanted tumors in animals. The study admitted that this effect takes place because cancer has many more glucose receptors on the cell surface than healthy normal cells. The researchers then assumed, but never found any evidence, that vitamin C should not be used in conjunction with chemo or radiation because the tumor was absorbing vitamin C to protect itself against the damaging effects of chemo and radiation. Any antioxidant by itself and/or in an anaerobic environment (such as a cancer cell) can become a prooxidant. Vitamin C in large doses in cancer patients is both protective of the patient and more selectively toxic to the tumor cells. We can exploit the differences in biochemistry between healthy and malignant cells by combining aggressive nutrition support with restrained cytotoxic therapies.

According to Charles Simone, an oncologist, "all studies show that vitamins and minerals do not interfere with the antitumor effects of chemotherapy or radiation therapy." In his book *Cancer and Nutrition*, he summarizes dozens of studies that support the use of supplements during chemotherapy. For example, studies performed at the National Cancer Institute showed that an antioxidant called N-acetyl cysteine protects the heart form Adriamycin, but did not interfere with the drug's ability to kill tumor cells in cancer patients. Cell studies and animal studies show that vitamins A, C, and E, and beta-carotene and selenium also protect healthy cells from this drug, and actually enhance its antitumor effects. Many other studies of these nutrients show the same results: they protect healthy cells while allowing chemo to kill cancer cells and often even improve the effectiveness of chemo, rather than lessen it. Several studies show that patients who took antioxidant supplements along with their chemo actually lived longer than patients who had chemo alone. As to the danger of folic acid supplements, he points out that folic acid itself does not reverse methotrexate's effects. "In order to reverse the effects of methotrexate, folinic acid (an analog of folic acid) has to be given in extremely high doses" available only with a doctor's prescription.

Before I began chemotherapy, my oncologist gave me a nutritional evaluation. Based on lab tests and dietary analysis, he suggested a few changes and added nutritional supplements. I took (and still take) a full-spectrum vitamin and mineral supplement that supplies me with doses much higher than the RDAs. Knowing I was doing something that was perhaps protecting me from some of the harmful effects of chemo helped put my mind at ease. It formed an integral part of my overall therapy and ability to tolerate the drugs psychologically and perhaps physically, too. Oncologists say that women on adjuvant chemotherapy for breast cancer typically have minimal side effects, as I did. But I also have met many women who were devastated by it. I have no way of knowing to which of these two groups I would have belonged and whether the handfuls of vitamin pills made any difference. But I think and hope they did; just as I took chemotherapy to help fight my cancer, my nutritional regimen meant I wasn't going to take chemo lying down. It made me feel more confident and secure and less afraid of the therapy and what it was doing to the rest of me while it killed the cancer cells.

CHAPTER NINE

Exercise

While many oncologists advise their patients to stay active and try to live as normal a life as possible, few recommend an exercise program as a specific support therapy for those on chemotherapy. This is surprising, since most of us by now know about at least some of the benefits we can derive from exercise. Regular exercise can play an important role in overall health, in our body image, body awareness, self-esteem, and self-sufficiency. It strengthens us and keeps us limber. It is a superb outlet for stress and tension and a proven nondrug antidote to the blues and the blahs. There's evidence that physically fit people have lower death rates from cancer and heart disease.

Linda E. Perkin, a registered physical therapist and exercise physiologist, is the former coordinator of the Oncology Fitness Program at Denver Presbyterian Medical Center. Ms. Perkin worked with cancer patients for six years at Presbyterian and is now in private practice. She says that though more oncologists are recommending that their patients get some exercise, some still think, "Oh don't bother them, just let them lie there. I think perhaps they focus so much on chemotherapy that they don't consider recommending generally healthy things like exercise."

In 1983 the Ohio State University Comprehensive Cancer Center conducted a formal pilot project to study the physical and psychological effects of an exercise program on women with breast cancer. This was the first formal study of this nature ever done and was designed to compare a relatively aggressive rehabilitation program with the standard conservative approach. Dr. James Neidhart, the former deputy director of the cancer center, says: "This project met with a fair amount of resistance from physicians and lay people on our Human Use Committee. They felt that people with this type of cancer on these drugs should not be subjected to exercise, that the drugs are too toxic to allow it."

The study, which consisted of ten to twelve weeks of a combination of twenty minutes of aerobic training on a stationary bicycle and stretching, demonstrated that some very positive results can be obtained by people receiving chemotherapy. Not only did the subjects not lose any of their fitness, they actually experienced an improvement of 20 percent. This was comparable to the control group of nonchemo subjects and may indicate that at least some chemo patients do not have to "just lie there." Maryl Winningham, exercise physiologist and director of the study, and others are very gratified by the result. In this and subsequent studies, Winningham and colleagues have found that exercise gives a psychological lift, reduces symptoms such as nausea, decreases fatigue, and improves patients' ability to continue normal day-to-day activities. She cites further evidence that the stereotype of the weak, sick cancer chemotherapy patient is not an inevitability. Dr. Winningham placed ads in *Runner's World*, *Nautilus* magazine, and *Bicycling*, asking that cancer patients who exercised contact Ohio State. She tells of the replies:

We got over two hundred and fifty responses—all ages, all types of cancers, all stages, from all over the country. These were people who said, "I am not going to sit down and die. I'm going to stay active as long as I can." One woman wrote us a letter about her husband, who was a runner. He ran on a Wednesday, entered the hospital on the next Sunday, and died on that Monday. That is not your typical picture of a cancer patient. You can carry on the fight as long as you live.

Ninety-two percent of the respondents claimed that they felt better both physically and emotionally as a result of their activity.

Dr. William Grace, chief of oncology at New York's St. Vincent's Hospital, feels:

> *Patients with cancer tend to baby themselves and they tend to get babied. It's good, I think, to emphasize that they remain very active, to emphasize their health rather than their illness. So we recommend a regular exercise program for most patients. There are people who run in races while on chemotherapy. Those high-performance folks do terrifically. People who are physically active seem to tolerate the chemotherapy. They tolerate more drugs, they have fewer side effects, and they often have a longer survival. Nobody knows why. It may be that they got more poison—but they do better.*

Recently, many fund-raising athletic events have been sponsored all over the country. For example, Race for the Cure for breast cancer—in which healthy people and cancer patients alike participate. And why not? We can't all be a Lance Armstrong, the world-class athlete who recovered from cancer and won the Tour de France, the multiday bicycle race famous for its grueling intensity—but we can emulate him at our own levels. These days it is fairly likely that you have been on some kind of exercise program before the diagnosis and treatment and would like to continue afterward. If you're an active person, you will want to remain as active as possible but may have questions about whether you should continue, what form of exercise is best, how much to do, whether it will hurt the action of the drugs or deplete the body of the energy it needs to fight the cancer and the side effects of chemotherapy. Whether you are already active or have been sedentary, you may be surprised to learn that many of the common side effects of chemotherapy can be minimized through the intelligent use of exercise.

The Benefits of Exercise

Exercise pays off in many ways before, during, and after chemotherapy. Before chemo, it can build up your strength, flexibility, energy stores, endurance, and balance and prepare you to withstand chemo better. If you are already physically active and fit before beginning chemo, you are ahead of the game. After chemo, exercise helps rebuild all of the above, improves your metabolism, normalizes your appetite, and helps your body rid itself of residual by-products of the drugs and encourages your body tissues to heal. In addition, both before and after chemotherapy, exercise is a superb tension reliever.

Perhaps most important to you is the news that regular exercise might prevent another cancer: women who exercised from one to three hours each week had a 20 to 30 percent lower risk of breast cancer, and those who worked out four or more times a week had a 60 percent lower risk than women who did not exercise. A study of men conducted at Harvard showed that frequent exercise lowered prostate cancer risk. We are not sure why this should be, but obesity and inactivity are related, and obesity is a risk factor for these cancers. Exercise may also normalize hormones because fat tissue increases production of estrogen in women and influences the length and frequency of the menstrual cycle, which may expose cells to less estrogen. Exercise also appears to reduce the incidence of colon cancer, perhaps because it speeds the rate at which food travels through the bowel. Exercise may also have an impact on prognosis once you have developed cancer. For example, researchers at the University of California at Los Angeles recently found that daily exercise, coupled with a low-fat, high-fiber diet slowed the growth rate of prostate cancer cells.

During chemo, exercise has many specific benefits, as shown in a more recent study out of Canada. In this study, 123 women undergoing adjuvant therapy for breast cancer were randomized into three groups. The control group was educated about exercise and instructed to exercise whenever they felt well enough. The self-directed group were instructed to educate on their own five times a week. The supervised group participated in a walking program led by an exercise specialist three times a week and exercised on their own twice a week. After 26 weeks, the differences in physical functioning, aerobic capacity, and body weight among the three groups were remarkable. The control group stayed the same or worsened. The supervised group and the self-directed group both increased physical functioning and aerobic capacity and lost weight, with those in the self-directed group improving the most. The lead author of the study, Roanne Segal, M.D., said, "I hope this study will change the standard of practice, which was in the past to advise patients in adjuvant therapy to rest."

INCREASE IN ENERGY

It is well known that rather than making you tired, exercise actually gives you more energy. Your muscles become stronger and more flexible; your body is able to do things with more ease and efficiency. With aerobic exercise especially, the heart and lungs get a workout. As a result, these systems are strengthened; the blood flow increases, as do the number of red blood cells that carry oxygen; and endurance improves. The more you do, the more you can do. Maryl Winningham says:

> We think the right kind of exercise helps maintain energy levels. If a person feels tired and just sits around, the enzymes that make energy in the body start going down the toilet—literally. The more you lie around, the worse you feel, and the more you lie around. People are just waiting to feel better, and they don't.

Studies show that about 70 percent of people being treated for cancer experience debilitating fatigue and loss of energy. According to a study published in 1997 and another in 1998, both aerobic exercise and weight training help improve energy—and significantly reduce pain.

A PSYCHOLOGICAL LIFT

Being physically capable and active is a positive step toward participating in your treatment and your life, especially if you have not been exercising much in the past. Regular exercise gives you a sense of vitality and physical accomplishment at the time you need it the most. It is well accepted that exercise can help you develop a clear, positive outlook.

Dr. Ward F. Cunningham-Rundles, an oncologist at Memorial Sloan-Kettering in New York who encourages many of his cancer patients to exercise regularly, reasons:

There's evidence to suggest that exercise tends to release endorphins, and that tends to make one feel better for many elaborate reasons. I also suspect that when a person exercises it tends to increase the amount of circulation to every part of the body, thus encouraging the turnover of end products from the tissues, and that tends to make one feel better.

Endorphins, the morphinelike compounds released by the brain during workouts, produce a "high" and are the body's own painkillers. With endorphins coursing through your bloodstream, you feel a sense of well-being, possibly even euphoria. Exercise can also help reduce anxiety and stress, and it provides a direct physical outlet for whatever frustrations and hostilities you may feel.

"Exercise lets cancer patients feel that they are maintaining control," says Maryl Winningham, pointing out another plus for chemo patients, "and this is of course a critical thing." The increase or maintenance in the level of self-care, independence, and economic productivity provides a real lift. In her survey, cancer patients felt that activity helped them cope with the stress of cancer and its treatment. Depression, which is one of the most common emotional states in a cancer patient, is relieved by exercise. Some doctors routinely prescribe exercise for depressed patients.

As healthy, attractive changes take place in your body and mind, you realize that your physical limitations are not what you thought they were. In addition, even a few minutes of exercise can be like a short vacation that takes your mind off cancer, chemotherapy, and how rotten you feel. One patient confesses:

I started jogging with a friend just after I stopped the chemo. I decided I had to do something to keep myself from feeling so blah. I just had no energy, and we thought that maybe jogging would help. And it did. I enjoyed it. If you stop thinking about the worst, you can do things that you didn't think you could do before—your job, keeping up with the other person. Maybe if I used my muscles a little more I wouldn't have felt so blah while I was on the chemo.

And if you indulge in sports it is especially enjoyable because of the company and because it's just plain fun.

I was a fitness nut before I got cancer, and I continued to exercise every chance I got. I wasn't up to running while on chemo, but I could swim and do calisthenics at home and at my gym. No one there except for one instructor knew I was on chemo. It was a great ego boost to see I could do just about everything that "normal" people could and in many cases even more. It made me feel less like a freak, less sorry for myself, and less that my life was a tragedy. I felt proud to be able to do as much as I did and relieved to be able to hold on to that part of the old me.

Physical exercise is an important symbol of health and vitality. If you have been exercising prior to your diagnosis and treatment, keeping physically active is an important affirmation of the continuity of your life and your lifestyle. In a time when so much may be changing, maintaining your exercise regimen as close to normal as possible assures you that your body and your life will go on and are not falling apart completely. If you can still swim laps, run around the park, dance, or touch your toes, things don't seem quite so bad.

DECREASE IN NAUSEA AND VOMITING

"Exercise seems to cause a decrease in the nausea and vomiting that chemotherapy patients suffer," says Lin Perkin. She continues:

> We haven't been able to come up with anything scientifically definitive as to the physiological mechanism, but it may be due to the fact that hypermotility in the gastrointestinal tract tends to make people more nauseated. When you exercise, blood is diverted from the digestive system and into the muscles. Since there's less action in the gut and more somewhere else, this could be one of the mechanisms of decreased nausea. Or it may just be part of the proven psychological benefits of exercise—the fact of being active, not sitting around and brooding about the way you feel, or anticipating the way you're going to feel.

Dr. Winningham says that the patients in her studies felt less nauseated within about five minutes of exercising and maintained this for the rest of the day. She suspects the improved circulation, muscle tone, and sense of achievement all play a role and cites the mind-body connection in minimizing physical and psychological stress.

I was plagued by a constant low-level queasiness for most of my time on chemo. Exercise made it better, and swimming made it vanish completely.

STIMULATION OF THE IMMUNE SYSTEM

There is evidence that vigorous exercise stimulates the immune system, possibly in many ways. This is important for the chemotherapy patient whose immune system is regularly being compromised. Some of the effects may be due to the stress-reducing ability of exercise, but this is not well documented. However, studies have shown that endurance (aerobic) exercise increases the number of circulating white blood cells in the body.

"People who exercise—particularly aerobically—tend to keep their white cells up," says Lin Perkin. She continues:

> *The count still drops, but it stays within a safer range. Not that you produce any more, but the turbulence of your blood brings them out of storage. So patients who have had a drop in their white count from chemotherapy can bring their immune systems back up by being active. This may help keep infections away and increase the effectiveness of chemotherapy by allowing the patient to accept a little more chemo, which might otherwise be held up or held back because of a low white blood cell count.*

Although there is general agreement that exercise can have a beneficial effect on the immune system and the white blood cell count, there is conflicting evidence as to the particulars and some doubt as to the implications. Maryl Winningham, for instance, points out that there is a temporary rise in the white blood cell count during and immediately following intense exercise and that patients probably should not exercise vigorously immediately before having a blood test. This could elevate the white blood cell count and result in misleading results of blood tests on which treatments are based. She cautions:

> We are unsure about how chronic exercise affects the white cell count. Our hunch is that it might help stabilize it. Studies by the Russians demonstrate instability of the white count as a result of inactivity—the count fluctuates and the cells break down. We can't say categorically that it improves the count, but we do know that a lack of exercise seems to have a negative effect.

Dr. Cunningham-Rundles says he has "every reason to believe that patients who exercise do better," but that there's some question as to the amount and duration of the exercise and its beneficial effect on the immune system. He explains:

> The situation is analogous to the relationship between alcohol and hypertension: A little bit will probably relax you a bit, but more will push your blood pressure up. In the same way, moderate exercise will likely improve immune function in many different ways. But if you've ever taken care of marathoners, you'll find they get sick all the time. The stress they put on their bodies is tremendous. It's important to get some exercise, but beyond a certain point, it uses up important body-building blocks.

OTHER BENEFITS

Exercise has many other effects on the body that should interest you before, during, and after chemo. It helps prevent osteoporosis (weakening of the bones that may accelerate because of chemo) and coronary-artery disease. It stimulates the process of digestion, absorption, metabolism, and elimination and so can help fight constipation. Recent studies suggest that exercise reduces the risk of breast and colon cancers.

It can help you sleep better on the one hand, and stimulate the brain on the other—endurance exercises may improve memory, mood, and attention span. It increases your sense of control and self-esteem, and gives you a sense of accomplishment and appreciation for your body at a time when you may not be on the best terms with it.

In addition, it is an invaluable tool for regulating weight. Many people lose weight while on chemotherapy; exercise can help you gain weight or prevent you from losing it because it can stimulate a waning appetite. Conversely, for people who gain weight from chemotherapy, activity helps prevent weight gain by burning up calories and raising your metabolism so calories are being burned even when you are not exercising. (Incidentally, Dr. Winningham comments on her study of women on chemotherapy for breast cancer: "The group as a whole did not gain any weight." In the Canadian study mentioned on page 297, women who exercised regularly lost an average of 1 to 3 pounds during the course of the study. And I didn't gain any weight, either; although I got a little bloated tummy from the prednisone, I actually lost seven pounds during chemo.) Also, exercise gives you a sense of well-being and relieves boredom, which you might otherwise be tempted to alleviate through overeating.

The Whats, Whens, and Hows of Exercise

Your exercise regimen depends on many factors, including your stage and type of cancer, the drugs and your reaction to them, your past and current fitness level, and, of course, your personal preference. No matter how weak and vulnerable you feel, you can do something that will in some way be beneficial. Cancer patients are capable of far more physical activity than most people usually assume. All that's needed sometimes is a little encouragement:

Before the chemo I used to run up to six miles a day. But while on it I couldn't run for five minutes. My husband encouraged me to try other exercise—he's the type of person who pushes to the limit, and in a lot of respects that paid off for me. I'd say to him, "What are you doing to me—I can't do this." But I accomplished a lot more than I would have. He'd say, "C'mon, you're going to go for a hike in the woods" or something like that. Physically I didn't feel any better after exercising, but psychologically I did.

It's important to rest when you need to, but unnecessary chair and bed rest results in progressive fatigue and weakness. During the first week of bed rest you lose about 3 percent of your strength each day. The longer you remain inactive, the harder it will be for you to regain strength. Even if you have been bedridden or inactive for some time, you should try to become as active as you were before the disease and its treatment took effect.

When lying in a bed, you can wiggle your toes, raise your arms and legs, sit up, do head circles, shrug your shoulders, and inhale and exhale deeply. Try the deep-breathing or the muscle-tensing/relaxing exercises in Chapter 11. Get up and walk around, even if it's just around the room. It's quite common these days to see cancer patients walking up and down hospital halls, IV pole and all. These gentle forms of activity will help you restore and maintain your bodily functions, increase your body awareness, and relax you.

With your doctor's permission, you can begin some form of exercise soon after surgery and continue during chemotherapy. A surgeon might give you recuperative exercises that relate specifically to restoring bodily function after your surgery or refer you to a physical therapist or a rehabilitation program, such as one of the ones offered to postmastectomy women at YMCAs and hospitals and through the American Cancer Society's Reach to Recovery. Women with breast cancer surgery need to ease into regular exercise and perhaps limit exercises that tax the upper body to avoid developing lymphedema, a swelling of the arm on the side of the surgery.

If you've been active, you will probably want to resume your regular regimen in some form as soon as possible. But if you're new to exercise, if you've had surgery, or if you have stopped exercising for any reason, many of the guidelines you should follow resemble those applicable to anyone who starts exercising: Start slowly, build up gradually, begin each session with a light warm-up and end with a cool-down, stop when it hurts, and

EASY DOES IT

There are many many books and videotapes on exercise for beginners or others who want to take it easy. If you haven't been exercising before chemo, or haven't been exercising for a while, try seated exercise. There are several videotapes and books of exercises you can do while safely and conveniently seated in a chair. For example:

Get Fit While You Sit by Charlene Torkelson provides a full hour of low-impact exercises.

Carol Dickman's Seated Yoga distributed by Yoga Enterprises
888-937-9642
www.stretch.com

Sitting Fit Anytime by Susan Winter Ward
800-558-9642
www.yogaheart.com

slow down when you become too winded to speak. You'll be amazed at how much you can do if you try.

For some, ordinary activities such as walking, shopping, cleaning, making the bed, climbing stairs, gardening, and playing with children might be enough. Others will want to continue or begin a more serious exercise program. There are many kinds of exercises that can improve your fitness level at all phases of your treatment, and there are dozens of books and classes. (It's wise for rookies to see a professional at first to learn the proper technique.)

Experts suggest that you do whatever you like and whatever you can manage. Jogging, alone or combined with walking, fast walking, rebounding on a trampoline, bike riding, climbing stairs, and aerobic dancing are all possibilities.

Dr. Winningham especially recommends "rhythmic walking" for cancer patients—walking briskly, arms swinging, so your whole body gets involved. In her book about the technique, she points out that it is inexpensive and requires no special clothes or equipment, except for sturdy, comfortable shoes. When the weather outside is too cold or hot or wet, look for enclosed shopping malls, many of which open early especially for people who want to walk.

After surgery or an infection, resist the temptation to begin exercising vigorously until the day after the first day you feel better. Lin Perkin also warns against taking dangerous risks involving balance, which may be off because of the drugs. Because I didn't trust my sense of balance, I avoided hopping on my beloved bicycle until after chemo was over. This was not the case with a friend of mine who fell off her bicycle and severely injured her jaw. "What if I had broken my jaw and they had to wire it shut? Can you imagine if the treatment made me throw up?" she wondered with typical chemo-induced black humor.

Both Dr. Winningham and Ms. Perkin warn that if you have metastases to the bone, high-concussive types of exercises such as running and jumping are dangerous; they recommend activities that put a minimum amount of force (from the body's own weight) on the skeleton, such as swimming, bicycling, and stretching. They also recommend modifying the usual formula for obtaining the target heart rate during aerobic exercise in some cases. Ms. Perkin says if patients are very debilitated, she begins with the figure 220, the maximum human heart rate, from which she subtracts the age, then the resting heart rate. She then multiplies by 60 or 70 percent. She finally adds in again the resting heart rate to obtain the target rate. In cardiotoxic therapies, she'll usually have patients use 50 to 60 percent rather the 60 to 70 percent in the above formula. Aim for at least thirty minutes of moderate physical activity every day.

Of course you may and should vary the intensity and frequency as needed during chemo; but this is your minimum goal once chemo is over and you are working on restoring your health and improving your level of

SPECIAL PRECAUTIONS

Check with your doctor about possible restrictions. For example, a less intensive exercise may be recommended if you are taking drugs that can be toxic to the heart or lungs or if your blood counts fall too low. Platelets below 50,000 increase the risk of bleeding, and hemoglobin below 10 deciliters precludes vigorous exercise. When white cell counts fall below 3,000, avoid crowded facilities, spas, pools, and hot tubs, which can pose a risk of infection. Stop exercising and consult your doctor if you notice exercise causes irregular heartbeat, dizziness or nausea, chest pain, leg pain or cramping, and difficulty breathing. In general, you should not exercise vigorously under the following conditions:

- Within at least twenty-four hours after having a chemotherapy treatment. You might divert the chemicals into the muscle cells, which don't normally get a large blood flow, and away from the tumor cells.
- If you have an irregular pulse. Some drugs can cause irregularities in heartbeat for hours after the treatment, which could prove dangerous during exercise.
- If your resting pulse is 100 or higher.
- If you have chest pain or feel short of breath.
- If you have nausea, fever, infection, or muscle weakness.
- If you feel dizzy or faint or nauseated when beginning to exercise.
- If you have recent and/or extreme pain in your bones, back, or neck.

fitness. In addition, you should do some sort of resistance training—most popularly known as weight lifting or weight training.

The American College of Sports Medicine guidelines recommend weight lifting or resistance training to maintain or enhance muscle strength. But because chemo can affect muscle control, gripping ability, tactile sense, and balance, this should be done using machines rather than free weights to reduce the risk of bruising or bone fractures. In addition, they recommend workouts that use low resistance and high repetition.

Many people find the practice of yoga to be particularly helpful because it systematically reduces stress and increases flexibility, mobility, and strength. There are several styles of yoga, all of which emphasize the benefits of deep breathing and some of which incorporate elements of meditation. Some forms are rather strenuous, so as with other forms of physical activity, use common sense, and refer to the general guidelines for exercise in this chapter.

Swimming is also excellent, and many chemotherapy patients report that plunging into the water feels "great." You don't have to know how to swim to reap the benefits of the water's buoyancy. Water therapy is especially useful after surgery to avoid injury and during chemotherapy, when your muscle strength is diminished. You can still safely perform movements in water that would be more difficult, and possibly injurious, on dry land. As soon as my surgeon gave me the go-ahead, I was back in the water. I began to do light water exercises and then swam a few laps. I eventually worked up to a mile, and it felt better than it ever had before. The moment I dived into the water, the nausea disappeared, and so did the rest of the world. If it were possible, I would have stayed in the pool the whole nine months of treatment.

In his book *Do Not Go Gentle,* Herbert Howe wrote that swimming in particular recharged him: "My pride in pulling against the water and rolling into a flip turn washed away any notions of defeat, dejection, and death." He remembered that Florence Chadwick, the marathon swimmer, had said, "Life in the water is less complicated."

Dr. William Grace says they often recommend the book *Royal Canadian Air Force Exercise Plans for Physical Fitness* at St. Vincent's because "the exercises start off at a very low level and build up gradually. They are also only twelve to fifteen minutes long," he points out, "and it's a very convenient way to judge progress or lack thereof. They're boring exercises, but they are good and they can be done without fancy equipment. A lot of people also walk or jog—and we recommend that."

Exercising for one hour three to four times a week is the goal in most programs, because anything less than that isn't as consistently beneficial. But if you can't attain this all the time, remember that something is better than nothing. Chemotherapy patients often have good days and bad days. When you are having a bad day, says Maryl Winningham, "do something moderate rather than nothing at all. Give your body a break."

If you are uncertain about your level of activity and there is no physical rehabilitation or exercise program at your hospital, a chemo patient's wife offers this tip: Hire a professional trainer to work with you and design two workouts—one higher-intensity workout for the days when you feel best and a second, lower-intensity one for the days when you feel less well. Although personal trainers aren't cheap, only one or two sessions are needed to set up a program, and she feels the money was well worth it.

CHAPTER TEN

Herbs, Botanicals, and Other Approaches

The complementary therapies covered in the other chapters of this book—nutritional therapy, exercise guidelines, mind-body therapies, and psychological support—may be all the help you need. Or you may want to go further and investigate the herbs and botanicals and energy-based approaches covered here. As with the other therapies, you may want to use them before, during, or after chemo. If you use them before you begin chemo, they may help to strengthen your immune and other systems. Starting them pre-chemo also allows you to establish a relationship with the practitioner early on, before you become swept up in the chemo life. During chemo, they may help you deal with side effects, protect your healthy cells, and help fight cancer themselves. After chemo, you may use them to help repair and rebalance your body and in particular restore your immune system. Many are also useful in treating any additional health problems that crop up as well as in helping with long-term side effects such as menopause symptoms or nervous system effects. Some also may help control or prevent cancer.

Although I have divided the therapies in this section into two groups—herbs and botanicals and energy-based approaches—these therapies do not always lend themselves to such strict categorization. There can be a great deal of overlap. And of course there are many more approaches other than those I have included here. Perhaps you want a more comprehensive system of complementary care and want to investigate independent, complete alternative health-care systems that incorporate both types of therapies. Many of these systems are part of a folk tradition belonging to a specific culture and present an entirely new way of seeing the world and living in it. For example, traditional Chinese medicine is an energy-based medicine that influences the life force (qi) through herbs, acupuncture, diet, exercise, and other lifestyle factors. Ayurveda means "science of life" and is the traditional healing system of India. Ayurveda includes diet, herbs, exercise, meditation, massage, breathing, and other lifestyle factors such as exposure to sunlight and moonlight. There are many other such systems including Tibetan medicine, Native American medicine, and macrobiotics.

The other therapies in this part of the book are relatively well researched and well accepted, and practitioners should be relatively easy to find. Even oncologists and cancer centers are offering these approaches. But the therapies in this chapter are less well accepted, especially in regard to cancer and combining them with conventional cancer treatment. Although some oncologists are knowledgeable about one or more of these therapies, such as herbs, it's likely you'll need to find specific practitioners outside your oncologist's office. They do not have to be medical doctors, but they should be trained, and certified or licensed, as is regulated by your state. In addition, they should be professionals who have had experience treating cancer patients who are getting chemotherapy and who can communicate with your oncologist.

Although these therapies are gentle and "natural," they can also be very powerful, and as someone who has been diagnosed with a serious disease and who has had toxic treatment, you want to work with a knowledgeable professional. The issue is not whether the therapies will interact—the question is: will they *interfere?* As naturopathic physician Dan Labriola writes in *Complementary Cancer Therapies,* "The last thing you want is for your combined therapies to interfere with each other, reducing the effectiveness of one or both. . . . The same herb that supports [one person's] cancer treatment might interfere with someone else's." Your best insurance that they will not interfere is to work with a knowledgeable professional who consults with your oncologist.

Herbs and Botanical Therapies

The practices in this category include herbal and other plant-based therapies. Herbs are used in many cultures and health systems (such as traditional Chinese medicine and European folk medicine), and many accepted conventional medicines are derived from herbs or plants. Herbs are available in many forms—tinctures or loose herbs to be made into teas, extracts, and pills. Herbalists usually make no claims that herbs can prevent or control cancer directly. Rather, these substances may generally protect and strengthen the body and help it to marshal its own healing forces. Many are excellent immune enhancers and may be valuable in particular between chemo treatments and during the aftermath. Herbs and botanicals are usually less toxic than drugs, but there can be side effects and allergic reactions. In addition, herbal preparations are not regulated in the United States and you therefore run the risk of contamination with undesirable substances (especially with Chinese herbs), and of preparations that can vary in potency unless you take a standardized form.

Herbs tend to work synergistically and therefore are rarely used individually. For example, Fu Zhen is a combination Chinese herbal treatment consisting of ginseng, astragalus, and several other herbs. In many studies, it has been shown to extend the life of people who receive it along with conventional cancer treatment. Fu Zhen is used as complementary therapy in many Chinese hospitals and has been shown to double the five-year survival rate and triple the three-year survival rate in certain cancers. Another herbal formula used in Ayruvedic medicine has also shown remarkable effects. Maharishi-4 and -5 (MAK-4 and MAK-5) have prevented cancer and caused tumor regression in animals. In other studies, patients who received Ayurvedic medicines along with chemotherapy lived two to three times long than those who received chemo alone.

An Ayurvedic formula called Amrit is continuing to be studied by Dr. Hari Sharma and researchers at the All India Institute of Medical Sciences in New Delhi. According to Dr. Sharma, whose results have not yet been published, the formula improved chemotherapy patients' overall well-being by reducing nausea, vomiting, diarrhea, insomnia, appetite loss, and fatigue. Sold by Maharishi Ayurveda Products International in Colorado Springs, Colorado, Amrit contains 44 herbs, minerals, and antioxidant vitamins. An ongoing study at the University of California at San Francisco is looking at a formula of Chinese herbs that is also designed to alleviate the side effects of chemotherapy. The lead researcher, Dr. Debu Tripathy, is a medical oncologist. "Most patients that go through chemotherapy at some point experience side effects [such as nausea and fatigue] that are not controlled by standard medications," he said in an Ivanhoe Broadcast News interview. Dr. Tripathy's team includes licensed acupuncturists and herbalists and collaborators who have chosen the herbs because they have been effective in their practices. However this is the first time the herbs are being studied formally. The study involves 60 women with early-stage breast cancer, half of whom are getting the herbal formula and half of whom are getting a placebo. The formula consists of 21 different herbs, most of which originate in China, and some of which also are traditionally used to boost the immune system. The study will not be complete until 2003, but so far the women have tolerated the herbs well and have not experienced any bad side effects.

Some herbs and botanicals used to treat cancer patients, along with their common uses, include:

- Ashwagandha: This Ayurvedic herb was studied by Indian researchers who found it improved immune system functioning in mice who were also given cyclophosphamide (Cytoxan).
- Astragalus: This herb seems to stimulate the immune system and have anticancer activity in human studies.
- Echinacea: Perhaps the most popular herb, it increases white blood cells, and is well studied for preventing and treating bacterial and viral infections. It may also have anticancer properties.

- Garlic: When eaten as part of the diet, garlic is associated with a lowered incidence of cancer, most likely due to its antioxidant abilities. It also increases white blood cells and has been shown to inhibit carcinogenic substances.
- Ginger: Fresh ginger in particular is an effective antinausea remedy.
- Goldenseal: This is another popular herb used to stimulate bone marrow to produce white blood cells. It has been shown to have antibiotic and anticancer abilities in animal studies.
- Green tea: This is primarily a potent antioxidant.
- Milk thistle: This herb is an antioxidant and in human studies has been shown to protect and help repair liver damage from many chemicals and drugs.
- Mistletoe: Many studies show that this herb has anticancer activity especially in breast cancer. It is usually administered by injection and is a popular cancer treatment in Europe.
- Mushrooms: Many mushrooms (the big three are shiitake, reishi, and maitaki) are believed to be cancer preventers, probably because of their potent antioxidant and bone marrow–stimulating abilities.
- Pau d'arco: Many anecdotes and studies suggest this herb has anticancer abilities in humans.
- Phytoestrogens: Many plants and herbs contain these plant chemicals that act like weak estrogens. The most popular sources are black cohosh, angelica, and soy. It is believed that phytoestrogens are taken up by the estrogen receptor sites on cells, and that this prevents stronger human estrogen from being taken up and stimulating cancer growth. Many foods and herbs with phytoestrogens also have antioxidants and some now theorize it may be the antioxidants, rather than the phytoestrogens, that hinder cancer. Studies using isolated phytoestrogens, without the accompanying plant constituents including antioxidants, have not had the expected results. It's possible that ingesting phytoestrogens alone might actually stimulate cancer, the same way our body's estrogen can, an effect that might be blocked by the antioxidants also present in the whole plant or food. Isolated phytoestrogen supplements and food products may not be a good idea, especially if you have estrogen-sensitive cancer.

- Siberian ginseng: This botanical is called an "adaptogen" and is used as an all-round health-building "tonic." It normalizes the functions of the body and mind—it calms them down when overstimulated and stimulates them when they are sluggish.
- Turmeric: This is a potent antioxidant; it is used as an antibiotic and studies suggest it has anticancer activity.
- Wheatgrass: Popularly taken as a juice, this herb is used to detox and fortify the body and reduce mutations in cells that might become cancerous.

Energy-Based Therapies

This group of approaches focuses on the energy field within and surrounding the body. Although the terminology and nuances differ among the various approaches, the basic principle is that a deranged life force may be at the root of the cancer and the side effects. Using energy-based medicines to restore balance and harmony to the life force helps lessen side effects and promotes the body's ability to control and fight cancer.

Some energy-based approaches seek to influence the energy by applying pressure or manipulating with the hands; others use substances such as herbs and specially prepared medicines to affect the energy quality and flow. Three popular examples are acupuncture, qi gong, and homeopathy, but there are many others.

ACUPUNCTURE

This technique is part of Traditional Chinese Medicine and seeks to manipulate your *qi* or energy flow by inserting thin needles at certain points on your body. These points lie along channels called meridians, pathways throughout your body along which the qi flows. The acupuncture points are where the meridians come closer to the surface of the body, thus allowing the needles the access to influence it. Acupuncture has been shown to be an effective treatment for chemo-induced nausea and vomiting, and for stimulating the immune system. It also is an effective pain and stress reliever. Many of these studies have been published in English, for example, in the *Chinese Journal of Integrated Traditional and Western Medicine*. The author of the definitive textbook on the subject writes: "Chinese medicine [can] minimize or control the side effects caused by radiation and chemotherapy, thus enabling the patient to complete their course of treatment more smoothly."

QI GONG

This beautiful art form is a component of traditional Chinese medicine. It combines movement, breathing, and meditation in order to enhance the flow of vital energy in the body, improve blood circulation, and enhance immune function. Qi gong can be a do-it-yourself treatment, but sometimes master qi gong practitioners use their hands and their own energy fields to affect yours.

HOMEOPATHY

This system uses extremely diluted doses of specially prepared herbs, minerals, animal tissues and products, and other substances. The treatment is highly individualized and is based on the principle that "like cures like" —the same substance that in large doses produces the symptoms of an illness in healthy people, in very minute or diluted doses will cure it in ill people. There are many homeopathic remedies on the market that people use to treat acute symptoms such as headache, insomnia, and nausea. Working with a homeopathic practitioner brings homeopathy to a new level, because they can individually prescribe more powerful doses of single or combination remedies that provide a deeper "constitutional" cure.

Bach flower remedies are a form of homeopathy that uses only flower essences and generally focuses on treating emotional states such as despair and lack of confidence. A combination flower remedy called Rescue Remedy is particularly popular for trauma and shock from a diagnosis of cancer or from surgery.

CHAPTER ELEVEN

Stress Management and Reduction

Whether stress plays a role in the development or growth of cancer is still an unanswered question. What is certain is that stress can affect your quality of life as well as the success you have in coping with cancer and its treatment. Many studies show that stress may affect our immune systems, but we don't know what effect this in turn may have on cancer. A strong immune system plays a role in controlling infections and perhaps cancer, but chemotherapy weakens our immune systems. While evidence is mounting that reducing stress may help bolster immunity, the evidence is far stronger that it may also help us tolerate the emotional and physical side effects of chemotherapy. Logic dictates, then, that we would be wise to pay attention to the negative stresses in our lives and learn techniques designed to reduce or manage stress.

But what is stress? And how can it have these effects on our well-being?

Stress can be positive or negative. Positive stress makes life interesting—it stimulates our minds and bodies to act purposefully in response to it. Positive stress occurs, we deal with it, and then it's over and we can relax and recover. Negative stress, however, increases our fears and makes us feel helpless and unable to function purposefully. Since we don't "take care of it," it's never-ending and we never relax or get the chance to recover.

As Malin Dollinger explains in her book *Everyone's Guide to Cancer Therapy*, people with cancer suffer negative stress from many sources. These include fear of dying, loss of the ability to work, pain, changes in appearance, changes in relationships, the need to make life-or-death decisions, and anxiety about the effects of cancer and chemo, such as fatigue, vomiting, and hair loss. Such stresses tend to be ongoing, and it's this unremitting negative stress that has been shown to affect many body systems, including our immune systems.

Recently a new field has emerged that studies some of the links between mind and body. This field of study is called psychoneuroimmunology (PNI), and it is dedicated to unraveling how the nervous system and the immune system communicate back and forth. While the complex interactions are mind-boggling, one key mechanism seems to be hormonal in nature. Studies have shown that the body releases "stress hormones," which in turn affect immune system responses. Hormones, for example, appear to reduce the ability of our body's natural killer cells to destroy cancer cells and control life-threatening infections. Other studies have shown that depression and anxiety make outbreaks of herpes more frequent and painful and that highly stressed people are more likely to get colds. What about cancer? A British study reported in 2001 produced rather startling results. Sixty-three patients who had either Hodgkin's disease or non-Hodgkin's lymphoma were followed for thirteen years after diagnosis, and those who practiced relaxation and hypnotherapy in addition to chemotherapy were more likely to survive than those who got only chemotherapy. These results need to be confirmed by more studies, but they do have important implications for all cancer patients.

In one of his movies Woody Allen said, "I can't express anger. That's one of the problems I have. I grow a tumor instead." While the neurotic character was joking (I think) and few scientists would subscribe to such a direct connection, fewer still would insist that the mind doesn't exert any influence on the body. Stress is widely acknowledged to contribute to many illnesses; estimates indicate that from 50 to 80 percent of illnesses are linked to stress. Fortunately, there are many stress-reduction techniques that have proven track records and are being used with increasing frequency by people undergoing chemotherapy.

Getting a Handle on Stress

Basically there are two things you can do to relieve stress. First, you can try to remove as much stress as possible. Second, you can try to learn how to deal with the necessary stress in a positive way. In order to accomplish either of these tasks, you must first be able to discern exactly what it is that is creating the stress. Sometimes just becoming aware of stress can begin to help; then you take it seriously and figure out ways to deal with it. Saying you are afraid of "cancer" or "chemotherapy" is not specific enough. For instance, if you are concerned about your prognosis, speak to your doctor, who may be able to help get your concerns more in line with reality so the unknown becomes known as much as possible. If you are afraid of being alone during treatments or afterward, ask a family member or close friend to stay with you. If you feel uncomfortable because you've lost all your hair, make the effort to find a natural-looking wig.

Emotional counseling, discussed in the next chapter, is another avenue to explore. With professional guidance, you can begin to fight back. Instead of bottling up frustrations and tensions and leaving them to bubble up inside, letting them out and letting go can reduce the harm that chronic tension can do. Feelings that are repressed or denied during treatment often crop up later as post-treatment depression. And you can help your body withstand stress better by maintaining general health—getting adequate nutrition, avoiding cigarettes, limiting your intake of coffee and alcohol and other drugs, and getting enough rest and exercise.

MIND-BODY TECHNIQUES

Another way to cope with stress is through specific stress-management/reduction techniques. Eastern medicine and philosophy have long recognized that the mind and the body are one and that people have the potential to control their minds and, through them, their bodies. This interrelationship between mind and body and the techniques used to exploit it have only recently begun to be appreciated by Western medicine. Though these techniques can be used by anyone, many of them are now being developed specifically and used as adjuvant treatments to relieve the physical and emotional side effects of cancer and chemotherapy.

These techniques, which range from simple relaxation methods to more advanced "mind-control" practices, include biofeedback, meditation, controlled deep breathing, progressive muscle relaxation, self-hypnosis, and creative imagery or visualization. Although they are relaxing, this form of relaxation is active. You do not merely sit back passively and do nothing. Therapists usually combine two or more into a unique package, in accordance with their style, training, and preferences and the requirements and abilities of the patient. Often the simpler techniques serve as stepping-stones for the more advanced methods. (In addition, there may be a psychotherapeutic element involved.)

Matthew Loscalzo, a social worker at Memorial Sloan-Kettering in New York who is trained in these techniques, stresses the importance of using an integrated approach:

Some people feel that self-hypnosis is a strong enough tool to use by itself to reach many goals. I do not share that view. I never do only one thing: Hypnotherapy is only part of my overall treatment plan. The issues going on are much too important and complex. We need to carefully tailor our treatments to meet the specific needs of our patients and their significant others.

Regardless of the name or level, such techniques are all based on the ability of the mind to directly control many of the bodily processes that the Western way of thinking has traditionally thought to be involuntary. These techniques "train" your mind to focus on your body with a minimum of distractions. Your mind becomes focused and relaxed, yet alert and aware. These techniques take time to learn, to use, and to show results. We don't know exactly why or how they work; and they do not work for everyone or always work to the same extent. But in many cases where drugs have failed to work their magic, and without adding any harmful side effects of their own, these techniques are achieving results in reducing stress and controlling the symptoms and side effects of cancer and chemotherapy. They have successfully reduced or eliminated anxiety, tension, insomnia, nausea, vomiting, diarrhea, lethargy, depression, feelings of helplessness and hopelessness, and pain in chemotherapy patients. They have increased patients' feelings of well-being, relaxation, and control over their lives.

DEEP BREATHING

This is a simple technique that you can do on your own, and is a good place for the novice to begin. It actually relaxes your muscles and can slow down your heartbeat, lower your blood pressure, and increase blood flow to your hands and feet. Matthew Loscalzo, who lectures and trains others in hypnosis, feels that slow or rhythmic breathing is especially helpful when you need to gain a sense of self-control quickly:

> *An example is with uncontrollable crying. It's amazing. The tears actually do stop flowing. The person will still feel the appropriate feelings of fear or sadness but will experience a greater sense of self-control and will stop crying. This in turn has an effect on one's self-esteem. All people need to feel they can maintain self-control, not just cancer patients. This in no ways means that people should not cry, which is a healthy and desirable human response, but rather that there are times when people need to control their emotions.*

Such a time may be during a meeting with your doctor, when you need to ask specific questions and listen to the answers. You can't do this if you're crying. Another example might be during a diagnostic test. I remember that during my bone scan I was sobbing so uncontrollably that it was interfering with the imaging. Perhaps if I had done deep rhythmic breathing, I could have controlled myself long enough to complete the test rather than having to come back again later in the day. Still another instance might be during a counseling session. As Mr. Loscalzo points out, "Sometimes these are the only times that people can cry, and we encourage them to do that. But if they can only cry, they can't get to what their fears and sadness are about."

To do deep breathing, sit or lie down in a comfortable position, preferably in a quiet place where you won't be disturbed for a while. Close your eyes. Place your hand over your abdomen and inhale through the nose, slowly, to the count of four, while puffing up your stomach and letting your diaphragm expand and the air travel up to the chest, back, and shoulders, and imagine it filling your entire body. When you feel as full of air as you can be, hold it a second. Then slowly, to the count of four, exhale through the mouth and feel the tension drain out of you along with the air. Repeat this, gradually slowing down the inhalation and exhalation to a count of ten and holding it for ten.

Mr. Loscalzo warns that if you do this incorrectly, you might hyperventilate. "Breathing too fast can make a person scare themselves more." He emphasizes that "the breathing needs to be slow and rhythmic so the brain gets the message that it's safe."

PROGRESSIVE MUSCLE RELAXATION

This technique has been around since the 1930s, when Dr. Edmund Jacobson, a psychophysiologist, developed it. Since then many variations have evolved, but they are all basically a way of systematically relaxing the body by alternately tensing and relaxing individual parts of it. It is easier to relax something that has been made very tense first: Using the principle of extremes, you first get to know how it feels to be really tense, then let go completely and thus get to know how it feels to be really relaxed. Here is an abbreviated form of progressive muscle relaxation you might want to try:

To do progressive muscle relaxation, lie or sit down (lying is best) in a comfortable position, wearing comfortable, loosened clothing. A quiet room where you won't be disturbed is preferable. Close your eyes and become aware of your body and your breath. You should breathe deeply, easily, and rhythmically throughout the exercise. Focus on your right foot and flex your toes back really hard; hold it this way for a few seconds and then let it go completely limp and relaxed. Work up your right leg by tensing each muscle group and then letting it go completely, making note of and enjoying the difference between the two sensations. Then do your left foot and leg. Then the hips, waist, back, chest, hands and arms, shoulders, neck, and scalp. Move to your face, open your mouth wide, raise your eyebrows, stare with wide open eyes. Next, scrunch your face and purse your lips as if you had just tasted something sour—and then completely relax those muscles. Stretch your arms overhead, point your toes, and stretch and tense every single muscle in your body at one time. Then relax. Return your focus to your breathing, gradually open your eyes, and bring your awareness back to your surroundings.

CREATIVE VISUALIZATION

Various forms of visualization have been used for many years in conjunction with hypnosis and relaxation to treat many ailments, complaints, and undesirable habits–pain, fears, overeating, and smoking. During visualization, you first enter a deeply relaxed state and then create a mental picture of a desired goal or outcome. Overweight people, for example, picture themselves as thin. When cancer patients use visualization, they often imagine their cancer cells as weak and confused, their treatment and white blood cells as destroying the cancer cells, and their bodies as recovering and being healthy.

Medical doctors, nurses, psychiatrists, psychologists, and social workers use visualization, usually after their patients have learned other relaxation techniques as a tool. A biofeedback technician told me that she begins with an education component. She explains to patients that chemotherapy is a stressful situation and helps them understand the way they are perceiving and reacting physically to the treatment. She uses biofeedback to measure the physical effects and point them out to the patients. Then she teaches them breathing and progressive relaxation, which they practice at home three times a day. "Once I see a patient is doing a lot of home practice and can really relax the body, I add visualization." She then uses visualization three ways:

I use it for rehearsal. The patients envision themselves getting the therapy, it coming into their bodies and killing the cancer cells. I have them picture themselves going through the treatment, feeling good, calm, relaxed, and in control. They feel themselves participating in their treatment process, seeing themselves healthy. We can start this a few days before the therapy is administered and then do it during the chemotherapy treatment itself, actually visualizing the drugs killing the confused cancer cells.

I also use it for manipulation, for pain reduction. I teach them how to manipulate pain by using some kind of symbol. For instance, they may assign a color and shape to areas of the body that are feeling pain; then the pain-free parts are assigned a light blue soothing color that gradually creeps into the colors where they feel the pain, slowly shrinking and easing the pain.

Finally, I use visualization as a minivacation. They visualize a safe, comfortable place that they enjoy going to and can relax in. Taking a vacation away from where you're at will create a relaxation response.

One patient describes her experiences with these techniques, which she became interested in because of her anxiety and nausea:

I felt kind of silly at first. It's a crazy thing to imagine your own cancer cells and create your own army of white cells to fight them. But believe it or not, you are able to visualize these things. As we get older, maybe we're stupid not to do things that are silly. Maybe we become too realistic.

I think the thing with this is it gives you a sense of control of yourself. It's like your own personal chemotherapy. It's something you can do for yourself. I think it is also a way of letting out hostilities. It takes me twenty-five minutes every day and it's hard to find the time to do it, but it's very relaxing and I feel such a sense of well-being. Even though I'm off chemo now, I'm continuing to do it.

Some proponents of visualization believe that the mind can actually control the cancer. There is no real proof of this in the form of the controlled studies that scientists have been trained to go by; there are only anecdotal material and uncontrolled studies. While the thought that we have the power within us to control our own minds and bodies to such an extent as to influence the course of our illness is an exhilarating one, it can also be frightening in its implications.

Critics of this view say it implies we somehow caused the disease in the first place. As Susan Sontag writes in *Illness as Metaphor*, it manages to "put the onus of the disease on the patient." This is "preposterous," she says; it is a punishment, a moralistic view of the disease. It seems to me that once you become sold on the idea that you have caused and can therefore "uncause" your cancer, you become solely responsible for your disease. Under these conditions, it may be more devastating when there is a setback. If the cancer is not controlled, it follows that you alone are guilty of failure, or weakness, of a lack of faith, of having the "wrong" feelings, of wanting to die no matter how much you really want to live—a tremendously unfair additional burden for a cancer patient to have to bear.

Matthew Loscalzo says, "I do visualization and all that stuff. The literature shows that white blood cell counts can be raised through these techniques, and I'm comfortable with that. But I'm very skeptical of people who take people's money and say they are curing cancer."

Of the many therapists who are trained in these techniques, few would go so far as to say that visualization alone can control cancer. Most use it in conjunction with other therapies, including conventional therapies such as chemotherapy, because it helps their patients feel more in control over their lives and because it helps them tolerate the therapy better and come to have faith in it as a friend, not an enemy.

RELAXATION TAPES

There are now many different audiocassette tapes designed specifically to help you relax. They may contain specific instructions for entering a relaxed state, usually some variation of progressive relaxation or visualization. Some, rather than being formal "relaxation tapes," are just recordings of pleasant music, natural sounds such as the ocean or rain or birds, or a combination of both.

"People use tapes for running and working out but don't think of using them for chemotherapy," says Rosemary Moynihan. "Yet developing a reverie from sound can be very helpful to people. It can help you center yourself, relax, sleep." You can try using tapes during the actual chemo treatment, during a hospital stay, or in the privacy of your own home.

Most experts feel it's ideal to have a tape individually made for you by a therapist. The images and sounds will be those you associate with feeling safe and comfortable, and the voice will belong to someone you have met. But this isn't always possible. Ready-made tapes are available from some cancer support organizations, through mail order, and at music stores, yoga schools, health-food stores, bookstores, drugstores, and libraries.

MEDITATION

In general, meditation aims to focus your attention inward by concentrating or reflecting on (meditating upon) the steady rhythm of your breathing or on a single object, thought, word, or sound. When you focus your concentration so intently, your body relaxes and your mind calms down and as a result, you feel a sense of well-being that can be quite profound.

Most forms of meditation are done while in a seated position, but there are also moving forms of meditation, such as tai chi, walking meditation, and qi gong, and the Japanese martial art aikido. Yoga can also be a type of moving meditation.

In the United States, transcendental meditation (TM) has been the most popular; in this form, you repeat a mantra such as "om" silently to calm your mind. Another form called mindful meditation, in which you focus your attention on the thoughts and sensations of the moment, is catching on rapidly.

Western science has shown that meditation has deep and measurable relaxing effects that are inherently pleasant and useful. Based on these studies, the National Institutes of Health (NIH) National Center for Complementary and Alternative Medicine reports that regular meditation can help you live longer and improve your quality of life. It can reduce chronic pain, anxiety, high blood pressure, cholesterol, health-care use, substance abuse, posttraumatic stress syndrome in Vietnam veterans, and blood cortisol levels initially brought on by stress. Studies show that meditation can lower respiration, lower the levels of certain stress hormones, and of the hormone DHEA, high levels of which are associated with breast cancer, heart disease, and osteoporosis. Meditation is one of several relaxation methods approved by an independent panel, convened by the National Institutes of Health, as a useful complementary therapy for treating chronic pain and insomnia. It may also improve immune functioning and enhance fertility. People who meditate regularly also say it improves their mood, increases mental efficiency and alertness, and raises self-awareness, which contributes to relaxation.

According to a Canadian study published in 2000, mindfulness meditation has been shown to help cancer patients reduce stress-related symptoms such as anxiety, depression, anger, fatigue, and confusion. After seven weeks of meditation, those who meditated reduced stress-related symptoms by 31 percent (compared with the control group's 11 percent), and their mood improved by 65 percent (compared with the control group's 12 percent improvement).

There are many other schools of meditation. You can learn how to meditate on your own, through studying books or listening to tapes. Or you can be guided by meditation instructors, doctors, psychiatrists, other mental-health professionals, and yoga masters.

BIOFEEDBACK

Some people have difficulty mastering the specific relaxation techniques on their own. To effect these changes, you learn to relax by trial and error, a process that takes considerable time, effort, and patience. In many cases, biofeedback is the first step in a total therapeutic package that utilizes a combination of several techniques. When you are under stress, your body reacts in several ways—muscles tense up, blood vessels constrict, blood pressure goes up, hand temperature goes down, and so on. Biofeedback (short for biological feedback) is a way of measuring and monitoring these bodily processes and feeding this information back to you visually or aurally so you can see or hear it. But having a direct line to your physiological responses is only a beginning. While you are hooked up to the machinery, the idea is to learn how to follow its signals and thus voluntarily change them.

HYPNOSIS

Sleeping and daydreaming are two altered states of consciousness; we enter these naturally and frequently. Hypnosis is thought to be an altered state, too—one that has been used in some form for many years. Lately, it has been increasingly used by the medical profession and related professions for a number of reasons, often to relax patients before anxiety-producing procedures, as drugless anesthesia, and as a means of controlling acute and chronic pain and discomfort. You can also use it for purposes related directly to chemotherapy. One patient told me, "The self-hypnosis helped me stop the anticipatory anxiety and vomiting; it also eliminated the metallic taste in my mouth from the drugs. The doctor tried to help me control the nausea after the chemotherapy, but that he couldn't do. I think that's because I didn't believe in it as much as I should have."

Matthew Loscalzo feels that though "this technique is becoming increasingly utilized, a lot of people still have a lot of ignorance and misconceptions about hypnosis. People fear that the hypnotist has power over the patient, rather than it being an extension of some everyday normal processes, such as daydreaming or fantasy. There is always a part of the self which is observing and protecting, regardless of the depth of the trance."

A hypnotist helps us enter the trance and may then go on to train us in self-hypnosis so we are no longer so dependent on the skills and time of another person. The hypnotic state has been compared to a meditative trance—both are valuable sources of relaxation and lead to a sense of well-being. But hypnosis is more than entering a relaxed state—it is a goal-oriented technique used to focus on specific problems that are usually stress-related. Self-hypnosis increases self-control. It is generally agreed that when a person is in a deeply relaxed state, he or she is more open to "suggestion"—the introduction of a believable idea, thought, or image into a person's mind. As Matthew Loscalzo continues:

Hypnosis is somewhat like a meditation technique. If people already know how to meditate, my work is half-done. I ask them to put themselves into a meditative trance, and we do the work in that state. But a trance itself doesn't do the work. It does nothing but put you in a relaxed state, which creates a medium for communication. Being in a relaxed state is not necessarily therapeutic in itself. It's a technique or a tool, or a way of thinking about treatment, it's not therapy.

Hypnosis and related techniques such as relaxation and desensitization help some patients cope with some of the side effects of chemotherapy and with some of the medical procedures that usually go along with it. Hypnosis can counteract conditioned aversions (such as anticipatory vomiting, which occurs before a chemotherapy treatment), posttreatment nausea and vomiting, phobic reactions (such as fear of a hypodermic or intravenous needle), acute or chronic anxiety (such as that surrounding a treatment or procedure or surrounding the diagnosis of cancer), and some types of acute and chronic pain. It can also be used to relieve depression by overcoming the "learned helplessness" common to many patients and imparting a generalized sense of self-control.

MASSAGE

A good massage is therapeutic for both the mind and the body. It is relaxing, it stimulates the circulation, it releases the joints, and it soothes away tension accumulated in the muscles. Massage is a particularly useful, though temporary, way of easing the discomfort of a particular physical problem, of physical exercise, or of everyday living. Though massage is not a cure, it can relieve aches and pains and thus reduce or eliminate the need for some medications.

Denver Presbyterian's Pam Felling says, "A lot of people in the cancer ward have a masseuse come in from outside. It is offered to them for relaxation, pain relief, improvement of circulation—all the normal things that massage is good for. They get the same benefits that anyone would— they're not that different."

One possible difference is the danger of massage spreading a cancer, a question that is brought up in massage textbooks. About this possibility, Lin Perkin says:

With really deep massage in the area of a tumor, you can actually physically break off tumor cells into the increased circulation. It used to be thought that the increased circulation itself was carrying off more tumor cells, but now doctors are using hyperthermia in conjunction with chemotherapy and rather than spread the cancer, the increased circulation enhances the effects of the drugs. So it's more the mechanical effects of massage that are dangerous. I don't think a light massage would do any harm; nor would a massage that avoids the area of the tumor or in cases where the tumor has been removed.

Concerned patients should still check with their oncologists to determine whether massage should be light or deep. Massage should not be painful, although in shiatsu the sensation has been described as "a good hurt." Communicate with the masseur or masseuse, too—let the therapist know whether you can tolerate only light stroking or a rubdown or whether you want something with more "oomph."

Your hospital may offer therapeutic touch (TT), as well as traditional forms of massage. Studies have shown that TT can cut the need for painkilling narcotics after surgery, speed healing, and possibly boost the immune system. There are now over thirty thousand practitioners in the United States, Canada, and dozens of other countries, and it is taught in more than eighty American universities.

Massage therapy is available from professionals whose skills and manners vary; some states require licensing to ensure a certain level of ability. Your doctor, nurse, or social worker may know of a practitioner or may refer you to a physical therapist who can give you a medical massage. When a massage is given by a family member or friend—no matter how amateur or brief—it can be a reassuring form of physical and emotional communication that closes any gaps between caring and doing. As one patient said, "Massage is one of the nicest things one person can do for another."

OTHER THERAPIES

There are many other therapies, disciplines, and practices that cancer patients have found help them cope with the mental and physical stresses of chemotherapy. Body work such as yoga and exercise, (in Chapter 9) are one type. Creative or expressive therapies such as dance therapy, music therapy, and art therapy are another—these enable people to be expressive in nonverbal ways. "People can be inhibited verbally—they can't talk about what's going on inside them," says M. L. Frohling. "But they can feel it. They might be able to move or draw and express it that way. When they do express it in some form, there is a sense of completeness and relaxation."

Music can be quite therapeutic, and is being offered as an option to cancer patients at a growing number of medical facilities all over the country. Soothing classical and/or harp music is often used in conjunction with the relaxation techniques described earlier to make chemotherapy treatments more bearable, to help patients sleep, or to ease anxiety in general. A lung cancer patient who discovered music early during the course of her very difficult therapy said using her small cassette player and earphones during and after each treatment got her over the roughest spots.

Music has indeed been shown to have direct effects on the mind and body, although we're not yet sure exactly how. Music can generate feelings of serenity and relaxation, cheerfulness and excitement, or gloom and melancholy; it can conjure up all sorts of mental images; it can affect our blood volume, our heart rate, and our blood pressure. Because it can affect us so powerfully, choose your playlist carefully. You may want to follow the advice of most music therapists, who recommend that people with medical problems work with professionals who will teach you how to use music specifically to reduce your perception of discomfort and create a positive state of mind.

A wonderful pilot study, published in 1996 in *Cancer Nursing*, confirms the power of music plus the voice of the patient's physician. Half of the participants received a tape of music and a message from their physicians during their chemotherapy treatments. After the fourth treatment, researchers found a significant difference between the levels of anxiety

PURE PLEASURE

Feeling pleasure is an important part of life, especially when you're undergoing something as unpleasant as chemotherapy. Yet it's easy to forget about pursuing pleasure when you're caught up in the whirlwind of treatments and its side effects. It may seem frivolous at a serious time. But experiencing pleasure helps restore a much-needed balance to your life and offers a well-needed break from chemo-related routines and stresses.

As Robert Ornstein and David Sobel show in their book *Healthy Pleasures,* feeling good not only enriches our lives, it can also extend them. "The human desire for enjoyment evolved to enhance our survival," they write. "What better way to assume that healthy, life-saving behaviors occur than to make them pleasurable?" The book then goes on to document how small, simple pleasures and "stolen moments" help absorb the everyday stresses of life, making them easier to bear. So go ahead and enjoy such healthy pleasures as a walk in the park, a hug, tasty food, a movie or a play, a good book, a fun game, collecting, creating, and immersing yourself in a favorite hobby.

A positive attitude, a will to live, optimism, and a fighting spirit are crucial elements in your treatment. Even though the part they play in actually fighting cancer is still uncertain and relatively minor, the part they play in your desire and ability to tolerate debilitating treatment may be major. A positive outlook that makes you feel more relaxed and in control will improve the quality of your life no matter how much time you have left. How much better it is to face everything with hope and equanimity than with helplessness and despair.

before and after the patients got the tapes, but the level of anxiety in the group who did not get the tape did not improve. The authors conclude that this is a simple and cost-effective way to decrease a patient's anxiety when getting chemotherapy.

Laughter therapy is a new addition to the menu of stress-reducing techniques. The idea may make you laugh, but laughter is one of the best coping mechanisms there is. Norman Cousins put laughter therapy on the map with his well-known book *Anatomy of an Illness,* which chronicles his use of humorous books, old episodes of *Candid Camera,* and old Marx Brothers movies to help him recover from a crippling degenerative disease.

There's nothing funny about having cancer, but we can still laugh at the world. Sometimes we can even laugh at ourselves or appreciate the absurdities involved with our disease and our treatment. It's hard to imagine laughing when you've been throwing up for three hours straight and know you'll be doing the same thing every two weeks for the next year, when you're so weak that you can barely drag yourself out of bed, when you're so pale and bald that even you don't want to be seen with you. And yet patients do find it within themselves to laugh. These things are so awful that people need to laugh—as an escape, as a defense, and as a release of tension. Patients often joke about looking like Kojak or majoring in advanced toilet bowl or how they might get arrested because their arms look like a junkie's. As one patient says, "It doesn't seem so awful when you laugh about it."

Your oncologist's attitude can encourage or discourage a healthy sense of humor about your situation. I sometimes spent more time joking and laughing than being treated. My doctor said I had the same type of humor you usually find in an oncologist. Dr. Charles Vogel of the Comprehensive Cancer Center for the state of Florida likens the atmosphere on some oncology services to that of the M*A*S*H unit of film and TV fame. Los Angeles oncologist Dr. Michael Van Scoy-Mosher is a firm believer in the value of laughter for his patients:

I think humor can be used—not that this isn't serious—but I found there's a real place for seeing it in an almost absurdist way. This view can be very useful. I remember, for example, I was treating a guy with a real sickening therapy for Hodgkin's disease. He happened to see me one day out in a store. The moment he saw me and his eyes met mine, he threw up. We both understood, but of course, nobody else in the store understood—they just saw this weird guy come in, throw up, and leave. We had a good laugh about it later.

Scientists actually have an explanation as to why laughter does us so much good. When you laugh, many parts of your body contract—your chest, abdominal muscles, diaphragm, and lungs. Your systolic blood pressure soars, your pulse rate can double, adrenaline is pumped into your blood, and endorphins (the body's natural painkillers) may be released. A good belly laugh is like a mini workout, an internal jogging. Afterward, everything goes back to normal or slightly below, which results in a release of tension and an all-around feeling of well-being.

CHAPTER TWELVE

Emotional Support

Beginning with the diagnosis and continuing throughout and after treatment, you need to make many psychological adjustments. Your new life has brought with it both intangible emotional reactions and concrete problems. Though many patients (and their families) manage somehow to cope well enough on their own, there is no reason not to call upon the many services and therapies that have been designed to make the coping process easier.

Ordinary life certainly has its stresses, and cancer and its treatment add more stress to the brew. Getting emotional support is one important way to deal with chemo-related stress. Some people believe that anything that helps reduce stress may also extend the life of a cancer patient. While this specific effect has not been proved, studies have suggested that stress can affect the immune system and thus perhaps can influence the course of a disease such as cancer. (The previous chapter discusses this and the many ways you can improve your quality of life using stress-reduction/relaxation techniques.)

Like the other support services for cancer patients, the field of psychosocial oncology, which deals with the way the patient and family react to the disease and its treatment, is fairly new. Grace Christ, the former director of social work at New York's Memorial Sloan-Kettering and editor of the *Journal of Psychosocial Oncology*, says, "It's taken time for people to appreciate some of the psychosocial consequences of cancer and its treatments. But as cancer patients live longer and the disease becomes long-term or chronic, or one from which people are cured, the social and emotional effects become much more visible."

Family and Friends as Support

Today, we may think "family" traditionally, in the sense of blood relatives. More likely, though, our "family" may be or include a circle of close friends.

Studies have shown that people who have strong relationships or support systems—whether family or friends—usually do better than those who go through it alone.

In his book *Living with Cancer*, Dr. Ernest Rosenbaum points out that as the traditional concept of the passive patient is becoming old hat, so is the idea that the family is an outside element. Both patient and family or close friends are able to contribute immeasurably to cancer care. He writes: "Having the family 'wait outside' wastes a great deal of valuable energy that could be available as additional 'people power' to facilitate a patient's recovery. Also, many family members need to do something to actively contribute to the patient's getting-well process."

How the family handles the crisis of cancer and chemotherapy usually depends on how well the family has functioned in the past. Good relationships often get even better. Many cancer patients report a learning, growing experience that brings them closer to their spouses, other family members, and friends.

You can let your friends and family know when their help is welcome in practical matters such as child care, cooking, shopping, phone calls, housework, and other errands and domestic chores. They can encourage healthful activities and low-key diversions such as taking a walk; going for a drive; taking in a movie, museum, or play; and visiting others or—keeping your physical limitations in mind—more strenuous activities such as swimming or bike riding. They can improve your sense of well-being through massage. They can act as researchers—by asking questions, writing letters, or going to the library—if you want additional information about your disease and its treatment.

Loved and loving family members often provide moral support and the motivation to continue treatment when one's own will falters:

Sometimes I didn't want to go for the chemo. Just as I was getting my system back together, it was time to go back for another treatment. My twenty-one-year-old daughter was with me through it all. When I got a little weak and didn't want to go, that little stinker said, "You'd better go and have those treatments because if I ever got breast cancer and I needed chemo, I'd go. But if you don't finish your treatments, Mom, I'm not going either." Blackmail! But she kept me going.

I don't know how many nights I spent sitting on the floor in the bathroom, my head bent over the toilet bowl, my husband patting my head, and my saying to him, "I'm quitting it. I've had enough. I don't need it. I don't want it." I might have quit—if I didn't have someone there stroking me saying, "You're going to be okay. You're going to see this through. You know you can. You know you have to."

Family members can help by accompanying you to the facility when you go for a checkup or a treatment. Having someone come along during a question-and-answer session or during a treatment is a simple yet important step in their understanding the treatment and lending their support.

Sometimes I'd feel so alone and vulnerable sitting in my doctor's waiting room and later on the bus ride home that I'd ask my husband to come with me. It wasn't that I felt sick after my shot or that I couldn't get home on my own. Sometimes I was just frightened and it felt good just having him there, holding my hand, or just reading magazines together while we waited. Once a friend asked me if I wanted her to go with me. I knew she was torn up over my having cancer and hated the fact that she couldn't do anything about it. I think she was just plain curious about the chemo, too. So even though it didn't make the cancer or the chemo go away, she came along. She felt better, and so did I.

And yet obstacles often prevent family and friends from living up to their full potential as helpers—the patient won't let them, or they don't know how, or they are having too much trouble coping themselves to help the patient cope. Cancer patients have said that a lack of communication within the family is one of the major problems they face in coping with their disease and its treatment. Of course communication is going to suffer if your family members find it difficult to discuss your illness, your treatment, and your prognosis. It's normal to be reluctant to face the unpleasant, and to want to protect one another. Furthermore, cancer and its treatment cause massive shifts in responsibilities, roles, and life patterns in addition to emotional upheavals. It is tempting for the family to focus exclusively on the patient's disease, so that friendships fade away and hobbies and interests fall by the wayside. Or they may feel that since you are in the hands of your doctors, there is nothing they can do. You may have trouble balancing a desire to assert your independence with the real need for help and the desire to let others feel useful.

Mimi Greenberg, a psychologist who specializes in counseling women with breast cancer, has written a book called *Invisible Scars*. In it, she advises that you ask yourself these key questions before reaching out to a family member:

- What has my history been with this person? (Has my husband, wife, mother, father, sister, or brother been able to support me emotionally during other times of crisis?)
- Are my expectations of the person realistic? (Am I asking too much or not enough?)
- Is this person "cancerphobic"? (And likely to hurt me by running away or being distant?)
- How does this person react to stress? (Will he or she be calm and reassuring or add to the stress and calamity?)
- Does this person encourage me to do the talking while he or she listens empathetically without interrupting or giving advice?
- When asked, will this person provide objective, sound advice?
- Will this person maintain my confidences and refrain from discussing my problems with others?

Support Outside the Family

Some families are able to solve their own problems and adapt to the new situation easily. But many others could benefit from some kind of assistance in adjusting to the new reality before they can effectively help one another. If help is not offered and you feel you and your family could use some assistance in getting back on the right track, ask for it. Meeting with your oncologist, oncology nurse, a social worker, a family therapist, or a family-oriented support group can make great strides in educating your family unit, helping its members communicate and sort out their feelings and realize they are normal, and encouraging them to develop their own coping strategies.

The idea of emotional counseling for the cancer patient and family has met with resistance from professionals and patients alike. On the patient's side, old taboos die hard: There is still some stigma attached to admitting that you might need a little help with your emotional problems. A social worker told me:

> *People tend, in our culture especially, to underappreciate the impact of the disease and the treatment. We tend to be a bit stoical in general and don't really understand how much we're being affected. Talking to someone, or using some outside help, doesn't mean we're weak, it doesn't mean we're coping poorly. It means we'd like to cope better, and this is one way to do that. Most people manage to cope reasonably well. But sometimes you can cope better and your whole experience can be of a different quality.*

Lari Wenzel, medical psychologist at The Long Beach Memorial Medical Center, says:

> *It is not unusual for people to have a need for support services during a time that is particularly stressful, regardless of what that stress is. Cancer as a chronic disease introduces particular stressors to the individual's life. Even people who normally handle stress well can*

*use a little help with problems that may arise as a result of this di-
agnosis.*

The whys and hows of getting information are discussed more fully in
Chapter 4. But this approach also bears mentioning here because we have
an emotional as well as practical need for information. Don't be afraid to
ask questions of your health-care team. Some people find that using books
and the information they contain helps them cope; in fact, the term "bib-
liotherapy" was coined to describe this option.

It's a good sign that community hospitals, agencies, and large medical
centers are sponsoring more and more educational conferences and workshops geared specifically to cancer patients and their families. I have been
a presenter at several and have found them to be excellent sources of information as well as an opportunity to meet other people who are going
though similar experiences. There are also an increasing number of individual classes and lectures that your health-care team or a community
agency should be able to refer you to.

Your oncologist, family doctor, or nurse may be able to help you and
your family get over some of the emotional hurdles you will face and perhaps all of them. However, physicians are often unaware of their patients'
need for emotional support; as patients, we want our doctors to be more
"human," but we are often reluctant to tell doctors about our emotional
needs. We may try to look like exceptional copers, afraid doctors will think
our emotions are too trivial. In addition, most doctors and nurses are not
trained as counselors or therapists. You may find yourself turning elsewhere for additional emotional support.

When shopping around for emotional assistance, be as choosy as when
looking for medical help. Some professionals are more skilled or have had
more experience with cancer patients than others, and some approaches
may be more comfortable for you than others. One bad or unproductive experience should not discourage you or prevent you from seeking another
more understanding or suitable source of therapy, as happened in my case.

The only person I spoke to about my cancer was the Reach to Recovery lady who just popped into my hospital room a few days after the mastectomy. She was so stiff and formal, I couldn't identify with her at all. She

just left me a ball, a booklet, a bra, and a boob made out of polyester. Sure, she wore a tight sweater to let me know that it is possible to look "normal" after a mastectomy. But she came before I was really ready to see anyone; I was still too shocked to think straight and ask questions. When I visited the Reach to Recovery office to look at prostheses, they were so grim about the whole thing. Maybe I'm nuts, but I saw some humor in opening up a whole filing cabinet drawer full of breasts. I wanted to talk to someone, but I knew I didn't want to talk to *them.*

I've since talked to many women who have had much more positive experiences with Reach to Recovery volunteers. Sometimes a successful match depends on location (as in any field, American Cancer Society chapters vary in style), or it could depend on timing and individual "chemistry."

Reach to Recovery did refer me to a prosthesis shop whose manager and salesperson had both had mastectomies many years earlier. Although neither had had chemo, both were wonderful women with whom I had an instant rapport. I and the friend who had accompanied me ended up spending hours there, having a terrific time, gabbing and laughing and trying on bras and breasts.

Grace Christ feels that "people should not hesitate to seek help. I think it can't hurt, even if it is just to stabilize yourself. But it's not always as accessible as it should be." Part of the problem, she feels, is that in the past people tended to think that support for cancer patients was either straight education—giving information—or intensive psychotherapy. Though it can include both of these, today psychosocial support comes in a wide variety of flavors (or "interventions"). Whatever your tastes and your needs, there is something for you, be it talking to your family and friends, reaching out to another patient, going to cancer-related talks and workshops, participating in a self-help or support group, or engaging in some form of individual counseling or psychotherapy. Sometimes one or two sessions with a social worker or psychiatric nurse will point the way for your problem solving, or a chat with a patient volunteer will help to put things in perspective and set your mind at ease.

Reputable sources for emotional support include your physician, nurses, hospital social workers, psychologists, psychiatrists, county health

departments, neighborhood mental-health clinics, and the various national, regional, and local cancer support organizations listed in the Resources section (Appendix B), such as the American Cancer Society and
the Cancer Information Service.

Social Workers

Social workers serve a wide variety of functions in our society but unfortunately are usually thought of in terms of the welfare system. Medical social workers, however, are the mainstay of the medical system in helping
cancer patients and their families find ways to get through it all. In their
basic roles of troubleshooters/problem solvers, social workers can help
you grasp the realities of living on chemotherapy and work to improve
those areas over which you have some control. To that end, they will fa-
miliarize themselves with your problems and concerns and work with you
to take care of them, be they medical, financial, emotional, religious, or related to your family or employment situation. Social workers can help you
communicate with the medical system, help you slice through red tape,
and help you and your family work together to detect and meet any emotional or practical needs. They can provide or help find useful items like
wheelchairs, prostheses, bedpans, bandages, transportation and financial
assistance if you need them. Social workers can help you fill out forms, or-
ganize your time around your treatment schedule, and arrange for housekeepers, child care, housing, or hospice service. Psychiatric social
workers who are specially trained in this field can provide psychotherapy
when emotional problems appear to keep you from functioning as well as
you might.

Social workers often engage in individual counseling with patients
alone, with patients and their families, or with families alone. They also
either run support groups or can put you in touch with support groups near
your home. Every hospital has social workers, but their availability and
usefulness vary. If you need help, a good way to start is to contact a staff
social worker at your community hospital or the hospital where you are being treated and see to what extent that person meets your needs. If their

time is limited (which is often the case), they are also good sources of information about other professionals who can offer ongoing treatment.

Peer and Group Support

Support groups have an overwhelming advantage over other forms of support in that they consist of your peers—other people like you who have cancer. Because of this common bond, many people feel more relaxed and find it easier to communicate with other cancer patients than with their families, friends, doctors, or nurses. "Because it reduces anxiety," says Grace Christ, "this kind of group is often the kind of forum in which people hear most easily." Many patients and professionals agree that a group is an ideal environment to exchange experiences and methods of dealing with both the practical and emotional issues surrounding cancer and its treatment.

The late Evelyn Ricki Dienst, Ph.D., was a cancer patient herself as well as consulting psychologist for the Cancer Support Community, an organization that provides psychological and educational support for cancer patients and their families in San Francisco. She told me:

> *People don't have to feel they are handling things poorly to join a support group. Many participants find their groups provide both social support and coping assistance. A group can be a good source of information and a place to talk about the experience with others who are interested and understand. It's especially good for those who find it awkward to talk much to family and friends. Often there can be a very useful lighter side to the group, and it can even be a humorous and uplifting experience . . . even if the sense of humor that develops might seem a bit strange to people without cancer. And, of course, participants often gain a great deal through what they are able to offer others in the group.*

A social worker and support group leader points out: "Groups help patients to make the decision to accept therapy, to continue it, to change it, to stop it. They help patients fill in gaps in their information or correct misinformation. We often try to help patients clarify their thoughts when they may be having trouble putting them into words."

However, another social worker observes: "Many people are shy of groups and given an option would avoid them. But once they get started, they find it's something that's very useful." Dr. Dienst found that men are often particularly reluctant to go to groups because they are afraid they will be too emotional. But when they go, they often find them helpful. People who participate in support groups say they sleep better, are less depressed, and feel more comfortable talking about their illness. For example:

The night after the first meeting, I went home and slept like a baby—fourteen, fifteen hours—better than I'd slept in a long time. I'd talked to people who understood. At first I thought it would be a waste of time, but it was very comforting. Now that I belong to a group, I can let out my feelings without burdening my friends with my concerns. I wish I had joined one earlier—I was one and a half years into cancer. I went through all those things you go through alone.

I think it's better to talk to other people who are having chemo because the doctor doesn't know how you feel. If you talk to patients, they have the same problems as you.

It's so good to talk to somebody who's been through it and is living a normal life again. I was so afraid of losing my hair, losing too much weight, not being able to take care of my children.

Kerry McGinn writes, in *Women's Cancers:*

Being in a group gave me a sense of perspective and progress. At first, others who were further along in treatment were cheering me on; later, I could lend a hand to those just beginning and could appreciate just how far I had come . . . I was also forewarned of com-

mon emotional potholes so I could avoid some completely and get through others more easily.

Support groups can help you keep or regain your self-esteem, your balance, and your self-worth. A good support group is made up of people who believe in one another, who offer one another optimistic, realistic help, encouragement, stimulation, meaningful advice, and valuable connections. When you belong to a group, you get help and give it, too.

Today, thank goodness, there are many more support groups, and many more types of them, than when I was undergoing chemo. Each has its own characteristics, its own pluses and minuses, so you are much more likely to find something that suits your needs and personality.

There are self-help groups that are organized and run by cancer patients themselves; some are local chapters of national organizations. Self-help groups can be extremely valuable, especially for people who are less vulnerable emotionally, such as those who are completing treatment and cancer survivors.

Support groups, by contrast, are generally led by specially trained individuals—social workers, psychotherapists, nurses, members of the clergy, and sometimes doctors or patient volunteers. This form is usually best for people who are actively dealing with their disease or treatment because there's a resource person to see that the information being relayed is appropriate and correct so that people aren't more upset by receiving confusing information. The leader helps keep the discussion going and protects people who might be more emotionally vulnerable.

As we gain in experience and as demand goes up, support groups are becoming more finely tuned and specialized. Support groups for patients may be heterogeneous and consist of people with a variety of cancers and prognoses and of people of different sexes and ages. Or they may be more specialized as to the type and stage of cancer. The more specific the group, the more individualized the support because the participants have more in common and can more closely compare experiences and share information and understanding.

According to Dr. Jimmie Holland, chief of psychiatry, Memorial Sloan-Kettering has a group that focuses specifically on support before as well as during chemotherapy. To help people control their anxiety, she says, "We're doing prechemo counseling, educating patients about what they can anticipate in terms of side effects and about relaxation, stress control, diet and nutrition, exercise, and anticipating what it will be like when the treatment is over."

Where a specific disease is concerned, breast cancer groups are becoming subspecialized, perhaps because the incidence is so high and because there are so many treatment-related and other issues involved. For example, there are groups for newly diagnosed women, women with metastatic disease, and women who have completed treatment. There are groups for men whose partners have cancer. There are groups for single women who are newly diagnosed to help women start a relationship and wrestle with issues such as "whom to tell" and "how to tell" a prospective partner. Support groups for spouses, children, and family members are becoming more available, as are survivors groups and bereavement groups.

Within these variations there are more variations. Groups may meet once a week or once a month. Some are ongoing, but most are time-limited. There also are "open" or drop-in groups with no registration or commitment. For some people, this is the perfect interim support until a more formal group opens up. Others may actually prefer the flexibility inherent in the drop-in arrangement; perhaps one or two visits to such a group may be all a person needs.

Or you may want to look into special workshops and retreats for cancer patients and their families, such as those offered by Commonweal and Exceptional Cancer Patients.

Support groups are being recognized as an integral part of the cancer patient's total medical care. Many people have learned firsthand that they can improve their quality of life by supplanting fear, anguish, alienation, helplessness, and hopelessness with hope, strength, productive activity, and a sense of community. As if this weren't enough, new evidence suggests that they can prolong life as well.

A study that stunned the cancer-care field was published in 1990 by David Spiegel and his colleagues at Stanford University and the University of California, San Francisco. The study involved two groups of women with advanced breast cancer. The group that received medical care and went to a support group experienced less pain and less anxiety, and they had more energy and slept better. What's more, they lived twice as long as did the group that received medical care only. Another 1990 study, by Dr. Fawzy Fawzy of University of California at Los Angeles, involved people with melanoma. Those who took part in a six-week mind-body program found that their moods and immune function improved, and they also lived longer than patients who did not participate did.

The Psychosocial Treatment Laboratory at the Stanford School of Medicine, headed by Dr. Spiegel, is currently engaged in numerous research projects designed to further study the mind-body relationship. One study in particular is designed to try to replicate the 1989 trial. Between 1991 and 1996, 125 women with metastatic breast cancer entered the study, which will continue for ten years. The primary goal is to assess the affect of group therapy on survival time, and the women are assessed at six-month intervals to measure relevant factors such as mood, social support, pain, sleep, diet and exercise, as well as immune and endocrine function.

With all these options, it makes sense to shop around for the type of group that's right for you. The quality of the groups and the degree to which you find them helpful will vary. It depends in part on the experience and capabilities of the leader, so ask about his or her credentials and training. Try to find someone who has been in the group and ask what that person liked and didn't like. Individual personalities, input, and group dynamics enter into the equation, too. These elements, of course, can't be completely assessed beforehand, but you can learn what the screening process is and whether the group is mixed or more specific as to cancer type, stage, and so on. Some groups focus on information or are action-oriented and focus on practical issues. Others are more introspective and may even incorporate music, poetry, or role playing to help participants explore their feelings. Some groups are time limited and others are ongoing. Some include families as well as patients. Ask whatever questions are important to *you*.

Most groups do not subscribe to a specific philosophy or belief system. But some do, and this may or may not appeal to you personally. As psychologist Ricki Dienst points out, David Spiegel's study notwithstanding, "there is little evidence that groups have a direct biological effect on the immune system or cancer cells. Some groups talk about the 'healing' properties of group support and positive attitudes. Patients often take this to mean physical healing, but many therapists really are talking about emotional healing." So make sure you understand the attitude and philosophy espoused by the sponsoring organization.

However, the whole idea of baring your innermost thoughts in front of a group of people may not be your style, or it may not be helpful. And it may be difficult to find the right group, as this patient comments:

> *The doctor got four of us together. It was nice in a way because I walked in feeling I was the only person in the world who had to wear a wig, and here were these two other girls in wigs looking perfectly normal. But part of it was depressing. One of them was only twenty-one years old, and I found it difficult to deal with somebody that young going through this. She was getting a more difficult chemo than I was—it really broke my heart; I really felt for her.*

Dr. Ward F. Cunningham-Rundles, an oncologist at Memorial Sloan-Kettering in New York, finds that groups may not be the answer for everyone: "One certainly has to have some kind of personal interaction; if people don't mesh, then they don't mesh. They have to be the right people, too. If you're in a protocol that causes you to be affected in a different way from the others in the group—if there are other patients with a very poor prognosis and one by one they do poorly, that can be difficult to take."

One-on-one peer support is an alternative to support groups that might suit your needs better. These are trained volunteers whom you can meet with personally or who are just a phone call away. Your hospital or physician or community cancer organization can put you in touch with a trained volunteer, or you can access an empathetic ear via the cancer hotlines scattered across the country, as this patient did:

> *Unless you have gone through the same type of situation, or are very close to someone who has, you just don't have the empathy, you don't understand. We have nobody to talk to. The day I called the Kansas City Hotline, I was crying, I was feeling so sorry for myself. But the*

woman I spoke to was so warm—and she was a living statistic. It made me feel so good. It cost me twelve dollars—we talked a long time—but it was worth every dime of it.

I wish I had been as smart as this patient. I think if I had just talked to even one other person who had had or who was having chemotherapy, I wouldn't have felt as terrified or as alone as I did at times. I wish that I had thought of it or that my oncologist had suggested it instead of mentioning psychiatrists, but we didn't.

Counseling and Psychotherapy

Sometimes it is helpful to explore your emotions more deeply with a person who is knowledgeable about cancer and experienced in helping others work out their feelings. Therapy goes beyond supporting the patient and family emotionally, beyond dealing with the common elements of the disease and its treatment, beyond encouraging you to talk about your feelings. Therapy looks into why you are feeling the way you do.

Psychotherapy deals with the unique issues that individual patients bring to the cancer experience and that may cause unique difficulties in facing common problems. Therapy is an intense experience, as it explores "old" issues that cancer has resurrected, such as self-esteem, self-worth, and relationships to parents. However, successful therapy frees patients from the burden of psychological ghosts that impose special meaning on cancer (such as thinking of cancer as some sort of punishment) so they can face the difficulties of cancer (which is tough enough) without this excess baggage. A therapist helps you understand feelings of guilt, resentment, and intense anger in a nonjudgmental way and helps you channel them more constructively.

Since cancer and its treatment affect the whole family, some families benefit from family counseling. Family counseling helps soften the shock and stresses of living with cancer; it opens up the lines of communication among family members, allowing participants to express the negative emotions and easing any resentment that may be part of the cancer package.

Therapy can be long-term or short-term; it may be one-on-one or take place in a group setting. Crisis intervention is short-term therapy specifically designed to get you through a tough time. Unlike support groups, which may be free or relatively inexpensive, there is generally a substantial fee for therapy. (However, many therapists will charge on a sliding scale, according to one's ability to pay.)

Religion and the Clergy

In times of trouble, religion is a refuge for many, be it drawn upon privately in the form of meditation and prayer or more publicly in the form of support and guidance from the clergy and/or fellow members of the congregation. A strong belief system can be a source of hope and comfort to a person who is undergoing treatment for cancer, as this patient explains: "I had a lot of help because I have a lot of faith. There's a psalm that goes 'Lift up your eyes into the hills from whence cometh my help. My help cometh from the Lord.' And oh, that verse really took me through it."

Severe stress may lead some people to revert to discarded religious beliefs. But you don't need to be a true believer to draw comfort from the rituals that you grew up with. As I say in my book *Rhythms and Cycles: Sacred Patterns in Everyday Life*, "Why pray, chant, recite scripture, or meditate? . . . These activities counterbalance the harrowing uncertainty of everyday life. They calm and shelter us in a world that is often without reason or peace, and that can shatter us without warning." They are symptoms of normality in a world gone wrong. And they may be even more. As Larry Dossey has so thoroughly explored in his book, *Healing Words*, prayer seems to have the power to affect our health in concrete ways. And several studies show that people who attend religious services regularly live longer than those who do not, while religious faith seems to help some people recover from depression and may also prevent it in the first place.

Even if you no longer have any religious affiliation and are not about to return to the fold, a member of the clergy—no matter what faith—can still be a welcome, sympathetic figure. It is part of the clergy's job and training to comfort the sick and troubled, to encourage people to unburden their souls. Today, increasing numbers of clergy are specially trained to counsel people with cancer and their families. If yours isn't one of them, you can ask to be referred to one who is. Members of the clergy can be very good listeners and, the trappings of religion aside, just having someone who is interested, who understands, and who has time for you can be very good for the soul.

Your Changing Needs

Whichever type of emotional support appeals to you, remember that you may need different approaches at different stages of the disease and treatment. What works for you now may not work two months from now, and what you would never consider now may start looking good in a year or so. Lari Wenzel advises that ultimately you need to know yourself well enough to know what is beneficial. Ask yourself whether a particular form of support is meeting your needs. Do you want immediate support or long-term reworking of the psyche? Is your anxiety increasing or decreasing? If it's increasing, why? Is it because you're dealing with a difficult issue on a particular day?

Before beginning treatment, you may want help absorbing the diagnosis and in getting information upon which you can make sound decisions. During chemotherapy, you may simply want the type of support that gets you through day by day. And after treatment is over, you may want more intensive work that reexamines life issues because you want to make changes in how you live your life, to live a more satisfying, less conflicted life.

CHAPTER THIRTEEN

The Aftermath

According to the National Cancer Institute, there are 7 million adult Americans who are living with cancer—nearly 4 percent of the adult population. Some are cured, some are in remission, and some have active disease.

If you are a survivor who is cured or in remission, and are off treatment, your life will be different from the lives of those who continue to battle active disease and need treatment either intermittently or perhaps for the rest of their lives. But all cancer patients share similar issues and concerns once the acute phase of diagnosis and treatment is over. Living with cancer, in the words of one research team, "is not trouble-free." It can, in fact, be the most challenging period of time you will face in your life.

Even if you are in remission or are probably cured, you face permanent life changes. As cancer survivor Susan Nessim writes, "Although I was cancer-free, I certainly wasn't free of cancer . . . there was more to overcoming this disease than surviving the hardships of treatment. Instead, the end of treatment marked the beginning of a new and unexpected challenge: adapting to life after cancer."

Adapting for me began with the end of chemo. As with most chemo patients, it would be an understatement to say I looked forward to my last treatment. Although chemotherapy wasn't as bad as I thought it would be,

I was very glad it was over. After giving me my last injection, my oncologist smiled, shook my hand, and said, "Congratulations. You made it. Now you can go out and play." In spite of the side effects and the misgivings, I had managed to see it through to the end. I felt a real sense of accomplishment. I was free at last! No more nausea, no more fatigue, no more jabbing needles. I did go out and play: My treatment ended on July 3, and the next day was my Independence Day. My husband and I left on a celebratory vacation to Montauk Beach. Next, I took off with a girlfriend on my first trip to Mexico. And after that I rented a Victorian mansion on Cape May, New Jersey, for me and my friends to play in. I felt high for weeks as I started to look and feel good again. I swam. I rode my bicycle. I ate and ate, regaining all the weight I had lost and then some.

After the first delirious weeks, however, I noticed a strange new feeling creeping in, a vague uneasiness. Playtime was, after all, over. It was time to return to real life. But I had changed; my life had changed. Somehow the old familiar pieces didn't quite fit together the way they used to. I began to realize I couldn't go back to life exactly the way it was. I wondered: What do I do now?

Though certainly happy to be off chemotherapy, many patients, like me, experience an unexpectedly bumpy transitional period. This process of "normalization" can be made more difficult by residual side effects, the need for follow-up care, and fear of recurrence. Our old "normal" lives may be beyond our grasp, but we can try to create new "normal" lives for ourselves. To varying degrees, life after chemo will be different, but in certain ways it can be better than life was before. Just as life on chemo is in part what you make it, how you handle the aftermath is up to you.

Dr. Michael Van Scoy-Mosher, an oncologist at Cedars-Sinai Medical Center in Los Angeles, believes that life after chemo is a matter of adaptation:

> There's a difference between coping and adapting. Coping, I think, is what you do in an acute situation. Adapting is what you do with a permanent change. In the long run you have to adapt to what has happened to you; it becomes a part of you, it gets incorporated for better or for worse.

Ingrid Bergman, who played two of her most demanding roles (in *Autumn Sonata* and *A Woman Called Golda*) during her eight-year battle with breast cancer, said in an interview that she was determined not to let her illness prevent her from enjoying the remainder of her life. "Cancer victims who don't learn to live with it," she said, "will only destroy what time they have left."

Making the Transition

Once the therapy is over, you will probably be exhilarated to see side effects subside. Who wouldn't be elated by their appetite, strength, and energy return, their hair growing back, their entire body gradually resuming its normal functions? One patient happily attests:

> *I was amazed at how quickly I bounced back. About two months after my last treatment, I was running two miles a day again. Unfortunately, I was also expected to cook and take care of the house just like in the old days. But I really didn't mind. It felt good to be me again.*

Although this period of normalization is for the most part suffused with relief and joy, it is sometimes tempered by the fact that like any time of transition, it is full of stresses of adaptation for the cancer patient and the family. As side effects diminish, everyone needs to stop thinking of the patient as being sick, to resume former roles and responsibilities, and to start thinking about and planning for the future, however uncertain that might be.

The former director of social services at New York's Memorial Sloan-Kettering enumerates some of the psychological and practical difficulties inherent in moving back into the community and normal life:

> *There are all kinds of problems and resistances. There may be job problems, insurance problems, problems with confronting an ongoing life or having to change your goals. Sometimes during treatment you have to constrict your time perspective: You learn to think*

day-to-day, which is a very useful way to manage a difficult experience. But then you learn to plan ahead, expand your time perspective, make long-range plans, and think more about the future.

After all that activity—treatments, blood tests, side effects, surprises—my life seemed somehow dull, a touch ordinary. So much time and energy had been focused on fighting the cancer, it felt strange to suddenly be doing nothing. I felt like a soldier coming home from active combat: battle-weary but let down by the unexpected absence of danger and excitement.

Sometimes such mixed feelings surface because stopping chemotherapy is anxiety-provoking. Much to everyone's—including the patients'—surprise, patients dread or regret the end of therapy because it means leaving the constant surveillance of the hospital, no longer being so closely monitored, and being out on their own. After you've been seeing a doctor every week or two, the security of knowing that if anything develops it will be picked up immediately is suddenly taken away. Some patients do not, in fact, want to go off their chemotherapy and ask their doctors to continue even though it is medically appropriate for them to be taken off it. As one health professional says, patients become so accustomed to doing something to control the illness, that "being without [chemo] is often really a downer for some people."

"Some people are so relieved that this is not an issue at all," comments Dr. Michael Van Scoy-Mosher. However, he is well aware that patients can have ambivalent feelings about ending the therapy:

I usually bring up the issue toward the end of the therapy. I'll mention the way some others have felt and try to get my patients to talk about it. Most of the time they have begun to feel that way themselves—I reassure them that they will still be seeing me, not as often perhaps—and discuss the fear of recurrence and why more therapy is not given. I give them a game plan for follow-up, so although they may not be getting more therapy, they will be closely observed. Beyond that, they just have to cope with it. First they have to cope with getting the therapy, then they have to cope with not getting it.

I have a patient whose adjuvant therapy I wanted to stop after six months. But she's fought with me to continue it for as long as I can. She's terrified of stopping. It's not as if she doesn't have any side effects, but she's more afraid of the cancer than she is of the side effects. But there are good reasons not to go on with the therapy.

As time goes on, so does the challenge. Cancer survivors continue their journey along a path that is strewn with physical, psychological, social, and economic changes, issues, and hurdles.

Long-Term and Delayed Effects

Most side effects subside rapidly after treatment is stopped; however, a few may take longer—months or years—and some never disappear completely. There are a few that may even crop up later on. Although these long-term side effects are usually just annoying or uncomfortable, a few may be debilitating or life-threatening. Researchers have begun to document the impact of cancer and its treatment on long-term survivors. The physiological fallout can occur in any organ system, causing problems such as infertility; menstrual irregularities and menopause symptoms; impotency; decreased lung capacity; lowered ability to exercise; chronic fatigue; increased infections; dry skin; constipation; transient heart attacks or strokes; bladder, kidney, and blood disorders; hearing loss; development of second or third cancers; and pain. In addition, you may need to live with changes caused by surgery or radiation. You may find yourself becoming very body- or symptom-conscious; so little is known about these long-range side effects that you can blame almost anything on chemotherapy.

Dr. Charles Vogel, director of the Comprehensive Cancer Center of Miami, admits that "the long-term sequelae of cancer and its treatments have only begun to be noted and understood." Yet they are important pieces of information for patients and doctors alike. The possibility of long-term effects needs to become part of the decisions made early on, when assessing risk versus benefit and treatment is being done. Knowledge of residual and late side effects also increases the likelihood that they will be recognized and treated when they occur and possibly prevented from occurring in the first place or at least minimized. Wherever possible, old drug regimens are being replaced by others with fewer short- and long-term effects.

It may be difficult to determine where psychological trauma ends and physical damage begins and whether a symptom is in fact due to chemotherapy or is a condition that might have developed anyway. One patient remarks:

> *I still have some nausea now and then, but I've gained back all the weight I lost anyway. People tell me how great I look. I almost feel guilty that I still feel tired all the time. People tend to judge too much how you are by how you look. It makes me feel strange because I don't feel as good as they think I look. People may really wonder if you really have been through all this.*

Although basically I'm well and functioning, it bothers me that no one can say for sure to what extent I've been permanently affected by chemotherapy. The nausea is gone, and my hair is thicker than ever. My blood levels are fine; even my white blood cell count, which remained below normal for years, has returned to the normal range. My menstrual cycle has reasserted itself, though with exasperating irregularity until I finally went through menopause twenty years after my diagnosis (see "A Word About Menopause" on page 359 for more on postchemo menopause). The foot and leg cramps I suffered during vincristine withdrawal gradually became less frequent, no doubt helped by the advice I got from a physical therapist and an addiction to yoga and aerobic exercise. These lingering effects, though tangible, are merely annoying, like gnats I can swat away.

The one thing the experience has left me with that I find not so easy to handle is a lingering "Chemo brain"—a residual intermittent fuzziness, a blunting of my physical and mental powers. I often—but not always—feel slightly slowed down, held back. My mind simply isn't quite as sharp and clear as it used to be. Although chemo's effect on mental function during treatment has been acknowledged, there is very little scientific research on chemo's long-term effects on the brain. Until recently, talking with other chemo patients has been the only way I could validate my own observations. We'd commiserate about having chemo brain, mush brain, or no brain. We'd make jokes about our memory problems and affectionately refer to this syndrome as CRS (can't remember shit). We share those magical moments during a conversation when, in the middle of a sentence, both talker and listener realize that the talker has lost all recollection of purpose ("Now, why am I telling this story?").

But because we patients complained to our doctors, the health profession has gradually begun to take notice. In 1992 Mary Wieneke, a doctoral candidate in clinical psychology at the California School of Professional Psychology, completed an exploratory study on the effects of chemotherapy in breast cancer patients. One month to one year after completing therapy, she found "statistically significant impairments in their mental flexibility, speed of processing, memory, and motor function." Those who had a longer course or greater amount of chemo were more affected.

A little more than a dozen studies including a follow-up study by Wieneke, have been conducted that have refined and confirmed this research. For example, a study from the Netherlands found that high doses of chemotherapy in women with breast cancer caused memory and concentration problems in 32 percent of the women receiving the therapy. Another study from Dartmouth Medical School found that people who got standard chemotherapy were twice as likely to score poorly on intelligence tests than other cancer patients, even ten years after their treatment.

Plus, my physical energy tends to fade earlier than before. It is subtle, but it is there. Sometimes I think these could be imagined changes: Maybe I wasn't really as smart and energetic as I like to think I was; maybe I'm getting older like everybody else; maybe I'm looking for an excuse for real or imagined shortcomings. Or my symptoms may be due to something other than the chemo. I must say it is a relief to watch my peers catching up with me, going through menopause and aging and complaining of the same cognitive "symptoms" and lack of energy.

Susan Nessim in her much-needed book *Cancervive: The Challenge of Life after Cancer* writes that instead of patients regaining energy after treatment ends, "months or even years later, they may find that they're still feeling run down, mustering all their reserves just to get through the day." According to a social worker and breast cancer survivor Nessim interviewed, chronic fatigue is just beginning to be recognized as a potentially debilitating long-term effect of cancer treatment. While chronic fatigue

A WORD ABOUT MENOPAUSE

Menopause and its immediate and long-term effects are a troubling issue for women in general. Menopause has additional issues for women with hormone-dependent cancers. Experiencing new symptoms while on chemo is one thing—we may be able to tough it out for a predetermined period of time. But once chemo is over, any woman who is going through natural or chemical menopause will need to make a decision about how to handle hormonal changes and their effects on her body and quality of life. This decision is hard enough for women who have not been diagnosed with hormone-dependent cancer because hormone replacement therapy (HRT) is linked with greater risk of endometiral cancer, breast cancer, heart attack, stroke, gallbladder disease, liver disease and type II diabetes. More chilling for us, it may also prod a quiescent hormone-dependent cancer into renewed growth.

Once we enter menopause, like most women, we are at higher risk for osteoporosis and heart disease, not to mention the uncomfortable day-to-day symptoms such as hot flashes. But because chemical (or surgical) menopause is much more abrupt than natural menopause, these symptoms can be more intense. In addition, some of us have taken or are taking steroid drugs and these can accelerate bone loss. What's a post-chemo woman to do? And what about younger women, who are thrown into early menopause because of chemo, and who are also likely to encounter osteoporosis earlier in life, and have a longer life ahead of them in which to deal with these issues?

This can be one of the most difficult postchemo issues we need to grapple with. Fortunately, there are many safe ways you may be able to manage symptoms until you have completed going through menopause. My main symptoms were hot flashes and irregular periods. In retrospect—now that I am pretty much over this transition and sleeping again—I realize insomnia and fatigue were also probably hormone related. I believe my diet, nutritional supplements, yoga, and exercise helped keep symptoms to a minimum. I have had a couple of bone-density tests and am relieved to find nothing alarming was happening. Still, it was hell watching my periods reassert themselves, and I had some of the worst pain and most bizarre menstrual symptoms I've every experienced. Once I was premenopausal for three months, and only acupuncture, moxibustion (the burning of herbs in addition to the needles), and Chinese herbs gave me relief. Later on, when I was writing a book on homeopathy, I tried an individually prescribed homeopathic remedy and that also seemed to even things out more. (Homeopathy also cured me of a lifelong eczema, but that's another story.) And now, all I am experiencing is some hot flashes, but adding extra vitamin E to my usual regimen works like a charm. Every time I drop my dosage, the hot flashes return. When I up the dosage again, they vanish. I don't take herbs with phytoestrogens in them, because the research is not certain what effect this might have in women with a history of breast cancer.

Not all doctors agree that women with hormone-related cancers should shun HRT, however, and there are several nonhormonal medications that are being used as alternatives. For example, fluoxetine (Prozac) was recently found to be more effective than a placebo (dummy pill) in relieving hot flashes in women aged 18 to 49. There are also nonestrogen drugs that appear to slow bone loss, so be sure to speak to your doctor about what might be considered for you.

used to be dismissed as a sign of mental depression, the likelihood of an organic origin is finally being acknowledged. The causes are still unknown, but some theorize that they include permanent bone marrow suppression of the red cells, which causes anemia, or of the white cells, which means the body needs to expend more energy to repair itself and fend off infections. Another possibility is that toxic byproducts from all the chemotherapy and support drugs used to treat your cancer are still lodged in your body. The primary detoxifying organ is your liver, and it's possible that it has been overworked and thereby has lost some of its ability to completely break down toxic substances so that your body can excrete them. You might want to try following a safe detoxification program to heal your liver and help rid your body of substances that are still poisoning your healthy tissues. The alternative therapy books and resources in Appendix B can help you find reputable practitioners who can design a program for you to follow. If you want to detox on your own—but of course under your doctor's supervision—there are several books available that provide information. A recent addition to this field is Ann Louise Gittleman's book *The Fat Flush Plan*. Gittleman, a certified nutrition specialist who worked with Pritikin, details a sound cleansing program that aims to detoxify the liver, help rid your body of harmful accumulated substances, restore energy, and improve your immune function.

As my oncologist told me, the experience does make a dent in you. I still feel "dented" and probably always will to some extent. Although I may never be "as good as new," time and effort continue to help straighten things out, and perhaps I'll ultimately end up better than new in some unexpected ways.

Psychological Effects

Cancer survivors also face a myriad of possible psychological effects. These include fear and anxiety about a cancer recurrence, death, depression, changes in body image, decreased interest in sex, and concern about the treatment's side effects (and feeling like a hypochondriac). Some people have lowered self-esteem, but others emerge with improved self-esteem. As with the physiological effects, these changes and issues have just begun to be studied.

An intriguing overview of the postchemo patient's plight comes from Ellen L. Maher of the Department of Sociology at Indiana University. Interviews with cancer survivors revealed that although they were in remission or possibly cured, all were not completely at ease with their good fortune. Ms. Maher describes their unease as *anomia*, a mental state characterized by confusion and anxiety, uncertainty, loss of purpose, and a sense of alienation.

Ms. Maher discusses the many factors that contribute to this strange, vague, unexpected discomfort that can occur when chemotherapy is stopped: the patient's initial perception of a poor prognosis and hence an unanticipated cure or remission; a sense of loss of purpose if a great deal of time and energy has gone into the treatment; uncertainty about the advisability of stopping treatment; the possibility of recurrence and its attendant insecurity and anxiety; the inability to make the switch from "living one day at a time" to thinking about future-oriented activities; ambivalent feelings toward the imperfect system to which patients nevertheless owe their lives; and the withdrawal of support from health-care givers and families who are convinced that "the healthiest thing is to put it all behind," even though the patient is not quite ready to do so.

Some of us may have doubts about whether we chose the "right" treatment. A year after surgery and six months after her last chemo treatment, a friend of mine who had recently been diagnosed with breast cancer continued to regret her decision to have a mastectomy rather than a lumpectomy. The fact that there were good medical reasons for a mastectomy, as confirmed by a second surgical opinion, didn't matter. She felt that she was rushed, that her surgeon pressured her into deciding, that he made the decision. She was beating herself up psychologically for allowing her breast to be removed: "How could I have done that to myself—to my beautiful, wonderful breast?"

Adjuvant chemotherapy, the type I had, poses other dilemmas. As I write this, twenty-two years after my diagnosis, I have no evidence of disease. Two medical oncologists have told me that since my disease-free survival is longer than chemo was expected to give me, it was probably the surgery that was responsible. In other words, there's a good chance I had chemo unnecessarily. On the other hand, I may be among the 10 percent of premenopausal women who do show an improvement in the ten-year survival rate if given adjuvant chemotherapy.

How does anyone really know how well he or she would have done with another form of therapy? Or with no therapy? How do you find answers where there are no answers? How do you give up wanting certainty when there is only uncertainty? We can never know if we made the "right decision"—we can only make the *best decision,* given the circumstances at the time.

Survivor's Syndrome

Perhaps the biggest, most frustrating obstacle to enjoying a full, happy postchemo life is the possibility of having a recurrence. Naturally, anyone who has been treated for cancer is concerned about a recurrence, and when chemotherapy was less effective than it is now, many people did indeed have recurrences, some quite soon after therapy. Some of course, still do, but now that long-term remissions and cures have become more common, a new medical phenomenon has been born: the survivor's syndrome. This anxious state of mind has also aptly been dubbed the Damocles syndrome, after the character in Greek mythology who sat at a banquet under a sword that was precariously suspended by a single hair. We, like Damocles, see that a sword hangs over us and never know how long we have until the hair breaks and the sword drops. A former mastectomy patient expresses this: "Sometimes I'm afraid to look at my other breast. I do self-examination, but I'm afraid I'll find something. I'll cover it up, or I'll take showers in the dark. It's not that I'm ashamed of the mastectomy—I'm afraid of something showing up in the other breast."

The necessity of follow-up care, with its frequent medical checkups and tests, places an additional stress on postchemo patients, with each serving as a reminder of a time in the past and of a possible future that most patients would prefer not to think about. Sometimes a physical crisis—any new symptom, no matter how minor—sets off an inner alarm:

Every time I go to the doctor for a follow-up, I am forced to remember why I am going and I think, "Oh God, will he find anything this time?"

My surgeon is very, very thorough when I go for exams. It scares me he's so thorough—you want him to find it if it's there, but you're hoping he doesn't.

Now I've turned into a very paranoid person. When any little thing goes wrong . . . One night I turned over on my stomach, and I felt a soreness in my rib. I kept pushing it and pushing it to see if it still hurt, and of course, the more I poked at it, the more it did hurt. It was only a month away from my regular time for a bone scan, mammogram, and chest X-ray, so my doctor suggested we do it then, just in case, rather than wait.

My husband came with me, and I waited around inside while they looked at the results quickly to see if they had to be done over. The nurse and a doctor came in, and I couldn't wait to ask them how they looked. They said, "Oh, fine, there's nothing abnormal." I can't tell you how relieved I was . . . I heaved a huge sigh and went out to see my husband, who looked at me and didn't know what to do—I broke out into this big smile and all I could say was "They're okay." He broke out in such a smile and began to cry. I never realized how frightened he was too. We both sat there—he was hugging me—just crying like a couple of idiots.

The frequency for follow-up tests and exams is being debated among experts. Some cancer survivors feel more secure when they have frequent checkups. But do routine follow-ups actually extend life? Maybe not, according to a study from the Netherlands, published in 2001. Dr. Marike Jacobs, the lead researcher, says that their study showed that "the impact of follow-up on life expectancy is very small." Using a mathematical model because it would be unethical to withhold standard treatment from patients, the team found that 45.4 percent of breast cancer patients with standard follow-up would die of breast cancer, compared with 45.8 percent of patients who got no follow-up. On the other hand, this may not hold true for everyone, says Carla Falkson, M.D., of the University of Alabama at Birmingham. She points out that patients who tend to disregard symptoms of recurrence might benefit from frequent routine follow-up.

Grace Christ has noticed that people may have strong reactive feelings on their "anniversaries"—the day of surgery, the day of diagnosis, or the start or end of treatment. Approaching benchmarks of one, two, five, or ten years can also cause considerable anxiety. In addition, she notes:

Sometimes normal life phases such as getting married or having children can be difficult for people because they're markers in their lives. They can remind someone who's had cancer of the whole traumatic experience.

Young people who have had Hodgkin's disease—when do they tell the people that they're dating? What do they say? If they're going to get married, then they have to confront the question of how long their lives will be. Are they going to be able to have children? There are a lot of uncertainties about that. What kind of sexual partners are they going to make? And if they are going to be able to have children, what impact will this have on their children?

In addition to a recurrence, you may be concerned about developing a second cancer in the years to come. Although the percentages vary, patients who have had one cancer are statistically at a higher risk of developing additional cancers than is the average person of getting an initial cancer. There are several theories as to why this may be so.

Possibly factors that led to the first malignancy are also responsible for allowing a second to arise and flourish. Regardless of the form of treatment, people who have had certain types of cancers seem to be more prone later to development of other specific types of cancers. Since heredity seems to play a role in the development of some cancers, you may be worried about other members of your family getting cancer. This issue is especially prominent when you are a woman with breast cancer and you are afraid your daughter might also get it.

Another group of statistics shows that people who have been treated with chemotherapy and/or radiation are more likely to develop cancer— usually leukemia—later on. This is usually associated with Hodgkin's disease patients and specific drugs that belong to the alkylating group. However, recent studies show that women who have had chemotherapy for breast cancer are also at a higher risk for leukemia. According to one study, published in 2000 in the *Journal of Clinical Oncology*, women treated with radiation and mitoxantrone (Novantrone) has twenty-eight times the risk of leukemia as the general population. Whether this is because the treatment has suppressed the immune system or is itself carcinogenic—or both—is not certain.

In general, people tend to either minimize the possibility of a relapse or exaggerate it. Some people think about it almost all the time, others almost never. Although they run the risk of ignoring real problems that could be successfully treated if they were acknowledged early, true minimizers are lucky. They seem to be able to absorb the shock and go on to live full, happy lives. The others, the worriers, seem to be unable to forget their cancer even for a moment. They are obsessed by their disease and their health; they anticipate the worst to such an extent that it taints the remainder of their lives by overshadowing and taking time away from the more pleasurable and positive pursuits that life has to offer. Dr. Richard Gralla, an oncologist, says about this:

> *Part of coping with chemotherapy is being well, being free of disease, doing the normal things, but still having that sword hang over you. Of course it's more real for the postchemo patient, but that same sword hangs over me. As a human being living in modern society I can get cancer, and I have to deal with it, too. I can ignore it—as can you—but that's probably not too healthy. I think it's better to come to grips with it rather than totally ignore the issue.*

Dr. Van Scoy-Mosher points out that fears of a recurrence generally recede as time goes by:

I find that although this concern never goes away completely, it does get better and patients are able to tolerate it. It depends on their capacity for denial: Some people are defenseless and don't have a capacity for denial—they can't push things back, and those are the people for whom it is worse.

Natalie Spingarn, a journalist, had been living with cancer for many years when she wrote *Hanging in There*. In her book, she eloquently and unflinchingly describes what it is like to be "hanging in there," to live the different life of the subculture of the "not well." It is tough for her to keep going, but keep going she does, helping herself lose her fear by keeping alive her hope in the future. She writes:

Unlike most "normal" people, we subculture members have to live with the persistent knowledge of our own mortality. "Background music" Stewart Alsop called that knowledge, and it is true that when I am occupied the fearful dark tones stay in the background. But they can blare forth, affecting my attitude and ability to get on with the business of living. I have found no skill more important (no matter how it's gained) than the ability to believe in my own survival.

The reasons for someone's uncertain health remaining subdued "background music" or becoming a full brass band may vary. Psychiatrist Judith Bukberg thinks that "people have certain styles of coping based on who they are. If you've had a life of bad things happening to you, then obviously you're going to have more of those thoughts than somebody who hasn't; similarly, some people are pessimistic by nature."

Social and Economic Issues

Being concerned about the cost of initial treatment and continuing care is stressful enough, but survivors also may have problems with continuing or getting medical insurance coverage or increasing life insurance coverage. Your medical benefits may change, or you may be concerned about changing jobs because you may lose insurance coverage. Eighty percent of people with cancer return to work, but one in four cancer survivors experiences some form of employment discrimination because of his or her history of cancer. Some are unable to work or need to change their type of work or reduce their workload because of the aftereffects of treatment. Some people get right back into the swing of things with or without the support of their employers and coworkers. Others may take a while longer to get up to speed or may run into misconceptions at the workplace that cause problems on the job.

Studies show that cancer survivors notice changes in their personal relationships—sometimes for the better, sometimes for the worse. Relationships may get better as the crisis of cancer brings people closer. Sometimes families and friends become overly protective, or you may feel they are uncomfortable about your cancer or feel pity for you.

You can contact the National Cancer Institute and the American Cancer Society (see Appendix B: Resources) for information to help you overcome insurance and employment problems.

Support for Survivors

As the number of cancer survivors increases, clearly more studies and support resources are needed if we are going to be able to live our hard-won time more fully rather than just "survive." And we need to recognize our own needs and have better access to the support that already exists. Dr. Bukberg says:

> It's useful for people to know that the survivor's syndrome exists, even though it's difficult to give specific solutions. I do think that continuing support groups are very important. So are hypnosis and other kinds of relaxation techniques. If you tend to be anxious about things, and you want to change that tendency, I'd say the best chance to do that is psychotherapy. Sometimes just by decreasing anxiety, obsessive thinking will stop. Sometimes cognitive approaches can help. It's a shame that more people don't enter psychotherapy if these techniques don't work.

Although a study published in 2002 suggests that breast cancer survivors who remain disease-free after primary treatment (mastectomy or lumpectomy plus radiation) have an excellent quality of life, women who also had adjuvant chemotherapy or hormone therapy have a different tale to tell. The prospective study, conducted by researchers at the University of California at Los Angeles Comprehensive Cancer Center, found that the adjuvant treatment was associated with a statistically significant decrease in physical functioning over time. However, the researchers also found that the social support the women received strongly affected their long-term post-treatment quality of life.

Lois Loescher's work also shows that the need for counseling and support doesn't end when treatment does. In addition, she found that cancer survivors feel it is helpful to hear about other survivors' experiences, talk about their own experiences, and participate in survivors programs. Fortunately, there are survivors programs cropping up, such as Cancervive (with chapters in several states). If you think a survivors group would be right for you, ask your doctor, nurse, social worker, or local cancer support organization to help you locate one. You might want to start (or continue) writing in a journal, a tried-and-true therapy. Or you might want to use the arts to express what you are feeling—painting, sculpture, dance, and music can sometimes express better than words what is going on inside you. A friend of mine began taking painting lessons after she completed treatment. She began with simple circles and progressed to more elaborate mandalas and then she painted other subjects with the joy and innocent exuberance of a child. We were all surprised and delighted at what came out of this sensible, somewhat somber woman who had only painted timid watercolors before.

I had had some dark moments while on chemo, but it seemed easy to dismiss them then—it seemed natural to feel anxious about so many things. I buried my feelings because I was sure that I could handle them for the duration and that things would be fine once I was off the therapy and I could put some time between me and the experience. But about two and a half years after I finished chemo I found it was still hard for me to live with intruding thoughts about my disease and worries about my prognosis. I'd be in the middle of something perfectly ordinary—grocery shopping, for instance—and find myself overcome with sadness. I would think, "What if the chemo didn't work?" I'd have to fight to keep back the tears as I fantasized the bleakest scenario: in pain, unable to work or take care of myself, completely miserable. That I was working on the first edition of this book, immersed in cancer facts and reliving my experiences daily, no doubt heightened my awareness and made my anxiety more acute. In a way, I am grateful for that: If my anxiety had stayed at a low level, I might never have decided that enough was enough and sought help from a psychotherapist. She incorporated hypnotherapy into the sessions, and I was able to resolve a lot of unfinished business. I must say the therapy allowed me to feel much better, much more relaxed about having had cancer.

I'm not a participant in a posttreatment cancer survivors' group, but I do have my own free-floating group of friends who have or have had cancer. Although I enjoy close relationships with other friends who are not cancer patients, as one cancer veteran put it, "It's different when you're talking to someone to whom you don't have to explain certain things."

Follow-up Care

Even though chemical therapy is finished, as cancer patients we will be getting follow-up medical care for the rest of our lives. Checkups and tests will be regularly scheduled, frequently at first and less frequently over the years as we remain well. Though the last thing we may want to do is spend more time in a hospital or waiting room, follow-up care is a useful and necessary part of postchemo life. It may be anxiety-provoking, but it is also reassuring.

For one thing, follow-up care may be able to address any problems with the residual effects of the therapy. Although our minds and bodies have remarkable resiliency and recuperative powers, sometimes medical support can strengthen us and hasten the recuperative process. Your doctors or other health practitioners may also be able to help you with any practical or psychological hurdles you face in living with cancer. If, for instance, you are preoccupied with your body and any symptoms—at one point I thought every cough might mean lung cancer, every bump or pim-

ple was melanoma, every little ache was a metastasis to the bone, every little bit of constipation was bowel obstruction, every headache was cancer
spreading to the brain—talking your fears over with your oncologist and
getting some facts and assurances may help. You can ask what the likelihood of spread is, where the metastases usually occur in your cancer, and
what the symptoms might be.

Regular contact with your oncologist is perhaps most advisable because as with primary cancer, the earlier recurrent cancer is detected and
treated, the better. As we have seen, cancer is not an automatic death sentence; neither is a recurrence. If you suspect your cancer has spread, do
not delay going to your oncologist. Make sure it is a recurrence. Get a
physical confirmation—blood tests, X-rays, and scans. Consider a second
opinion. Diagnosis can be inaccurate at any stage of this disease. There
are many cases where a patient was presumed to have a metastasis and
treated as if he or she were terminal but was in fact found to be metastasis-
free later on.

If there's a recurrence, it may make even more sense than before to
turn to psychological support to help deal with feelings of shock, anger,
and disbelief; with fears of pain, disability, and death; and with physical
and psychological inadequacies. Patients may blame themselves or their
families or feel betrayed by their bodies and their doctors. Bitterness and
a mistrust of the medical system are not unusual. A mental-health worker
speaks about her awareness of the devastating impact recurrence can have
on patients:

> *This is a very big crisis for people who kind of thought they were go-
> ing to do all right, and they were all right for a while, and then sud-
> denly . . . it's a very big crisis for the staff, too.*

As before, be aware of your treatment options. There is usually some
form of treatment available, be it standard or investigational. Radiation is
often used effectively at this point to reduce pain from metastases; in some
cases, surgical removal of metastases is successful. It is important for patients to have realistic expectations: Usually no more than a temporary
halt to the progression of cancer and/or the palliation of symptoms can be

expected when chemo is being used for a second or third time. However, even though additional treatment usually does not offer the chance for a cure, it still may prolong life significantly and can make it more comfortable.

Dr. William Grace at New York's St. Vincent's Hospital, for example, says:

> *Sometimes oncologists just run out of therapeutic options and don't have access to newer drugs and methodologies. So it may be fruitful to explore investigational drugs, treatments, and combinations at larger cancer care facilities. Even old drugs may be administered so they are effective. I had a patient with breast cancer who had been through all the medications. We finally decided to give her a drug that had no longer worked for her, and we used it in a new way, called continuous infusion. She had a marvelous response.*
>
> *So there are always things to do, although we don't always know exactly what to do in every case. The problem is the combinations and permutations of different cancers, their different sensitivities, the different types of agents—the variables are astronomical. You just do the best you can. If you're lucky, you'll pull the ace out of the deck.*

You especially need to weigh the cost against the benefits of treatment for recurrent cancer because the primary goal is to keep you free of pain and as productive and able to enjoy life as possible. If the side effects are too severe, your quality of life is not being improved. Some people feel that once is enough; having been there, they feel they know what is in store and are reluctant to go through it again.

It is especially important for a patient with progressive disease to have a good relationship with an oncologist capable of seeing patients through the tough times that lie ahead. As always, you have the right to get a second opinion or to refuse or stop toxic treatment altogether.

For some patients, unorthodox treatments may seem more attractive at this point than at the time of original diagnosis and therapy. Many feel that if conventional medical treatment has little or nothing to offer, it may be better to pursue an alternative therapy because it keeps their hopes and sense of control alive. Although some alternative therapies are very rigorous and the cost-benefit ratio may be high, many people do opt to have them. See Appendices B and C for sources of information about alternative cancer therapies.

Even if all therapies fail or become inappropriate and the end draws near, you can still try to maintain a degree of control over your life. There is still reason to hope that the rest of your life will be as full of dignity and comfort as possible for you and your loved ones. Within the last couple of decades, real strides have been made in understanding and coping with this final phase of life. The works of Elisabeth Kubler-Ross and the hospice movements may prove enlightening and comforting (see the Bibliography and Suggested Reading section: Appendix C).

A Better Life

Whatever time we have left—be it months, years, or a full lifetime—it can be high-quality time if we let it. There's a growing survivorship movement, with individuals, treatment centers, professional societies, and groups such as the National Coalition for Cancer Survivorship working to develop resources to support people living in the aftermath of cancer. And the National Cancer Institute has established an Office of Cancer survivorship.

Many patients have discovered that just because life is different, that doesn't mean it has to be worse. Life after chemo can be an improvement over life before. Although shaken, they emerge from the cancer/chemotherapy experience strengthened, with a fresh perspective and a heightened appreciation for the big and little things in life that they used to take for granted and that others still do. Although the experience may have imposed its share of difficulties, they find it has made them learn about themselves, about others, and about how precious life is. They have learned that the extent to which they can take control over their lives and the way they feel is greater than they ever imagined. Although they may look back wistfully at a more innocent time, they realize one can't go back, one can go only forward, toward a life that may not be normal but may be better than normal in many ways. Ask them their philosophy and they might tell you, "When life hands you a lemon, make lemonade."

In fact, it seems that these people—those who are able to pull something positive out of having had cancer and chemotherapy—*are* able to cope better. It is important for them to feel that it wasn't all for nothing, that it wasn't all bad. There's even a name for it now—"posttraumatic growth" and it is the flip side of posttraumatic stress. Dr. Van Scoy-Mosher has seen this in many patients:

> *I've noticed again and again from personal observation that people who seem to cope better than others are able to extract something positive from their experiences. It may be a change in their value systems, their motivations, their family structures, their interests. It may be writing a book about chemotherapy. Often levels of intimacy in a family that were good before are intensified. Even the motivation to adopt a healthier lifestyle—to stop smoking, to be more careful about your diet—is a good thing.*

Dr. Gralla has witnessed this same phenomenon:

> *A young patient of mine was on chemo for Hodgkin's. He said, "You know, as much as I hated the whole horrible experience, it's been about the most important and maturing experience in my life, and it's made a better person of me." In almost every aspect, from athletics, which were important to this fellow, to his life with his wife, to his career, it's made a not very mature adult into a quite mature, quite introspective, and thinking young adult.*

Barbara Carter, a San Francisco nurse, published a study in 1989 of the long-term psychosocial adjustments of a group of women who survived breast cancer beyond five years. Carter feels that the study highlights the importance of understanding that survivors go through a process involving many phases of recovery that persist for many years after recovery. During this time, her subjects felt that they had moved "from something to something"—and emerged from the experience with a clearer sense of self, a gratitude for life, and strength and confidence in their ability to manage life crises.

The ways people find to express this change are varied. Many choose, for example, to make changes in their diets and lifestyles. They may adopt a cancer-prevention lifestyle because it might prevent a recurrence or another cancer from developing. They might begin or resume an exercise regimen because it may also prevent certain types of cancer, as well as heart disease and osteoporosis as well as diabetes. Some swing in the other direction and react by plunging into a kind of live-for-today hedonism and deny themselves no pleasure. Still others make no changes. Most, however, probably fall somewhere in the middle.

No matter when you begin—before, during, or after chemo—making constructive, health-building changes can be a very useful, positive step: Becoming involved in creating better health has many benefits, some directly related to cancer. It improves the quality of your life because you feel better, have more energy, and are able to fight illness of all kinds. When you participate in positive health building, you help reduce some of the anxiety and letdown about stopping chemotherapy or any active medical treatment. Optimizing the strength of your immune system and all your organ systems may inhibit the growth of any residual cancer or secondary cancer. This is a very important possible benefit, given the fact that we are at such high risk. Additionally, the healthier you are, the better you will be able to cope with a relapse should one occur.

My oncologist believes that "what one does after chemotherapy needs to be individualized," just as is the case with what one does while on chemo. He stresses common sense and moderation:

Obviously one doesn't get into the situation where one is going to be tantalizing the system any more than is necessary. Does a person go out and smoke cigarettes because now he or she is as free as a bird? No, that would be foolish—nicotine is an immune suppressant. Does one go out and drink barrels of coffee? I don't think so; coffee is a growth stimulant. But does one say that one will never drink a cup of coffee? No, that's not human.

I think it makes sense to do the things that are the least likely to

*create second malignancies, since the incidence of second malig-
nancies is high in people who have had one. For instance, it's important to have a fairly high fiber diet that's going to include plenty
of good things. Modest intake of vitamins is a good idea. Being involved with things that are life-building is a good idea, and getting
back into the mainstream is terribly important.*

Dr. Michael Schachter, who treats cancer patients who are receiving
chemotherapy from their oncologists, feels strongly about postchemo care.
He bases his recommendations on "years of long-term observation, which
have made it pretty clear that nutritional and life-style changes are crucial
over the long haul in terms of quality of life and survival time during and
after chemo."

Because the evidence linking diet, stress, and exercise with overall
health (and cancer) is building every day, I have made several changes in
the way I live. I have reduced my intake of fats and refined carbohydrates
and have increased my intake of fiber. I keep potentially harmful chemicals to a minimum and continue to take the vitamin/mineral supplements
recommended to me while I was on chemo. I make a continual effort to improve the way I handle stress, and I exercise almost daily. I don't smoke,
and because of the dangers of secondhand smoke, I try to avoid smoke-
filled places, although my penchant for blues music admittedly makes this
difficult. For several years I had a monthly acupuncture treatment. It
proved to be marvelously relaxing and has miraculously straightened out
my menstrual cycle, which had been totally unpredictable ever since chemo.

There are no guarantees, but these practices don't compromise my
quality of life; they enhance it. Not only do they support good general
health (how ironic it would be to beat cancer and succumb early to some
other condition such as heart disease that I could have easily prevented),
they may have a direct bearing on my chances of avoiding a recurrence or
another cancer. I can't be on chemo all my life, but I can continue in a
lifestyle that may affect any cancer cells the chemo left behind as well as
any new ones that might be produced.

Patients notice and cultivate spiritual and intellectual differences in
the postchemo life, too. Natalie Spingarn found that having cancer can be

a challenge that forces people to grow and search for personal meaning, to set priorities, to view life more critically and intensively, to sort out the things they really want to do and do their best to do them. The prospect of death, she says, can teach you what life is all about. These patients agree:

I don't think my life will ever be the same. But that's not a bad thing. It's not even the cancer at this point. It's just the idea—this brush with death—I look at life now and I see how tenuous it is, how very short it is. You have only your moment. Not just me, but all of life. Most of the time you don't recognize how insignificant your life is, or how short. After something like this you realize that nothing is forever.

A couple of good things came out of this whole mess. My relationship with my husband is even better than it had been. People are more important. Relationships are more important. Things that people do that would bother me before don't bother me anymore. I think about something, "Is this worth the time and energy?" Things get put in their proper perspective when you're faced with something like cancer.

Since my diagnosis and treatment, the quality of my life and the way I look at things have changed in many ways. I have learned to be more assertive, to ask questions. I have learned to be less accepting of the way some things are and more accepting of others. A former perfectionist, I've become more tolerant of my failings, and therefore of other people's too. Reaching out and helping others has given meaning to my experience— that's why I wrote this book and speak to cancer groups and individual patients. I have learned how to sit still—every moment, though precious, does not have to be jam-packed with activity; some moments it's okay just to "be," to merely enjoy the fact of existence. I have become more philosophical, and see illness and tragedy and challenge as part of the rhythms and cycles of life.

Many cancer patients find meaning and purpose in their experience by voluntarily sharing it with other cancer patients by becoming peer counselors:

People ask me, "How can you be doing this? Doesn't it bother you to be constantly reminded of old memories?" I say it doesn't really, that I was in their position once—I didn't have anybody to talk to. If I can pass something on, I feel good inside; talking to them is soothing to me, too. Out of all of the years I've been nursing, those that I've been counseling cancer patients have been the most rewarding. I was looking for a reason why this happened to me—now I kind of have an idea why it did. If you can just get to somebody— if I can just reach one in five—if they're happy and can adjust to their lives, it can make it all worthwhile.

There are many opportunities to volunteer your knowledge and insights to people who are going through cancer and chemotherapy. Your local hospital, chapters of the American Cancer Society, and the other support groups listed in the back of this book will be able to guide you in finding a situation that is satisfying and helpful to both you and the uninformed patients who need you. You can let your oncologist and friends know that you are available to talk with newly diagnosed cancer patients. Some people prefer to make financial contributions to cancer foundations or help raise funds for cancer care and research. One woman with malignant melanoma started a newsletter; many others have started local self-help groups. Others find meaning and purpose by becoming cancer activists, either starting grassroots organizations or joining them. The National Coalition of Cancer Survivors, Breast Cancer Action, and Cancervive are just a few of the advocacy organizations founded by cancer patients. Cancervive's Susan Nessim writes:

While the camaraderie of other survivors may be our greatest source of comfort and support, education and advocacy are our greatest weapons against fear and discrimination. We need to band together to make a difference.

Admittedly, this type of activism isn't for everyone. Although exhilarating, it is hard work and takes a certain personality and commitment that not everyone will be able to offer. Some of us are simply not suited for it and never will be. Others need a certain amount of time to heal themselves and come to terms with cancer before reaching the point where they are ready to assume an activist role. Some prefer to do their part as an individual, to educate themselves about cancer prevention and pass that knowledge on to others. Many people find it liberating and therapeutic to talk openly with friends or in front of small groups or to write an article for the local newspaper or club newsletter. The more people we reach, the easier the path will be for everyone.

On the other hand, some choose to contribute in other ways not so directly related to cancer. In addition to joining cancer organizations, I became an active member of one environmental organization and started donating money to others. I simply couldn't ignore the connections between the fragility of the health of the earth and my own health and that of other living things. And what is life worth if there's only a battered world to enjoy? A Hodgkin's disease survivor once wrote about how he labored to establish an income source for charitable organizations that provide food, clothing, or shelter for the poor. What drove him to such an undertaking? He wanted to make his life count, but he also felt "survivor's debt"—the need to somehow repay for being cured.

No matter how it is expressed, the positive changes that many post-chemo patients have made signify an affirmation of life and a commitment toward improving and maintaining their health and happiness. Death has tapped them on the shoulder, and they have said, "Not yet," first by taking chemotherapy, and then by continuing to do everything in their power to continue to improve their prognosis and quality of life. They want to give themselves every chance there is by making positive changes in their lifestyles, attitudes, and priorities. These may include the complementary therapies I explore in this book, and more: improving their diets, avoiding known harmful substances such as tobacco, getting more exercise, reducing and managing stress, dealing openly and honestly with their emotions, relaxing and enjoying hobbies and friends, having fun, getting rest and sleep, helping others, being productive, and enjoying sexual expression. Rather than wasting time and energy worrying about things they can't control, they prefer to deal with the things they can control.

Many cancer patients are able to make some of these moves toward living better lives while they are on chemotherapy. For those for whom it was too difficult to initiate and maintain such changes: It is not too late now to turn over a new leaf! Whether you have chemotherapy only once or it becomes an intermittent part of your continuing care, you can still live life to the fullest while continuing a multifaceted program to stay in the best possible health.

Dr. Michael Van Scoy-Mosher ended my interview with him with these encouraging words we can all live by:

> *There are two components of health. One consists of the aspects that we have some control over; the other of things we don't, like genetics or things that just happen. And I think we have a certain responsibility to at least control what we can. It's not going to answer it all, but I, for one, don't want to lie on my deathbed and say that I could have delayed death or avoided it but I didn't because of certain things I did or didn't do. With chemotherapy, you have to resolve the conflict of the intellectual side—understanding the need for treatment—and the emotional aversion to it in favor of rational thought. You just have to know in your heart of hearts that you did what you could. And you should see that as a source of pride, that you were able to understand it, cope with it, tolerate it, and get it done with. Even though we know it's no guarantee, at least you know you did all you could do.*

It took some time and the writing of this book to realize it fully, but in some sense I am proud I underwent chemotherapy. Though I have mixed feelings about it, I have no regrets. Chemotherapy is not an easy undertaking no matter how you look at it. It has its ups and downs, its imperfections and uncertainties. Yes, I experienced side effects while on chemotherapy, and some have yet to subside completely. But chemo was worth it, and this is true whether it ultimately has given me only a few extra years or a normal life span. Because of chemo, I at least have a better chance of survival; I'm also a different person, a better person, a more knowledgeable person. I walk around during the day and go to sleep at night knowing I gave cancer my best shot. I hope I have helped you to give it your best shot, too, and to make your best even better.

Glossary

Acute: Occurring suddenly or over a short period of time.

Adenocarcinoma: Cancer that originates in glandular tissues such as the breast, lung, thyroid, colon, and pancreas.

Adjuvant chemotherapy: Anticancer drugs used in combination with either surgery or radiation as part of the initial treatment of cancer, before detectable spread, in order to prevent or delay a recurrence. Neoadjuvant chemotherapy is given before surgery.

Allogeneic transplant: Transfer of a tissue, usually bone marrow, from one person to another.

Alopecia: Hair loss, a common side effect of chemotherapy drugs.

Alternative medicine: Practices not generally recognized by the medical community as standard or conventional medical approaches and used instead of standard treatments such as surgery, chemotherapy, and radiation. Compare with "Complementary medicine."

Amenorrhea: Abnormal absence or stoppage of menstruation, a side effect of chemotherapy.

Angiogenesis: Blood vessel formation. Tumors release certain chemicals that stimulate the growth of blood vessels that supply the tumor with nutrients so it can grow.

Angiogenesis inhibitor: A substance that helps prevent the formation of blood vessels. In anticancer therapy, an angiogenesis inhibitor prevents the growth of blood vessels from surrounding tissue to a solid tumor, thus "starving" the tumor of nutrients and slowing or stopping the tumor's growth.

Anorexia: Loss of appetite, a common side effect of chemotherapy.

Anti-emetic: A drug used to reduce nausea and vomiting.

Aspiration: Removal of fluid or tissue with a hollow needle or tube.

Autologous transplant: Removal of a patient's own tissue, usually bone marrow, which is returned to the patient after chemotherapy.

Benign: Not cancerous.

Biopsy: Removal and microscopic examination of tissue from the body for the purpose of diagnosis. An exisional biopsy removes the entire suspicious tissue; an incisional biopsy removes only a small portion.

Bone marrow: The spongy inner core of the bone that produces blood cells, usually affected by chemotherapy.

Bone marrow transplantation: A procedure that replaces bone marrow destroyed by treatment with high doses of anticancer drugs or radiation. Transplantation may be autologous (an individual's own marrow saved before treatment), allogenec (marrow donated by someone else), or syngeneic (marrow donated by an identical twin).

Bone scan: A picture of the bones taken after a radioactive dye has been injected; causes abnormalities to show up as "hot spots." Helps determine if cancer has spread to the bones.

Cachexia: The wasting away of the body often seen in advanced cancer.

Cancer: A general term used for more than a hundred different diseases characterized by abnormal, uncontrolled cell growth.

Carcinogen: A cancer-causing agent. Carinogenesis is the cause of cancer.

Carcinoma: Cancer that originates in the epithelial tissue (glands and lining of the internal organs) of the body. Most cancers are carcinomas (80 to 90 percent).

Catheter: A rubber or plastic tube that is inserted into the body to drain fluids or deliver fluids or medication such as chemotherapy.

CEA (carcinoembryonic antigen): A tumor marker that may indicate the presence or growth of certain cancers.

Chemoprevention: Attempt to prevent cancer by giving drugs, vitamins, or minerals, or other chemicals.

Chemosensitivity assay: A laboratory test that analyzes the responsiveness of a tumor to a specific drug.

Chemotherapy: The treatment of disease, especially cancer, with chemicals or drugs.

Chronic: Lasting a long time (as opposed to acute); said of a condition.

Chronobiology: The study of body cycles that govern our susceptibility to disease and our response to medications.

Clinical: Pertaining to direct observation and care of patients, as opposed to research.

Clinical trials: Studies of new cancer drugs in humans; done after studies in animals.

Combination chemotherapy: Use of two or more anticancer drugs together or sequentially.

Complementary medicine: Practices used to enhance or complement the standard treatments. Complementary medicine includes taking dietary supplements, megadoses of vitamins, and herbs; and practices such as massage therapy, spiritual healing, and meditation.

Complete blood count (CBC): A laboratory procedure that determines the number of red cells, white cells, and platelets in a sample of blood.

Cooperative group: A group of physicians and hospitals that together take part in clinical trials, increasing the number of patients enrolled.

CT scan (computerized tomography): A type of X-ray that creates cross-sectional images of the body and may show metastases better than other methods.

Cytology: Scientific study of the origin, structure, and functions of cells. Cytotoxic drugs are drugs that inhibit or kill cells in the body, such as anticancer drugs.

Differentiation: Characteristic of a cancer cell; the more differentiated the cell, the more it resembles a normal cell.

Dose limiting: When the amount of some drugs that can safely be given is limited by certain risks or side effects, such as heart damage with Adriamycin.

Edema: An abnormal accumulation of fluid in tissues of the body that causes swelling; a side effect of hormone therapy.

Emesis: Vomiting; an emetic is a substance that causes vomiting; an antiemetic blocks or minimizes this reaction.

Epidemiology: The study of factors that influence the frequency and distribution of diseases, such as cancer, in an effort to find the causes and therefore prevent them.

Extravasation: Leakage of an intravenous drug into the surrounding tissue.

Flow cytometry: A test done on cancer cells to determine the aggressiveness of the tumor; used to decide whether chemotherapy should be considered.

Hematologist: A physician who specializes in blood diseases and may also specialize in cancer.

Hematoma: A lump of clotted blood under the skin.

Hormonal therapy: The manipulation of hormone levels in the body; can cause a tumor to stabilize or shrink.

Immunotherapy: An experimental therapy used to stimulate the body's own defense mechanism to control cancer.

Informed consent: A legal standard (put in writing for experimental therapies) that states how much a patient must know about the potential risks and benefits of a therapy before being able to undergo it knowledgeably.

Infusion: Administration of drugs or fluids into a vein or artery over a period of time. Infusion pumps are sometimes used to infuse intravenous chemotherapy for a specific amount of time.

Intra-arterial: Administered into an artery through a catheter.

Intramuscular: Injected into a muscle.

Intraperitoneal: Administered into the abdominal cavity.

Intrapleural: Administered into the space around the lungs.

Intrathecal: Administered into the spinal fluid.

Intravenous: Administered into a vein.

Investigational new drug (IND): A drug that has been licensed by the Food and Drug Administration (FDA) for use in clinical trials but not yet approved by the FDA for commercial marketing.

Lesion: A change in the structure of part of an organ or tissue as a result of disease or injury; a tumor is often referred to as a lesion.

Leukopenia: A decrease in the number of white blood cells in the blood.

Lymph nodes: Small, bean-shaped structures in the body that act as filters, collecting bacteria and cancer cells that may travel through the lymphatic system, a part of the immune system. When infection or cancer is present, lymph nodes may become enlarged and are commonly called "swollen glands." Nodal involvement in cancer means that cancer cells have spread from the primary tumor site to nearby nodes.

Lymphedema: Swelling of an arm or leg as a result of damage to lymphatic vessels that connect to lymph nodes; caused by surgery or radiation.

Malabsorption syndrome: A group of symptoms such as gas, bloating, abdominal pain, and diarrhea resulting from the body's inability to properly absorb nutrients, and which may result from cancer or its treatment.

Malaise: A state of feeling tired, with no "oomph."

Malignant: Life-threatening. In medical terminology, it usually means cancerous as opposed to benign.

Metastasis: The migration of cancer cells from the primary tumor site to other parts of the body, producing cancer spread. Metastatic cancer occurs when cancer has spread from its original site to one or more distant sites.

Modality: A method of treatment, such as surgery, radiation, chemotherapy, or immunotherapy.

Monoclonal antibodies: Substances that meet with a specific type of cancer and are currently being researched to deliver drugs exclusively to tumor cells.

MRI (magnetic resonance imaging): Creates images of the body using a magnetic field and radio waves, rather than X-rays, from the top, bottom, and side.

Mucositis: Inflammation and soreness of the mucous membranes of the mouth.

Myelosuppresion: A decrease in the bone marrow's production of blood cells.

Nadir: The lowest point of the white cell or platelet count after chemo.

Neoplasm: A new, abnormal growth of cells, also called a tumor, which may be benign or malignant.

Oncologist: A physician who specializes in cancer. Oncology is the study of tumors, especially cancerous ones.

Palliation: The act of relieving or soothing a symptom, such as pain, without actually curing the cause. Chemotherapy is sometimes used for this purpose.

Pathologist: A doctor who is specially trained to interpret and diagnose the changes in body tissues caused by disease.

Perfusion: a treatment technique that involves bathing an organ or tissue with a fluid. In regional perfusion, a specific area of the body (usually an arm or a leg) receives high doses of anticancer drugs through a blood vessel.

Prognosis: The expected or probable outcome of an illness or disease.

Prophylactic: A treatment to prevent a disease or complication that has not yet occurred but is likely to occur, such as antibiotics to prevent a bacterial infection.

Protocol: The outline or plan for a cancer treatment.

Recurrence: The return of cancer after its apparently complete disappearance.

Regression: The shrinkage or disappearance of a cancer.

Remission: The decrease or disappearance of detectable disease.

Scans: Procedures that help detect cancer or metastases of internal organs such as liver, brain, and bone.

Side effect: A second, unintentional, and usually undesirable effect from a drug or other treatment, besides the primary therapeutic effect. The primary effect of chemotherapy is to control or kill cancer cells; side effects may be hair loss or nausea.

Single-agent chemotherapy: Treatment of cancer using one drug rather than a combination of several drugs.

Staging: System for classifying cancer as to how far it has spread; helps determine the prognosis and treatment.

Stomatitis: Inflammation and sores in the mouth; a common side effect of chemotherapy.

Thrombocytopenia: A decrease in the number of platelets in the blood.

Titration: A method used to determine the smallest amount of a drug that is required to bring about a desired effect. In chemotherapy, this balancing keeps the toxicity and side effects to a minimum and the antitumor activity to a maximum.

Toxic: Poisonous.

Tumor: An abnormal mass of tissue that results from excessive cell division and performs no useful function; may be benign or malignant.

Appendix A

Guide to
Anticancer Drugs

There are three categories of drugs or substances used against cancer: cytotoxic drugs, hormones, and biologicals. This section contains specific information about how they work and their known side effects. The drugs listed here are all approved by the Food and Drug Administration (FDA) for commercial use (sometimes referred to as "standard" drugs); other drugs are available on an experimental basis but have not yet been approved, and they are not included here. The drugs used in hormone therapy that are listed here are also FDA-approved. Although very few biological therapies have been approved for use outside of a clinical trial as of this writing, more are in the pipeline and will no doubt be approved soon.

Experience with these drugs has shown that some cancers respond well to a single drug (single-agent chemotherapy); these include some chronic leukemias and some lymphomas. Most cancers, however, respond much better when several drugs are used (combination chemotherapy). From the dozens of drugs available, oncologists choose two, three, four, five, or six drugs—and sometimes as many as a total of twelve—to be given concurrently or in a certain sequence. Most protocols consist of at least three drugs, which can triple or even quadruple single-agent response rates while minimizing toxicity. This is possible because:

- The drugs used have different mechanisms of action, so various phases of growth are affected.
- Using several drugs reduces the likelihood of drug resistance.
- The drugs are chosen to work synergistically, with one enhancing the effect of the other.
- The drugs are chosen to produce different kinds of toxicity at different times, so the harm to the tumor remains high without increasing the harm to the cells in any one organ or system.
- The doses are timed far enough apart, so the normal cells have time to recover but the cancer cells don't.

In addition to their desired effects, anticancer drugs have unwanted side effects. The list that follows gives the standard (that is, not experimental) anticancer drugs along with their known possible side effects. As you look up the drugs in your treatment plan, remember that these are the side effects that might happen—not the ones that necessarily *will* happen. It is highly unlikely that you will experience all or even most of them. A few side effects are not listed because they are so unusual that they occur in only a handful of the people taking the drug. (It is also possible for a drug taken in combination with others to produce side effects different from the ones that occur when it is taken alone.) In most drugs, the rare side effects far outnumber the common side effects. Whatever the potential side effects of the drugs you are taking, a skillful, caring oncologist will be able to avert or minimize the risks. There are many measures that both you and your doctor can take to prevent most side effects and make others more tolerable.

If you want more information about your drugs and their side effects, ask your doctor, nurse, or pharmacist. Many hospitals make available to their patients individual drug information cards that list the major common side effects and ways to alleviate them. The package insert that comes with the drug is daunting but very informative; your oncologist or pharmacist will supply these upon request. In addition, there are several reference books with detailed information on anticancer and other drugs. *The Physicians' Desk Reference (PDR)* has been a standard source for drug information, but its text can be hard for the average person to decipher. A good alternative for lay readers is *The PDR Family Guide to Prescription Drugs.* Also available is the *United States Pharmacopeia Dispensing Information* (USP DI), published by the United States Pharmacopeial Convention, or its *Physicians' and Pharmacists' Guide to Your Medicines,* which is written for a general audience. For the most current list of anticancer drugs approved by the FDA, call 1-888-INFO FDA or see http:// www.fda.gov/cder/cancer/approved.htm. for these materials. This listing is in chart form and does not include side effects.

If you have a specific drug in mind and want to look up the side effects, here are some other Internet sources:

New Drugs Approved for Cancer Indications: http://www.fda.gov/ oashi/cancer/cdrug.html

Oncology Page: http://www.fda.gov/cder/cancer/index.htm

New and Generic Drug Approvals: http://www.fda.gov/cder/ approval/index.htm

FDA Drug Approvals: http://www.fda.gov/cder/da/da.htm

Cancer Clinical Trials Directory: http://www.fda.gov/oashi/cancer/ trials.html

Cancer Liaison Program: http://www.fda.gov/oashi/cancer/ cancer.html

Phrma has a site about new drugs in development for cancer: http://www.phrma.org/searchcures/newmeds/cancer2001/cancer01.pdf. When you reach the Web site click on "New Medicines in Development" and select "New Medicines in Cancer." The drugs are listed by tumor type.

Cytotoxic Drugs

Cytotoxic anticancer drugs (or antineoplastic drugs) kill cancer cells by interfering with their ability to grow and reproduce. They do this either by blocking the cells' supply of essential building blocks for growth or by interrupting the reproductive cycle. These anticancer drugs fall into three main groups, depending on the way in which they work.

- *Alkylating agents* are the oldest chemotherapeutic chemicals we have. These compounds cross-link with DNA—they grab the strands of DNA, which then cannot pull apart during cell division. When the cell tries to divide, it self-destructs.
- *Antimetabolites* work because they resemble substances that the cell needs in order to grow. The cell mistakes an antimetabolite for the needed substance, absorbs it, and tries to use it during division and growth. Because antimetabolites are not really usable, the cell dies. Drugs belonging to this group were the first to be designed specifically to combat cancer.
- *Antibiotics* are derived from naturally occurring soil fungi, as is the case with the antibiotics used against bacterial infections. They are believed to act by blocking cell growth by slipping between the strands of DNA and thus preventing it from copying itself.
- *Miscellaneous drugs* include *mitotic inhibitors* such as vincristine and vinblastine derived from the periwinkle plant; they destroy cells by halting a particular mechanism (mitosis) necessary for the physical process of division. Other miscellaneous drugs are L-asparaginase, an *enzyme* that breaks down the amino acids needed for cancer cells to grow, and cisplatin.

Hormones and Antihormones

Hormone treatment is used mostly in cancers of the reproductive system such as breast and prostate cancer. They act against cancer by changing the balance of hormones upon which tumors depend for growth. In many cancers, the adrenocorticoids are widely used in addition to anticancer drugs because of their ability to help patients tolerate the therapy better.

- *Adrenocorticoids* are cortisonelike hormones; they include prednisone, Decadron, Hexadrol, fluoxymesterone (Halotestin), and Medrol. Aminoglutethimide (Cytadren) is an antiadrenal.
- *Estrogens* are "female hormones" and include estradiol, DES (diethylstilbestrol), Stilphostrol, Zoladex, and Tace.
- *Anti-estrogens,* such as tamoxifen (Nolvadex) and nafoxidine block the effects of a natural estrogen.
- *Aromatase inhibitors* are a relatively new class of drugs that reduces the effects of estrogen by inhibiting the enzyme needed to produce them. These include letrozole (Femara), anastrozole, and exemestane.
- *Androgens,* are "male hormones" and include Depo-testosterone, Deca-Durabolin, and flutamide (Eulexin).
- *Anti-androgens* block the effects of androgens such as testosterone and include goserelin acetate (Zoladex), ketoconazole (Nizoral), and Lupron.
- *Progestins* mimic the effects of progesterone; they are available as Delalutin, Depo-Provera, Megace, and medroxyprogesterone.

Biologicals

This term is used to describe many of the new wave of anticancer drugs that represent a more targeted approach in that they aim to affect only the cancer cells themselves and leave the healthy cells unharmed. Many are still being tested and are available only in a clinical trial or through the FDA compassionate use program. The main categories of biologicals are:

- Immunotherapy aims to assist the immune system to recognize and destroy cancer cells. Immunotherapy agents include interferon, vaccines, and monoclonal antibodies.

- Genetic therapy aims to get at the very heart of cancer by affecting the genes responsible for cancer. Agents include Gleevec and herceptin.
- Anti-angiogenesis therapy aims to cut off the tumor's blood supply; examples are endostatin and angiostatin.

Alphabetical Listing
of Anticancer Drugs

actinomycin D. *See* actinomycin.

adrenocorticoids (prednisone, Decadron, Hexadrol, Medrol)
   Side effects: increased appetite and sense of well-being, sleeplessness and agitation, fluid retention and weight gain, diabetes, high blood pressure, increased risk of infection, acnelike skin condition, stomach and intestinal ulcers, loss of potassium, muscle weakness, muscle cramps, muscle pain, hirsutism (abonormal hairiness), decreased or blurry vision, frequent urination, mood changes, menstrual problems, sterility, irregular heartbeat, and osteoporosis (weakening of bones).

adriamycin. *See* doxorubicin.

Adrucil. *See* 5-fluorouracil.

Alkeran. *See* melphalan.

altretamine (Hexalen, Hexastat, hexamethylamine)
   More common side effects: nausea, and vomiting.
   Less common or rare side effects: anxiety, clumsiness, confusion, dizziness, depression, weakness, and numbness in limbs.

aminoglutethimide (Cytadren)

More common side effects: drowsiness, skin rash, nausea and loss of appetite, and dizziness.

Less common or rare side effects: headaches, low blood pressure, clumsiness, and lack of energy.

amsacrine (m-AMSA)

More common side effects: nausea, vomiting, diarrhea, pain at injection site, allergic reaction, and low blood counts.

Less common or rare side effects: hair loss, liver problems, heart problems, and nerve problems.

androgens (Halotestin, Depo-testosterone, Deca-Durabolin, Flutamide, Eulexin)

Side effects: nausea, vomiting, liver problems, lowering of voice, skin changes, water retention and weight gain, changes in libido, constipation, diarrhea, bladder problems, and liver problems.

In women: changes in menstruation; hot flashes; and itchy, burning vagina.

In males: impotence, enlarged breasts, and low sperm counts.

anti-androgens (triptorelin pamoate, estramustine, leuprolide [Lupron])

Side effects: breast enlargement and tenderness, heart problems, heart failure, leg cramps, nausea, vomiting, diarrhea, loss of appetite, lethargy, insomnia, low white cell count, liver abnormalities, water retention, trouble breathing, blood clots, and stroke.

anti-estrogens (tamoxifen, Nolvadex, nafoxidine)

Side effects: transient nausea and vomiting, hot flashes, loss of appetite, vaginal discharge, itching, bleeding, headache, blurred vision, confusion, weakness, sleepiness, increased fertility, bone pain, pain or swelling in legs, skin rash, weight gain, and shortness of breath.

Ara-C. *See* cytarabine

aromatase inhibitors (Femara [letrozole], anastrozole, and exemestane)

Side effects: hot flashes, nausea and vomiting, weight gain, hair loss, hirsutism, blood clots, and shortness of breath.

asparaginase (Elspar)

More common side effects: abdominal pain, nausea, vomiting, skin rash, itching, difficulty breathing, joint pain, light-headedness, slow blood clotting, liver problems, headache, irritability, loss of appetite, weight loss, and puffy face.

Less common or rare side effects: diabetes, risk of infection, shaky body movements, mouth sores, mental depression, drowsiness, confusion, hallucinations, nervousness, and tiredness.

5-Azacytidine (5-AzaC)

More common side effects: nausea, vomiting, low blood counts, liver damage, and diarrhea

Less common or rare side effects: lethargy, weakness, confusion, skin rash, mouth sores, and fever.

BCNU. *See* carmustine.

Blenoxane. *See* bleomycin.

bleomycin

More common side effects: fever, chills, cough, and breathing problems.

Less common or rare side effects: nausea, vomiting, fainting, weakness, hair loss, mental confusion, loss of appetite, change in taste perception, skin rash, discoloration, swollen and painful legs or fingers, headache, and changes in fingernails.

busulfan

More common side effects: slow blood clotting, risk of infection, and tiredness.

Less common or rare side effects: lung problems, cough, skin darkening, acne, loss of appetite, hair loss, dizziness, fatigue, impotence, nausea, vomiting, menstrual irregularities, mental confusion, breast enlargement (men), stomach pain, joint pain, and swollen feet.

Campath (alemtuzumab)

Side effects: neurotropenia, fever, anemia, thrombocytopenia, sepsis, pneumonia, nausea, vomiting, rash, and hypotension.

carboplatin (Paraplatin)

More common side effects: low blood counts, risk of infection, anemia, nausea, vomiting, and pain.

Less common or rare side effects: hearing problems, neuropathy, central nervous system problems, liver abnormalities, heart problems, breathing problems, allergic reactions, hair loss, skin rash, and itching.

carmustine (nitrosourea) (BCNU)

More common side effects: nausea, vomiting, risk of infection, and slow blood clotting.

Less common side effects: lung problems, cough, liver problems, loss of appetite, pain at infusion site, mouth sores, tiredness, weakness, diarrhea, hair loss, skin rash, and itching.

CCNU. *See* lomustine.

chlorambucil (nitrogen mustard) (Leukeran)

More common side effects: slow blood clotting, risk of infection, and tiredness.

Less common or rare side effects: hair loss, nausea, vomiting, stomach pains, skin rash, itching, lung problems, cough, menstrual irregularities, joint pain, swollen feet, and mouth sores.

cisplatin (Platinol)

More common side effects: nausea, vomiting, hearing problems and ringing in ears, sore throat, diarrhea, stomach pains, risk of infection, joint pain, swollen feet, and slow blood clotting.

Less common or rare side effects: tiredness, kidney problems, loss of appetite, loss of taste perception, numbness/tingling in fingers or toes, tremors, rapid heartbeat, and loss of balance.

cisplatinum. *See* cisplatin.

cosmegen. *See* dactinomycin.

cyclophosphamide (Cytoxan)
More common side effects: nausea, vomiting, loss of appetite, menstrual irregularities, risk of infection, and hair loss.
Less common or rare side effects: tiredness, cough, painful urination, bloody urine, liver problems, joint pain, swollen feet, rapid heartbeat, slow blood clotting, dizziness, confusion, stomach pain, skin darkening, flushing, headache, mouth sores, and sterility.

cytarabine (Ara-C)
More common side effects: nausea, vomiting, tiredness, weakness, risk of infection, slow blood clotting, fainting, headache, and irregular heartbeat.
Less common or rare side effects: stomach pain, liver problems, mouth sores, joint pain, swollen feet, diarrhea, and skin rash.

Cytosar-U. *See* cytarabine.

Cytoxan. *See* cyclophosphamide.

dacarbazine (DTIC-Dome)
More common side effects: nausea, vomiting, loss of appetite, redness, pain at injection site, risk of infection, and slow blood clotting.
Less common or rare side effects: blurred vision, confusion, uneasiness, headache, hair loss, and joint/muscle pain.

dactinomycin (Cosmegen)
More common side effects: nausea, vomiting, tiredness, vein inflammation at IV site, risk of infection, and slow blood clotting.

Less common or rare side effects: hair loss, stomach pain, mouth sores, skin rash, discoloration, acnelike condition, and loss of appetite.

daunomycin. *See* daunorubicin.

daunorubicin (Cerubidine)
More common side effects: nausea, vomiting, hair loss, risk of infection, and shortness of breath.
Less common or rare side effects: stomach pain, heart problems, mouth and throat sores, diarrhea, loss of appetite, skin darkening, joint pain, pain at injection site, red urine (not bloody), and slow blood clotting.

docetaxel (Taxotere)
Side effects: low blood counts, weakness or pain in limbs, tingling or burning sensations in hands or feet, diarrhea, nausea, skin rash, and mouth sores.

doxorubicin (Adriamycin)
More common side effects: nausea, vomiting, risk of infection, mouth sores, shortness of breath, hair loss, and slow blood clotting.
Less common or rare side effects: stomach pain, diarrhea, swollen feet, joint pain, red urine (not bloody), pain at injection site, skin and nail darkening, liver problems, and heart problems.

DTIC-Dome. *See* dacarbazine.

Elspar. *See* asparaginase.

Endoxan. *See* cyclophosphamide.

estrogens (DES [diethylstilbestrol], Stilphostrol, Tace, estradiol)
Side effects: nausea, vomiting, fluid retention and weight gain, swollen, tender breasts, headache, dizziness, depression, lethargy, lowered blood calcium, heart and circulation problems, worsening of near-

sightedness or astigmatism, difficulty wearing contact lenses, abdominal cramps, diarrhea, constipation, changes in menstruation, sterility, loss of potassium, vaginal infections, cervical secretions, skin changes, and excess body hair. In males: impotence and enlarged breasts.

etoposide (a derivative of epipodophyllotoxin; *also* VP-16, Vepesid)
More common side effects: nausea and vomiting, loss of appetite, diarrhea, and mouth sores.
Less common or rare side effects: low blood count, hair loss, headache, and fever.

floxuridine (FUDR)
More common side effects: nausea, vomiting, diarrhea, stomach cramps, pain, and mouth sores.
Less common or rare side effects: risk of infection, vertigo, slow blood clotting, skin rash, sores, depression, and lethargy.

5-fluorouracil (5-FU or Adrucil)
More common side effects: nausea, vomiting, and diarrhea.
Less common or rare side effects: risk of infection, hair loss, mouth sores, skin darkening, skin rash, nail problems, and weakness and clumsiness.

Foex. *See* methotrexate.

5-FU. *See* 5-fluorouracil.

gemcitabine (Gemzar)
More common side effects: low blood counts, constipation, diarrhea, general malaise, loss of appetite, muscle pain, nausea and vomiting, sweating, and sleep disturbances.
Less common or rare side effects: shortness of breath, cough, headache, problems urinating, pain in side or lower back, and change in color of skin.

Gleevec (imatinib mesylate)

Side effects: nausea, fluid retention, muscle cramps, diarrhea, vomiting, hemorrhage, musculoskeletal pain, skin rash, headache, and fatigue.

Herceptin. *See* trastuzumab.

Hexalen or Hexastat. *See* altretamine.

Hycamtin. *See* Topotecan.

Hydrea. *See* hydroxyurea.

Hydroxyurea (Hydrea)

More common side effects: nausea, vomiting, risk of infection, and slow blood clotting.

Less common or rare side effects: diarrhea, mouth sores, skin rash, skin darkening, drowsiness, dizziness, loss of appetite, and constipation.

Ifosfamide (IFEX)

More common side effects: bladder problems (irritation, loss of control, blood in urine), hair loss, nausea, vomiting, low blood counts, slow wound healing, and slow blood clotting.

Less common or rare side effects: central nervous system problems, drowsiness, confusion, hallucinations, depression, dizziness, forgetfulness, kidney problems, liver abnormalities, fever, heart problems, and mouth sores.

interferons

Side effects: achy muscles, changes in taste of food, metallic taste, fever, chills, other flulike symptoms, headache, loss of appetite, nausea and vomiting, skin rash, and fatigue.

interleukin

Side effects: agitation, confusion, diarrhea, dizziness, drowsiness, depression, nausea and vomiting, mouth sores, tingling hands or feet, fatigue, decreased urination, weight gain, anemia, heart problems, liver problems, kidney problems, low white blood cell counts, dry skin, skin rash, fever, chills, and shortness of breath.

irinotecan (Camptosar, CPT-II)
Side effects: low blood counts, abdominal cramps, fever, nausea, diarrhea, constipation, and weight loss.

l-asparaginase. *See* asparaginase.

Leukeran. *See* chlorambucil.

lomustine (nitrosourea, CeeNu, CCNU)
More common side effects: nausea, vomiting, risk of infection, slow blood clotting, and loss of appetite.
Less common or rare side effects: tiredness, weakness, hair loss, mouth sores, kidney problems, confusion, skin darkening, and skin rash.

L-PAM. *See* melphalan.

Matulane. *See* procarbazine.

mechlorethamine (Mustargen)
More common side effects: nausea and vomiting, risk of infection, slow blood clotting, menstrual irregularities, and metallic taste.
Less common or rare side effects: loss of appetite, hair loss, hearing problems, pain/redness at injection site, dizziness, drowsiness, headache, and weakness.

Megace (megestrolacetate)
Side effects: fluid retention, weight gain, increased fat deposits, hair loss or thinning, liver damage, fatigue, nausea, vomiting, and carpal tunnel syndrome.

Melphalan (nitrogen mustard) (L-PAM)

More common side effects: nausea and vomiting, risk of infection, and slow blood clotting.

Less common or rare side effects: loss of appetite, stomach pain, joint pain, mouth sores, and hair loss.

6-mercaptopurine (Purinethol, 6-MP)

More common side effects: nausea and vomiting, risk of infection, and slow blood clotting.

Less common or rare side effects: stomach pain, loss of appetite, mouth sores, weakness, skin rash, liver problems, headache, dizziness, and drowsiness.

mediotrexate (Folex, Mexate)

More common side effects: nausea, vomiting, diarrhea, loss of appetite, mouth sores, stomach pain, risk of infection, and slow blood clotting.

Less common or rare side effects: hair loss, headache, liver problems, joint pain, acne, skin rash or darkening, shortness of breath, cough, tiredness, weakness, bloody or dark urine, and blurred vision.

Mithracin. *See* mithramycin.

Mithramycin (plicamycin)

More common side effects: nausea and vomiting, diarrhea, mouth sores, loss of appetite, slow blood clotting, and risk of infection.

Less common or rare side effects: drowsiness, fever, headache, tiredness, weakness, and depression.

mitomycin (Mutamycin)

More common side effects: nausea and vomiting, pain at IV site, risk of infection, and slow blood clotting.

Less common or rare side effects: blood in urine, loss of appetite, mouth sores, hair loss, skin rash, tingling skin, and tingling fingers and/or toes.

mitotane
>*More common side effects:* nausea and vomiting, diarrhea, mental depression, drowsiness, dizziness, tiredness, and aching or twitching muscles.
>
>*Less common or rare side effects:* loss of appetite, skin rash or darkening, fever, and visual problems.

mitoxantrone (Novantrone)
>*More common side effects:* low blood counts, skin bruises, fatigue, nausea, vomiting, diarrhea, heart problems, mouth sores, risk of infection, fever, lung problems, central nervous system problems (seizures, headache), and hair loss.
>
>*Less common or rare side effects:* gastrointestinal bleeding, mucositis, heart failure, abdominal pain, liver abnormalities, kidney failure, and blue discoloration of nails and urine.

6-MP. *See* 6-mercaptopurine.

Mustargen. *See* mechlorethamine.

Mutamycin. *See* mitomycin.

Myleran. *See* busulfan.

Navelbine. *See* Vinorelbine tartrate.

Novantrone. *See* mitoxantrone.

Oncovin. *See* vincristine.

paclitaxel. *See* Taxol.

Paraplatin. *See* carboplatin.

Platinol. *See* cisplatin.

procarbazine (Matulane)

> *More common side effects:* nausea and vomiting, diarrhea, slow blood clotting, risk of infection, loss of appetite, low sperm counts, tiredness, weakness, cough, shortness of breath, drowsiness, and muscle or joint pain.
>
> *Less common or rare side effects:* mental depression, agitation, muscle twitching, mouth sores, skin rash, itching, darkening, nervousness, insomnia, nightmares, hallucinations, confusion, clumsiness, headache, hair loss, constipation, and tingling or numbness in fingers or toes.

progestins (Delalutin, Depo-Provera, Megace, medroxyprogesterone)

> *Side effects:* fluid retention, weight gain, nausea, vomiting, abdominal cramps, dizziness, headache, lethargy, depression, heart and circulatory problems, changes in menstruation, cervical secretions, vaginal infections, decreased libido, skin rash, and breast enlargement or tenderness.

Purinethol. *See* 6-mercaptopurine.

rituximab (Rituxan)

> *Side effects:* flulike symptoms of chills and fever, and low white blood cell counts.

rubidomycin. *See* daunorubicin.

streptozocin (Zanosar)

> *Side effects:* nausea and vomiting, and pain at IV site.
>
> *Less common or rare side effects:* kidney, liver, and blood problems.

Taxol (paclitaxel)

> *More common side effects:* low blood counts, hair loss, mucositis (sores in mouth and esophagus), muscle and joint pain, nerve damage (numbness and tingling in hands and feet, difficulty moving), and allergic reactions (low blood pressure, breathing difficulties, and skin rash).

Less common or rare side effects: cough, fever, anemia, chills, nausea, vomiting, diarrhea, fatigue, headache, pain in lower side or back, difficult urination, flushing, increase in blood triglycerides, and heartbeat irregularities.

Taxotere. *See* docetaxel.

6-TG. *See* 6-thioguanine.

6-thioguanine (6-TG)

More common side effects: nausea and vomiting, diarrhea, risk of infection, and slow blood clotting.

Less common or rare side effects: stomach pain, skin rash, liver problems, loss of appetite, mouth sores, and joint pain.

thiotepa

More common side effects: nausea and vomiting, pain at IV site, risk of infection, and slow blood clotting.

Less common or rare side effects: stomach pain, loss of appetite, menstrual irregularities, low sperm counts, skin rash, headache, hair loss, dizziness, and tightness in the throat.

topotecan (Hycamtin)

More common side effects: low blood counts, pain in abdomen, constipation, diarrhea, headache, loss of appetite, nausea and vomiting, hair loss, weakness in arms and legs, numbness, and tingling or burning in fingers or toes.

Less common or rare side effects: black stools, cough, difficult or painful urination, fever, chills, pain in side or lower back, mouth sores, bruising, and generalized weakness and fatigue.

trastuzumab (Herceptin)

Side effects: fever and chills; heart failure (risk is increased when taken with other chemotherapy drugs).

Triethylenethiophosphoramide. *See* thiotepa.

TSPA. *See* thiotepa.

Velban. *See* Vinblastine.

vinblastine (Velban)
  More common side effects: nausea and vomiting, pain at IV site if drug leaks, risk of infection, and hair loss.
  Less common or rare side effects: headache, jaw pain, mouth sores, constipation, mental depression, tingling and numbness of fingers and toes, muscle pain, weakness, loss of reflexes, loss of appetite, stomach pain, low sperm counts, and skin rash.

vincristine (Oncovin)
  More common side effects: pain at IV site if drug leaks, constipation, difficulty walking, hair loss, headache, jaw pain, joint pain, tingling and numbness in fingers and toes, and weakness.
  Less common or rare side effects: confusion, agitation, dizziness, hallucinations, depression, insomnia, loss of reflexes, bloating, diarrhea, skin rash, loss of appetite, and mouth sores.

vinorelbine tartrate (Navelbine)
  More common side effects: low blood counts, nausea, fatigue, diarrhea, skin rash, hair loss, irritation or swelling at injection site, cough, fever, chills, pain in side or lower back, and difficulties with urination.
  Less common or rare side effects: constipation, numbness or tingling in fingers and toes, mouth sores, and shortness of breath.

VP-16. *See* etoposide.

Xeloda
  Side effects: diarrhea, nausea, vomiting, mouth sores, dermatitis, and fatigue.

Zanosar. *See* streptozocin.

Appendix B

Resources

Information and Support Services

Your local hospital is the best place to start looking for support services in your community. Looking in the telephone directory under "Cancer" (in the White Pages) or "Social Service Organizations" (in the Yellow Pages) will also help you find what you need.

This listing includes the national and regional organizations that are the largest and that will be able to refer you to their chapters near you or to other similar local resources.

American Cancer Society (ACS)
1599 Clifton Road NE
Atlanta, GA 30329
800-ACS-2345
www.cancer.org
(Check telephone directory for your local office.)

Local units offer patient education and information, counseling information on home health care, community services, psychological support, physical rehabilitation, transportation to and from treatment, financial counseling, employment assistance, equipment, loans, and wigs and prostheses. ACS has a variety of programs for cancer patients and their families. *I Can Cope* is a hospital-based program that provides education and psychological support for patient and family. *CanSurmount* is a short-term visitor program that provides patient and family education and information. *Reach to Recovery*'s trained volunteers have had breast cancer themselves and provide practical information and support to women with breast cancer. The *Look Good ... Feel Better* program provides education and consultation with volunteer salons to evaluate skin and hair needs and help deal with the appearance-related side effects of cancer treatments. The three sponsoring partners work together to provide patient education through group or individual sessions, free program materials that include videos and pamphlets, and free makeup kits for patients in group workshop. Call (800) ACS-2345 or www.lookgoodfeelbetter.org.

American Association of Acupuncture and Oriental Medicine
433 Front Street
Catasauqua, PA 18032
610-264-2768
www.aaom.org

For referral to qualified practitioners of traditional Chinese medicine and acupuncture.

American Association of Marriage and Family Counselors
225 Yale Avenue
Claremont, CA 91711

American Association of Sex Educators, Counselors, and Therapists
5010 Wisconsin Avenue NW
Washington, DC 20016

American Society of Clinical Hypnosis
130 East Elm Court, Suite 201
Roselle, IL 60172-2000
630-980-4740
info@asch.net orwww.asch.net

Contact them for a directory of professionals practicing hypnotherapy near you. Another source for practitioners is the Society for Clinical and Experimental Hypnosis

sunsite.utk.edu/IJCEH/scehframe.htm or by phone at 509-332-7555.

American Society of Clinical Oncology
435 N. Michigan Avenue, Suite 1717
Chicago, IL 60611
312-644-0828

Anderson Network
MD Anderson Cancer Center
1515 Holcomb Boulevard, Box 216
Houston, TX 77030
800-345-6324
713-792-2558 (Texas)
www.mdanderson.org

This telephone and web service matches callers with patients and care givers who have had a similar cancer or treatment.

The Association for Applied Psychology and Biofeedback (AAPB)
10200 W. 44th Avenue, Suite 304,
Wheat Ridge, CO 80033-2840
800-477-8892
www.aapb.org

This is the national membership association for professionals using biofeedback; contact them for a list or directory of qualified biofeedback practitioners in your area.

Association of Cancer Online Resources

www.acor.org

Hosts and manages a large number of online information resources and support groups geared specifically toward cancer and its treatment.

Association of Oncology Social Work

1233 York Avenue, Suite 4P
New York, NY 10021
212-734-8891
www.aosw.org

A national organization whose members are trained to deal with the emotional issues and concerns of cancer patients.

Cancer Care, Inc. (National Office)

275 7th Avenue
New York, NY 10001
212-302-2400 • 1-800-813-HOPE (4673)
info@cancercare.org
www.cancercare.org

A social service agency that provides professional counseling and planning for patients and families. Consultation, education, nursing care, home health care, homemakers and housekeepers, and financial assistance are provided. They will refer you to appropriate resources in your geographic area if you live outside the New York area.

Cancer Consultation Service

237 Thompson Street
New York, NY 10012
212-254-5031

A regional resource for emotional/supportive counseling to help people think through treatment options as well as deal with the emotional, spiritual, and psychological issues of those options.

Cancer Hope Network

Provides free, confidential, one-on-one support to people with cancer and their families. Matches patients with trained volunteers who have themselves undergone a similar experience.

877-HOPE-NET (toll free)

www.cancerhopenetwork.org

Cancer Hopefuls United for Mutual Support (CHUMS)

3310 Rochambeau Avenue

New York, NY 10467

212-655-7566

A national self-help organization that includes crisis intervention, information, self-help rap sessions, educational meetings, and a newsletter. Founded by a psychologist.

Cancer Hotline

Kansas City, MO

800-433-0464

www.blochcancer.org

A service that provides "phone mates" for cancer patients.

Cancer Info

www.cancer-info.com

Cancer Information Service (CIS)

1-800-4-CANCER

Hawaii: 808-524-1234; Washington, D.C.: 202-636-5700; Alaska: 800-638-6070

www.cancernet.nci.nhi.gov

Supplies information about local and regional resources and programs for those interested in psychological, emotional, medical, physical, financial, and employment assistance, support, and education. Publishes printed educational material. Most chapters are affiliated with a Comprehensive

Cancer Center. This will also get you access to PDQ (Physician Data Query), a computerized listing for patients and health professionals that provides the latest treatment information, including clinical trials of promising new cancer treatments.

Cancer Supportive Care Programs

Based on the book *Supportive Cancer Care* by Ernest H. Rosenbaum, M.D. and Isadora R. Rosenbaum. The mission of the *Cancer Supportive Care Program* (CSCP) for Total Supportive Care is to provide multidisciplinary information and services for cancer patients and their families and friends. This program for patients undergoing radiation therapy, surgery, chemotherapy, or immunotherapy is currently a part of the Stanford Complementary Medicine Clinic (Stanford Health Care), Kaiser Permanente in Oakland and San Francisco. It has been proposed for supportive care in cancer centers and hospitals.
650-498-5566, Fax: 650-498-5640
www.cancersupportivecare.com

Cancervive, Inc.
11636 Chayote Street
Los Angeles, CA 90049
310-203-9232
800-4-TO-CURE
cancervive@aol.com
www.cancervive.org

Support groups that deal with issues involving cancer survivors and the disease itself. Face-to-face counseling is offered; you can be referred to local resources if you live outside of their region.

Center for Attitudinal Healing
33 Buchanan Drive
Sausalito, CA 94965
415-331-6161
www.healingcenter.org

Helps patients with life-threatening illnesses cope by changing their perceptions about illness and its related problems. Groups, programs, books, and tapes are available.

The Center for Mind-Body Medicine
5225 Connecticut Avenue NW, Suite 414
Washington, DC 20005
202-966-7388
www.cmbm.org

Commonweal
P.O. Box 316
Bolinas, CA 94924
415-868-0970
www.commonweal.org

Offers weeklong retreats designed to help you reduce the stress of cancer, explore better health habits, be in the company of others in similar situations, and consider information about mainstream and complementary therapies.

Exceptional Cancer Patients (ECaP)
522 Jackson Park Drive
Meadville, PA 16335
814-337-8192
www.ecap-online.org

Provides individual and group counseling for patients, families, and cancer survivors.

Gilda's Club
www.gildasclub.org

Provides supportive services to center patients and their families.

The Health Resource, Inc.
933 Faulkner
Conway, AZ 72032
501-329-5272 · 800-949-0090
Fax: 501-329-8700
www.thehealthresource.com

Founded by a cancer patient who provides individualized, in-depth research reports on specific health problems; includes both traditional and alternative treatments, new treatments, self-help measures, and physicians who specialize in the specific disease.

Leukemia Lymphoma Society
1311 Mamaroneck Avenue
White Plains, NY 10605
914-949-6691
800-955-4572
www.leukemia.org

Provides referral to local support services. Gives support and information for patients with blood-related cancers and their care givers to improve their quality of life.

National Alliance of Breast Cancer Organizations (NABCO)
9 East 37th Street, 10th Floor
New York, NY 10016
888-80-NABCO
www.nabco.org

A central breast cancer information network and publisher of a newsletter and resource list.

National Center for Homeopathy
801 N. Fairfax Street, Suite 306
Alexandria, VA 22314
703-548-7790
www.homeopathic.org

National Cancer Institute (NCI)
Cancer Information Service
6116 Executive Blvd.
Rm. 3036A
Bethesda, MD 20892-8322
800-4CANCER (800-422-6237)
www.cancer.gov

Coordinates a national research program on cause, prevention, detection, diagnosis, treatment, rehabilitation, and control of cancer.

National Coalition for Cancer Survivorship (NCCS)
1010 Wayne Avenue, Suite 770
Silver Spring, MD 20910
301-650-9127
www.cansearch.org

A network of groups and individuals concerned with survivorship and support of cancer survivors; acts as a clearinghouse for information, advocates for the rights of cancer survivors, and publishes a newsletter.

National Lymphedema Network
Latham Square
1611 Telegraph Avenue, Suite 1111
Oakland, CA 94612
800-541-3259
www.lymphnet.org

Provides information and treatment for people suffering from lymphedema, a common but underrecognized complication from lymph node surgery and radiation therapy.

National Prostate Cancer Coalition
1300 19th Street NW, Suite 400
Washington, DC 20036
202-463-9455
www.4npcc.org

National Self-Help Clearinghouse

Graduate Center and University Center of the City University
of New York
365 Fifth Avenue, Suite 3300
New York, NY 10016
212-817-1822
www.selfhelpweb.org

Helps people locate self-help groups in their region.

National Women's Health Network

514 10th Street NW, Suite 400
Washington, DC 20004
202-347-1140
www.womenshealthnetwork.org

A national consumer rights group concerned with women's health needs,
including those related to cancer. Publishes brochures and an informative
newsletter.

North American Menopause Society (NAMS)

P.O. Box 94527
Cleveland, OH 44101
216-844-3348
www.menopause.org

For information about soy and other natural methods of managing menopause symptoms during and after chemotherapy for reproductive cancers.

Oncology Nursing Society

501 Holiday Drive
Pittsburgh, PA 15220
412-921-7373
www.ons.org

They have a patient information and education resource section and a link
to cancerfatigue.org.

Planetree Health Resource Center
California Pacific Medical Center
2040 Webster Street
San Francisco, CA 94115
415-600-3681

San Jose Medical Center
98 North 17th Street
San Jose, CA 95112
408-977-4549

Offers research packets by mail tailored to specific medical problems. Researchers draw on medical texts and computer databases as well as on printed material geared toward the general public. Both traditional and alternative approaches are covered.

R.A. Bloch Cancer Foundation Hotline
4410 Main Street
Kansas City, MO 64111
800-433-0464
www.blochcancer.org

Will refer you to hospitals that provide multidisciplinary second opinions and to support organizations; ask for free books on cancer for patients and care givers.

United Ostomy Association, Inc.
19772 MacArthur Blvd., Suite 200
Irvine, CA 92612
800-826-0826
www.uoa.org

Has 500 nationwide chapters. Offers information, peer support, and new techniques and equipment; has an insurance plan for members.

Vital Options International
15821 Ventura Blvd., Suite 645
Encino, CA 91436
818-788-5225
www.vitaloptions.org

Facilitates global cancer dialogue via communications technology. Sponsors a weekly radio show.

Wellness Community
2716 Ocean Park Boulevard, Suite 1040
Santa Monica, CA 90405
310-314-2555
www.wellness-community.org

A national network of support centers that offer a variety of support groups as well as classes in relaxation and other mind-body therapies. Their programs promote active participation by patients in their treatment and quality of life.

Y-Me Breast Cancer Support Program
18220 Harwood Avenue
Homewood, IL 60430
800-221-2141 (9 A.M. to 5 P.M. CST)
312-799-8228 (24 hours)

Provides support and counseling through its telephone hotline. Publishes a newsletter.

Y-Me WIG
800-221-2141
www.y-me.org

Provides wigs free of charge.

Magazines and Catalogs

Living Arts: The Catalog for Well-Being
800-254-8464
www.gaiam.com

A beautiful catalog with products that help you live a healthier lifestyle—yoga, tai chi, qi-gong, pilates, ballanceball, and other exercise supplies, massage, meditation, aromatherapy supplies, audiotapes, and videotapes.

Coping: Living with Cancer **magazine**
P.O. Box 1700
Franklin, TN 37065

A quarterly magazine published for patients and their families.

General Internet Sources

More and more people are turning to the Internet for medical information. In 2000, an estimated 60 million Americans visited the thousands of medically oriented Web sites. Where to begin? How reliable is the information? For background information on cancer or any other disease, a good starting point is the Merck Manual of Medical Information. The information in this site is written by medical experts. It offers an interactive edition with animation and photos of disease as well as a text version for people with a slower computer connection.

MEDLINE plus
http://www.medlineplus.gov/

A service of the National Library of Medicine, which provides disease information as well as drug information.

Merck Manual of Medical Information
http://www.merckhomeedition.com/

The National Guideline Clearinghouse
http://www.guideline.gov

Offers treatment recommendations based on the latest scientific evidence.

Oncolink
www.Oncolink.upenn.edu

A Web site sponsored by the University of Pennsylvania that provides cancer information for patients and health-care professionals.

WebMD
www.Webmd.com

A large health-oriented Web site.

For Terminally Ill Patients

Choice in Dying
1035 30th Street NW
Washington, DC 20007
202-338-9790
www.choice.org

A nonprofit organization that distributes information about and forms for the living will, which records the patient's wishes concerning treatment, and durable power of attorney for health care.

Hospice Foundation of America
800-854-3402
www.hospicefoundation.org

National Hospice Organization
1901 North Moore Street, #901
Arlington, VA 22209
703-243-5900 for professionals; 800-658-8898 for patients and families.
www.nho.org

Provides general information on the hospice concept, philosophy, and services and referral to local hospice programs. Publishes an informative booklet.

If you would like more information about hospices, refer to *The Hospice Movement: A Better Way of Caring for the Dying* by Sandol Stoddard (Briarcliff Manor, N.Y.: Stein & Day, 1977); *Hospice* by Parker Rossman (New York: Fawcett Columbine, 1979); *A Consumer Guide to Hospice Care* by Barbara Coleman, National Consumers League, 815 15th Street, NW, #516, Washington, DC (1985); *On Death and Dying* by Elisabeth Kubler-Ross (New York: Macmillan, 1978). For those who wish to die at home, read *Coming Home: A Guide to Dying at Home with Dignity* by Deborah Duda (Santa Fe: Aurora Press, 1987).

Oncologists Who Combine Conventional and Complementary Therapies

It's not easy to find board-certified medical oncologists who also are knowledgeable in complementary therapies. The following are a few of them. With some research, you may be able to find one in your area or within convenient traveling distance.

Keith Block, M.D.
1800 Sherman Avenue, Suite 515
Evanston, IL 60201
708-492-3045
www.blockmd.com

Keith Block is Medical Director of the Cancer Treatment Program and Medical Chief of Nutritional and Behavioral Oncology at the Edgewater

Medical Center in Chicago. He offers conventional treatment along with nutrition, body maintenance, stress care, and psychological support.

William Buchholz, M.D.
1174 Castro Street, Suite 275
Mountainview, CA 94040
650-988-8011
www.buchholzmedgroup.com

William Bucholz is an internist, hematologist, and oncologist in private practice. He offers conventional Western medicine as well as complementary therapies that support patients and their families physically, emotionally, and spiritually.

Rudy Falk, M.D.
Falk Oncology Centre Limited
890 Yonge Street, 2nd Floor
Toronto, Ontario M4W 3P4, Canada
416-921-2525

Rudy Falk is a professor in the Department of Surgery at the University of Toronto. He offers "combination therapy" that consists of low doses of chemotherapy, hyperthermia, and psychological and nutritional support, including intravenous vitamin C to help rid the body of broken down cells.

Charles B. Simone, M.D.
Simone Cancer Center
123 Franklin Corner Road
Lawrenceville, NJ 08648
609-896-2646

Charles B. Simone is a cancer specialist (in breast cancer, in particular) who has trained in medical oncology and clinical immunology at the National Cancer Institute. His cancer center is a multifunctional facility dedicated to comprehensive patient care. He is the author of *Cancer and Nutrition: A Ten-Point Plan to Reduce Your Chances of Getting Cancer.*

Alternative Therapy Books and Resources

An Introduction to Complementary and Alternative Therapies. Pittsburgh: Oncology Nursing Press, 1999.

Can Help
3111 Paradise Bay Road
Port Ludlow, WA 98365-9771
360-437-2291
www.canhelp.com

Patrick McGrady, Jr., the founder, will send a personal computer printout of up-to-date information regarding cutting-edge, conventional, and alternative therapies, tailored to your specific case. (Requires that medical records be sent.) Send SASE for information and fees.

Fink, John. *Third Opinion: An International Directory to Alternative Therapy Centers for the Treatment and Prevention of Cancer,* revised edition. Garden City Park, N.Y.: Avery Publishing Group, 1992. For people who want to make informed decisions about alternative cancer-care programs, support groups, and informational services.

Office of Alternative Medicine, *Alternative Medicine: Expanding Medical Horizons.* (Washington D.C.: Government Printing Office, 1994.) GPO stock number: 017-040-00537-7. Available from Government Printing Office, Superintendent of Documents, P.O. Box 371954, Pittsburgh, PA 15250-7954. 202-512-2250. This is not about cancer treatments per se; however, the OAM does fund its own cancer studies, the results of which you will find at their Web site. Go to http://nccam.nih.gov

Gordon, James S., and Sharon Curtin. *Comprehensive Cancer Care: Integrating Alternative, Complementary, and Conventional Therapies.* Boulder, CO: Perseus Books, 2001. This book is based on the findings of the annual conference cosponsored by the Center for Mind-Body Medicine and the National Cancer Institute. It is an authoritative guide to the integration of conventional, complementary, and alternative medicines for cancer. It provides the latest research and simple, powerful tools to help you make wise decisions and sensible choices to both treat and prevent cancer.

Lerner, Michael. *Choices in Cancer: Integrating the Best of Conventional and Complementary Approaches to Cancer.* Cambridge: MIT Press, 1994. The most thoughtful and respected compendium you'll find, written by the president of Commonweal who is also one of the country's leading authorities on complementary cancer treatments. This comprehensive book covers choices in healing, mainstream therapies, complementary therapies, pain control, and dying. The main focus is on complementary therapies, with major sections on spiritual, pharmacological, nutritional, and various specific unconventional treatments. Also available from Commonweal (see page 413) are tapes on complementary medicine.

People Against Cancer
515-972-4444, Fax: 515-972-4415
www.peopleagainstcancer.com

A grassroots, nonprofit, public benefit organization dedicated to new directions in the war on cancer; members are people with cancer, their loved ones, and citizens working together to protect and enhance medical freedom of choice. They distribute a wide range of educational materials about nontoxic innovative forms of cancer prevention, diagnosis, and therapy.

Ralph Moss on Cancer
800-980-1234
www.ralphmoss.com
www.cancerdecisions.com

At this Web site you will find a wealth of information on complementary and alternative cancer treatments. It contains the archives of ten years of *The Cancer Chronicles.* It also includes a list of the many types of cancers for which there are Moss Reports; sample sections from some of the Moss Reports now online; frequently asked questions about the Moss Reports; a comprehensive list of links to treatment and research Web sites; use of an informative on-line newsletter, *The Cancer Chronicles.*

The University of Texas Center for Alternative Medicine in Houston, which houses the center that specializes in alternative cancer treatment studies, also has a Web site: www.sph.uth.tmc.edu/utcam. Information includes summaries of the scientific evidence for various nontraditional cancer therapies such as herbs, traditional Chinese Medicine, biologic/organic therapies, and special regimens/integrated systems.

U.S. Congress, Office of Technology Assessment. *Unconventional Cancer Treatments.* (Washington D.C.: U.S. Government Printing Office, 1990). Report OTA-H-405. Available from Government Printing Office, Superintendent of Documents, P.O. Box 371954, Pittsburgh, PA 15250-7954. 202-512-2250. A landmark government investigation of alternative cancer treatments that is considered to be a remarkably fair assessment of the major alternative therapies, although the report is not without its detractors.

Walters, Richard. *Options: The Alternative Cancer Therapy Book.* Garden City Park, NY: Avery Publishing Group, 1993.

Zhang, Dai-zhao. *The Treatment of Cancer by Integrated Chinese-Western Medicine.* Boulder: Blue Poppy Press, 1989. Zhang is a specialist in the treatment of cancer in Beijing. Since the mid-1970s, he has been working with integrated ChineseWestern medicine. "Since neither modern Western nor traditional Chinese medicines in themselves treat cancer totally satisfactorily, attempting to combine the two approaches offers the possibility of capitalizing on the strengths of each system as well as using one system to neutralize or ameliorate the shortcomings of the other" (from editor's preface).

Help With the Cost of Chemotherapy

The cost of chemo varies tremendously—from a few thousand dollars to hundreds of thousands of dollars. The drugs themselves account for a good portion of the cost: Some are inherently more expensive than others, but the dosages, the frequency and length of treatment, and the facility at which you receive them can also influence the cost. In addition to the drugs, you will be charged for the administration of the drugs, the doctor's time and examination fees, and frequent tests used to monitor your condition. Add to this any hospital charges if you are admitted for chemotherapy or any serious side effects caused by chemotherapy—plus any support services that you will require, such as additional drugs, nutritional supplements, hairpieces, psychosocial counseling, and home-care personnel. Transportation and accommodations for you and/or your companions may also be a part of the total bill.

Some medical insurance policies cover chemotherapy, and some don't. Some cover chemotherapy only when administered in a hospital, not in a private doctor's office. Some cover only a percentage, some cover 100 percent, and others cover only up to a certain amount. Insurance policies do not cover transportation or accommodations, and some may not cover all the support services you need.

In some cases the reactions to chemotherapy are so severe that the patients cannot work or cannot work well while having treatment. Some must follow a reduced work schedule or work performance suffers, or prejudice and fear may cause the loss of a job. Even with medical insurance and sometimes even in spite of disability insurance, chemotherapy can be a very heavy financial burden to bear.

You can begin to cope with your financial concerns by discussing them openly with your doctor, nurse, social worker, or health-insurance representative. Find out exactly what your insurance covers and how to get maximum coverage. Reading the fine print may reveal that your policy covers chemotherapy only when administered in a hospital, not in your doctor's office, and you may want to adjust your treatment plan. Make sure to keep a careful record of all your expenses and claims. Chemo can leave you exhausted and confused. If you need to, enlist the aid of your family, friends, or a social worker in filing claims and keeping records. If any claim is refused, ask why. You may need to ask your doctor to talk or write to the representative to explain why your claim meets their requirements. Discuss with your doctor the way the office submits the paperwork; sometimes the way your treatment is described influences the degree of coverage. It pays to ask questions and get what you deserve. For example, you may have problems with reimbursement if your doctor has prescribed a treatment that is "off label," in other words, a use that is not specifically approved by the Food and Drug Administration and so not listed on the label for that purpose. Your doctor can help you by documenting that the labeled uses of a drug are not all-inclusive and that the usage of the claimed drug is appropriate. Another example of procedures and drugs that your insurance carrier may be unwilling to cover is the use of high-dose chemo with autologous bone marrow transplant.

If you are having trouble with reimbursement, you can contact the Association of Community Cancer Centers at 301-984-9496 to find out if there is an association chapter in your state that is involved in solving these problems. As a last resort, some cancer patients are suing insurance companies to pay for treatments, and in many cases, they are winning.

Consult with an accountant, if necessary, to receive all the federal income tax deductions allowed, including gas mileage for transportation to and from medical treatment and insurance deductibles and out-of-pocket expenses not covered by your policy.

Make every effort to continue to work. You may want to discuss the possibility of modifying your therapy so you are less debilitated. Thoroughly utilize any support services or therapies you need to keep you physically and emotionally as strong as possible.

If you have no insurance or inadequate insurance, there are several ways to get help. For instance, you can ask a social worker about Social Security disability and about obtaining Medicare or Medicaid or some other form of public assistance to help pay your bills. The American Cancer Society, the Leukemia Society of America, and Cancer Care, Inc., are examples of sources of financial help with drugs, home-care expenses such as housekeepers and nurses, transportation, equipment, and blood transfusions. Other sources of free transportation include local volunteer ambulance and fire departments, the American Red Cross, and local religious organizations. The Corporate Angels Network (914-328-6962 or www.corporateangelnetwork.org) provides free air transportation on corporate planes to and from treatment centers when flights are available.

If you cannot afford chemotherapy, there are many ways to reduce or at least begin to whittle down the cost. One patient I spoke to had had several operations, had been misdiagnosed, and was emotionally and financially depleted. She found an oncologist who finally got her diagnosis right, and for her inoperable tumor she was put on maintenance chemotherapy that will last the rest of her life. She says: "I wrote to the company who makes my drug and pleaded my case. I said I could no longer afford my cancer. They now send me the drug for free." Her oncologist allowed his fees to accumulate and let her pay him off (very) gradually. Many pharmaceutical companies have patient assistance programs for indigent patients. Ask your doctor to contact the Pharmaceutical Research and Manufacturer's Association at 800-PMA-INFO for their Directory of Prescription Drug Patient Assistance Program, or a representative of the company or companies that supply your drug(s). Those with known programs include Adria Laboratories, Bristol-Myers, ICI Pharmaceuticals, Lederle Laboratories, Eli Lilly and Company, Merck Sharpe & Dohme Inc., F. Hoffman-La Roche, Ltd., and Miles Inc.

Chemotherapy is available at some institutions for free. Veterans Administration hospitals give free treatments to veterans; Public Health Service hospitals give free treatments to former Merchant Marines and to Native Americans. The National Cancer Institute and some other cancer centers give treatments that are wholly or partly paid for by the institution. Sometimes, but not always, the treatment is experimental. Even if you have financial problems, you will rest easier if you do your homework: Investigate the treatment, the doctor, and the institution to find out if this is a situation in which you feel comfortable.

Diana Bryan has generously allowed me to reproduce her system for keeping track of bills and making sure she gets reimbursed properly. The following is her 10-step plan for submitting and collecting claims.

1. Make and label a folder for each quarter year of the insurance claims you have submitted. On the outside of the folder list all bills submitted, including the date submitted and the amount and date of the invoice. Put all bills (duplicates) inside the folder; each submission should be stapled together with a file card on top showing the date of submission.
2. Make and label another folder for insurance claims that have been processed and put all the paperwork accompanying the checks inside.

3. Compare submitted claims with processed claims to make sure all bills were received.

4. Try to find out what the codes on processed bills stand for. Check all rejected bills for code numbers to see if they exceed the deductible.

5. As checks come in, cross off the paid bills or bills applied to the deductible on the outside of the folder containing submitted claims.

6. Make a third folder for out-of-pocket expenses.

7. Make a fourth folder for all correspondence and notes taken during phone calls to the insurance company and your doctor. Put dates on everything; try to get the names of everyone you speak to on the phone.

8. Write or call the insurance company about uncovered bills or other discrepancies.

9. Resubmit the claim, if necessary.

10. As checks for resubmitted claims come in, cross them off the folder.

Appendix C

Bibliography and Suggested Reading

Books on Cancer and Its Treatment

Ahmed, Paul, ed. *Living and Dying with Cancer.* New York: Elsevier North Holland, 1981.

American Cancer Society's Guide to Complementary and Alternative Cancer Methods. Atlanta: American Cancer Society, 2000.

Anderson, Greg. *50 Essential Things to Do When the Doctor Says It's Cancer.* New York: Plume, 1999.

Beattie, Edward J., Jr. *Toward the Conquest of Cancer.* New York: Crown, 1980.

Benjamin, Harold H. *From Victim to Victor: The Wellness Community Guide to Fighting for Recovery.* Los Angeles: J. P. Tarcher, 1987.

Benson, Herbert. *The Relaxation Response.* New York: William Morrow, 1975.

Bognar, David. *Cancer: Increasing Your Odds for Survival.* Alameda, CA: Hunter House Publishing, 1998. (A resource guide for integrating mainstream, alternative, and complementary therapies.)

Bohannon, R., et al. *Food for Life: The Cancer Prevention Cookbook.* Chicago: Contemporary Books, 1987.

Brody, Jane. *You Can Fight Cancer and Win.* New York: Quadrangle/ Times Books, 1977.

Bursztajn, Harold, et al. *Medical Choices, Medical Chances.* New York: Delta Books/Dell, 1981.

Cancer Care, Inc. *A Helping Hand.* New York: Cancer Care Inc., 1998.

Canfield, Jack, et al. *Chicken Soup for the Surviving Soul: 101 Stories to Comfort Cancer Patients and Their Loved Ones.* Deerfield Beach, FL: Health Communications: 2001.

Clegg, Holly B., and Gerald Miletello. *Eating Well Through Cancer.* Holly B Clegg, 2001. www.Hollyclegg.com

Coleman, Norman. *Understanding Cancer: A Patient's Guide to Diagnosis, Prognosis and Treatment.* Baltimore, MD: Johns Hopkins University Press, 1998.

Cornacchia, Harold J., ed. *Shopping for Health Care.* New York: New American Library, 1982.

Dodd, Marylin. *Managing the Side Effects of Chemotherapy and Radiation Therapy,* third edition. San Francisco, CA: University of California San Francisco Nursing Press, 1996. (A consumer's guide written by an oncology nurse.)

Dollinger, Malin, Ernest Rosenbaum, and Greg Cable. *Everyone's Guide to Cancer Therapy.* Kansas City: Andrews and McMeel, 1994.

Drum, David E., *Making the Chemotherapy Decision.* New York: McGraw Hill, 1998.

Epstein, Samuel S. *The Politics of Cancer Revisited.* Chicago: East Ridge Press, 1998.

Fiore, Neil A. *The Road Back to Health—Coping with the Emotional Side of Cancer.* Berkeley: Celestial Arts, 1990. (Based on a psychologist's personal and professional experiences.)

Fishman, Joan, and Barbara Anrod. *Something's Got to Taste Good: The Cancer Patient's Cookbook.* New York: New American Library, 1981.

Foote, Patricia. *How Are You?: Manage Your Own Medical Journey.* San Luis Obispo, CA: Medical Journeys Network, 1998.

Glassman, Judith. *The Cancer Survivors—and How They Did It.* New York: Dial Press, 1983. (Inner and outer resources: alternative therapies.)

Greenberg, Mimi. *Invisible Scars: A Guide to Coping with the Emotional Impact of Breast Cancer.* New York: Walker and Co., 1987.

Harpham, Wendy Schlessel. *After Cancer: A Guide to Your New Life.* New York: HarperPerennial, 1995.

Haylock, Pamela and Carol Curtiss. *Cancer Doesn't Have to Hurt.* Alameda, CA: Hunter House Publishers, 1997.

Inlander, Charles. *Take This Book to the Hospital with You.* New York: Pantheon, 1991.

Johnson, Judi, and Linda Klein. *I Can Cope: Staying Healthy with Cancer.* Minneapolis: DCI, 1988.

Kahane, Deborah. *No Less a Woman: Ten Women Shatter the Myths about Breast Cancer.* New York: Prentice Hall, 1990. (An educational and inspirational account of ten women with breast cancer, written by an educator and breast cancer survivor.)

Kauffman, Danette. *Surviving Cancer: A Practical Guide for Those Fighting to Win!* Washington, D.C.: Acropolis Books, 1989. (Resources for managing the medical, emotional, and financial aspects of cancer.)

Keane, Maureen B., and Daniella Chace. *What to Eat if You Have Cancer: A Guide to Adding Nutritional Therapy to Your Treatment Plan.* New York: McGraw Hill, 1996.

———. *The What to Eat If You Have Cancer Cookbook: Over 100 Easy-to-Prepare Recipes for Patients and Their Families and Caregivers.* New York: McGraw Hill, 1997.

Kleinman, Arthur. *The Illness Narratives.* New York: Basic Books, 1988.

Kushner, Rose. *Alternatives—New Developments in the War on Breast Cancer.* New York: Warner Books, 1985.

Labriola, Dan. *Complementary Cancer Therapies: Combining Traditional and Alternative Approaches for the Best Possible Outcome.* New York: Prima Publishing, 2000.

LeShan, Lawrence. *You Can Fight for Your Life: Emotional Factors in the Causation of Cancer.* New York: M. Evans and Company, 1977.

———. *Cancer as a Turning Point.* New York: Penguin Books, 1990.

Levine, Stephen. *Healing into Life and Death.* Garden City, NY: Doubleday, 1987.

———. *Meetings at the Edge: Dialogues with the Grieving and the Dying, the Healing and the Healed.* Garden City, NY: Anchor Press, 1984.

Locke, Stephen. *The Healer Within.* New York: New American Library, 1987. (The new science of psychoneuroimmunology and the ways emotions can affect your health.)

Love, Susan M., with Karen Lindsey. *Dr. Susan Love's Breast Book.* Reading, Mass.: Addison-Wesley, 1990. (Good general reference for breast cancer patients by a well-respected breast surgeon and feminist.)

MacDonald, John A. *When Cancer Strikes: A Book for Patients, Family, and Friends.* Englewood Cliffs, NJ: Prentice Hall, 1981.

Matthews-Simonton, Stephanie. *The Healing Family: The Simonton Approach for Families Facing Illness.* New York: Bantam Books, 1984.

McGinn, Kerry, and Pamela Haylock. *Women's Cancers.* Alameda, CA: Hunter House Publishing, 1998.

McGinn. *The Informed Woman's Guide to Breast Health.* Palo Alto, CA: Bull Publishing, 1992.

Moore, Katen, and Schmais, Libby. *Living Well with Cancer: A Nurse Tells You Everything You Need to Know About Managing the Side Effects of Your Treatment.* New York: G. P. Putnam's Sons, 2001.

Morra, Marion, and Eve Potts. *Choices: Realistic Alternatives in Cancer Treatment,* revised edition. New York: Avon Books, 1987.

———. *Triumph—Getting Back to Normal When You Have Cancer.* New York: Avon, 1990.

Moss, Ralph W. *Cancer Therapy: The Independent Consumer's Guide to Non-Toxic Treatment and Prevention.* New York: Equinox Press, 1993.

———. *Questioning Chemotherapy: A Critique of the Use of Toxic Drugs in the Treatment of Cancer.* New York: Equinox Press, 1995.

———. *The Cancer Industry: The Classic Exposé on the Cancer Establishment.* New York: Equinox Press, 1996.

Mullan, Fitzhugh, and Barbara Hoffman. *Charting the Journey: An Almanac of Practical Resources for Cancer Survivors.* Mount Vernon, NY: Consumer Reports Books, 1990.

Nessim, Susan. *Can Survive: Reclaiming Your Life After Cancer.* New York: Houghton Mifflin, 2000.

Noyes, Diane Doan, and Peggy Mellody. *Beauty and Cancer.* Dallas: Taylor Publishing Co., 1992. (How to look better while on chemotherapy or radiation or after surgery.)

Quillen, Patrick, and Noreen Quillen. *Beating Cancer with Nutrition: Clinically Proven and Easy-to-Follow Strategies to Dramatically Improve Your Quality and Quantity of Life and Chances for a Complete Remission.* Salina, OK. Nutrition Times Press, 2000.

Ramstack, Janet L., and Ernest H. Rosenbaum. *Nutrition for the Chemotherapy Patient.* Palo Alto: Bull Publishing, 1990.

Reich, Paul R., M.D. *The Facts about Chemotherapy: The Essential Guide for Cancer Patients and Their Families.* Consumer Reports Books, 1991.

Reingold, Carmel Berman. *The Lifelong Anti-Cancer Diet.* New York: New American Library, 1982.

Rosenbaum, Ernest. *Living with Cancer.* St. Louis: C V Mosby Medical Library, 1982.

Rosenbaum, Ernest H., and Isadora R. Rosenbaum. *A Comprehensive Guide for Cancer Patients and Their Families.* Palo Alto: Bull Publishing, 1980.

Rosenfeld, Isadore. *Second Opinion: Your Medical Alternatives.* New York: Simon & Schuster, 1981.

Roth, J. S. *All about Cancer.* Philadelphia: George F. Stickley, 1985.

Rothman, Roger A. *Using Marijuana in the Redaction of Nausea Associated with Chemotherapy.* Seattle: Murray Publishing Company.

Salsbury, Kathryn H., and Eleanor L. Johnson. *The Indispensable Cancer Handbook.* New York: Seaview, 1981.

Siegel, Bernie S. *Love, Medicine and Miracles.* New York: Harper & Row, 1986.

Siegel, Mary-Ellen. *The Cancer Patient's Handbook.* New York: Walker and Co., 1986. (By an oncology social worker.)

Silffer, Bill. *Life in the Shadow: Living with Cancer.* San Francisco: Chronicle Books, 1991.

Simone, Charles. *Cancer & Nutrition: A Ten-Point Plan to Reduce Your Risk of Getting Cancer.* Garden City Park, NY: Avery Publishing Group, 1994.

Simonton, Carl O., and Stephanie Matthews-Simonton. *Getting Well Again: A Step-by-Step Guide to Overcoming Cancer.* Los Angeles: J. P. Tarcher, 1978. (Visualization.)

Sontag, Susan. *Illness as Metaphor.* New York: Farrar, Straus & Giroux, 1977.

Stoddard, Standol. *The Hospice Movement: A Better Way of Caring for the Dying.* New York: Vintage/Random House, 1978.

Tache, Jean, Hans Selye, and Stacey B. Dan, eds. *Cancer, Stress, and Death.* New York: Plenum, 1979.

Weihofen, Donna L., and Christina Marino. *The Cancer Survival Cookbook: 200 Quick and Easy Recipes with Helpful Eating Hints.* New York: John Wiley & Sons, 1997.

Nutrition and General Health

Balch, James, and Phyllis A. Balch. *Prescription for Nutritional Healing,* 3rd ed., 2001. New York: Avery, 1998.

Borysenko, Joan. *Minding the Body, Mending the Mind.* New York: Bantam Books, 1988. (Practical exercises to promote physical and emotional well-being and an active role in healing.)

Brody, Jane. *Good Food Book: Living the High Carbohydrate Way.* New York: Bantam Books, 1987.

Cousins, Norman. *Anatomy of an Illness.* New York: W W Norton, 1979.

Dadd, Debra Lynn. *Nontoxic, Natural and Earthwise.* Los Angeles: Jeremy P. Tarcher, 1990. (How to select products that are safe for you and the environment.)

Dossey, Larry. *Healing Words.* New York: HarperCollins, 1997.

Downing, George. *Massage Book.* New York: Random House, 1972. (A classic how-to.)

Gittleman, Ann Louise. *Fat Flush Plan.* New York: McGraw Hill, 2002.

Goodhart, Robert S., and Maurice E. Shils. *Modern Nutrition in Health and Disease,* sixth edition. Philadelphia: Lea & Febiger, 1980.

Haller, James. *What to Eat When You Don't Feel Like Eating.* Hansport, Nova Scotia: Lancelot Press Limited, 1994.

Hofer, Jack. *Total Massage.* New York: Grosset & Dunlap, 1976.

Lieberman, Shari, and Nancy Bruning. *The Real Vitamin and Mineral Book,* Second edition. Garden City Park: Avery Publishing, 1997. (How to create your own vitamin and mineral program to supplement a wholesome diet.)

Northrup, Christiane. *Women's Bodies, Women's Wisdom.* New York: Bantam Books, 1998.

Ornstein, Robert, and David Sobel. *The Healing Brain: Breakthrough Discoveries about How the Brain Keeps Us Healthy.* New York: Simon & Schuster, 1997.

————. *Healthy Pleasures.* Reading, Mass.: Addison-Wesley, 1989.

Torkelson, Charlene. *Get Fit While You Sit: Easy Workouts from Your Chair.* Alameda, California: Hunter House Publishers, 1999.

Weil, Andrew. *Natural Health, Natural Medicine.* Boston: Houghton Mifflin, 1990.

Personal Accounts

Reading other people's personal accounts gives you a reassuring glimpse at what other individuals have gone through, although these experiences may or may not resemble your own. Many of these stories also contain medical and practical information and can give you a sense of not being alone, which you may find helpful.

Armstrong, Lance. *It's Not About the Bike: My Journey Back to Life.* New York: Berkley Pub Group, 2001.

Blumberg, Rena. *Headstrong.* New York: Crown, 1982.

Brady, Judy, ed. *1 in 3: Women with Cancer Confront an Epidemic.* Pittsburgh: Cleis Press, 1991. (The social, interpersonal, environmental, and political dimensions of cancer.)

Brinker, Nancy, with Catherine McEvily Harris. *The Race Is Run One Step at a Time: My Personal Struggle—and Every Woman's Guide—to Taking Charge of Breast Cancer.* New York: Simon & Schuster, 1990.

Burton, Scott. *A Life in the Balance: A Professional Juggler and Comic's Story of Surviving Cancer with Laughter and a Passion for Living.* Inconvenience Productions, 1997.

Frahm, Anne with David Frahm. *A Cancer Battle Plan: Six Strategies for Beating Cancer, from a Recovered "Hopeless Case."* New York: Jeremy P. Tarcher, 1997.

Frank, Arthur. *At the Will of the Body: Reflections on Illness.* Boston: Houghton Mifflin, 1991.

Gunther, John. *Death Be Not Proud.* New York: Harper & Row, 1949.

Hargrove, Ann. *Getting Better.* Irvine, Calif.: CompCare, 1988.

Howe, Herbert M. *Do Not Go Gentle.* New York: W. W. Norton, 1981.

Ireland, Jill. *Lifewish.* New York: June, 1988.

Kelly, Orville E. *Until Tomorrow Comes.* New York: Everest House, 1979.

Mullan, Fitzhugh. *Vital Signs: A Young Doctor's Struggle with Cancer.* New York: Farrar, Straus & Giroux, 1983.

Murcia, Andy, and Bob Stewart. *Man to Man: When the Woman You Love Has Breast Cancer.* New York: St. Martin's Press, 1988. (By men who are married to women with breast cancer.)

Photopulos, Georgia. *Of Tears and Triumph.* New York: Cogden & Weed, 1988.

Radner, Gilda. *It's Always Something.* New York: Simon & Schuster, 1989. (Comedienne Gilda Radner tells about her experience with ovarian cancer.)

Rollin, Betty. *First, You Cry.* New York: Signet, 1978.

Ryan, Cornelius, and Kathryn Morgan Ryan. *A Private Battle.* New York: Simon & Schuster, 1979.

Sattilaro, Anthony J., with Tom Monte. *Recalled by Life.* Boston: Houghton Mifflin, 1982. (Personal account of cancer treatment with a macrobiotic diet.)

Smith, Gregory White, and Steven W. Naifeh. *Making Miracles Happen.* New York: Little Brown & Company, 1997.

Spingarn, Natalie Davis. *Hanging in There: Living Well on Borrowed Time.* Briarcliff Manor, N.Y.: Stein & Day, 1982.

Stevens, Barbara F. *Not Just One in Eight: Stories of Breast Cancer Survivors and Their Families.* Deerfield Beach, FL: Health Communications, 2000.

Articles

Averette, H. E., et al. "Effects of Cancer Chemotherapy on Gonadal Function and Reproductive Capacity." *CA* 40 (4): 199–209 (1990).

Bailar, John C. III. "Rethinking the War on Cancer" *Issues in Science and Technology:* 16–21 (Fall 1987).

Bailar, John C. III, and Elaine Smith. "Progress Against Cancer?" *New England Journal of Medicine* 314:1226–1232 (May 8, 1986).

Begg, Colin B., et al. "Participation of Community Hospitals in Clinical Trials." *New England Journal of Medicine* 1076–80 (May 6, 1982).

Blair, Steven. "Low Fitness Levels Associated with Increased Mortality." *Journal of the American Medical Association* 263: Nov. 3, 1989.

Boffy, Philip. "Cancer Progress: Are the Statistics Telling the Truth?" *The New York Times*, Sept. 18, 1984, page C-1.

Cairns, John, and Peter Boyle. "Cancer Chemotherapy." *Science* 220:254–256 (1983). (Criticisms of cancer mortality statistics, with a reply.)

"Cancer Survivor Advocacy." *Health Facts*, newsletter of the Center for Medical Consumers. February 1991, page 1. (Includes criticisms of the "war on cancer.")

Carl, William. "Oral Complications in Cancer Patients." *American Family Physician* 27 (2): 161–170 (Feb. 1983).

Carta, Barbara J. "Going Through: A Critical Theme in Surviving Breast Cancer." *Innovations in Oncology Nursing* 5(4): 2–4 (1989).

"Chemotherapy: A Dull Weapon." *Innovation*, health letter of the Foundation for the Advancement of Innovative Medicine. Spring/Summer 1991, page 26. (Translation of an article in the German magazine *Der Speigel* about Ulrich Abel's findings.)

Christ, Grace H. "A Psychosocial Assessment Framework for Cancer Patients and their Families." *Health and Social Work* 8(1): 57–64 (Winter 1983).

Dreizen, Samuel. "Nutritional Deficiencies in Patients Receiving Cancer Chemotherapy." *Postgraduate Medicine.* 87(1): 163–170 (Jan. 1990).

Fawzy, Fawzy, et al. "A structured psychiatric intervention for cancer patients." *Archives of General Psychiatry* 47:720–25, 729–35 (1990).

Frenster J. H., "Phase 2 Clinical Study of Low-Dose Combination Chemotherapy of Unusual Human Neoplasms," *Cancer Chemotherapy Reports* 57:89 (February 1973).

Gold, Joseph. "Hydrazine Sulfate: A Current Perspective" (review article). *Nutrition and Cancer* 9: 59–66 (1987). (Interrupts the wasting away of advanced cancer cachexia.)

Hanson, P. G., and D. K. Flaherty. "Immunologic Responses to Training in Conditioned Runners." *Clinical Science* 60(2): 225–228 (Feb. 1981).

Hegsted, D. M. "Optional Nutrition." *Cancer* 43(5): 1996–2003 (May 1979).

Hrushesky, W. M. J. "Circadian Timing of Cancer Chemotherapy." *Science* 228: 73–75 (April 5, 1985).

Loescher, Lois, et al. "The Impact of the Cancer Experience on Long-Term Survivors." *Oncology Nursing Forum* 17(2): 223–229 (1990).

———. "Surviving Adult Cancers (part I): Physiological effects." *Annals of Internal Medicine.* III(5): 411–432 (1989).

Lokich, Jacob. "Improved Cancer Chemotherapy: Benefits of Delivery by Infusion." *Postgraduate Medicine* 87(2): 239–246 (Feb. 1, 1990).

Mahler, Ellen L. "Anomic Aspects of Recovery from Cancer." *Social Science Medicine* 16: 907–912 (1982).

Maule, W. F., and M. C. Perry. "Management of Chemotherapy-Induced Nausea and Emesis." *American Family Physician* 27 (1): 226–234 (January 1983).

Maxwell, Mary B. "Scalp Tourniquets for Chemotherapy-Induced Alopecia." *American Journal of Nursing* 80(5): 900–903 (May 1980).

McPhail, G. and Smith, L. N. "Acute menopause symptoms during adjuvant systemic treatment for breast cancer: a case-control study." *Cancer Nursing* 23(6):430–43 (2000).

Melzak, Ronald. "The Tragedy of Needless Pain." *Scientific American.* 262(2): 27–33 (Feb. 1990).

Morrow, Gary R., and Christine Morrel. "Behavioral Treatment for the Anticipatory Nausea and Warning Induced by Cancer Chemotherapy." *New England Journal of Medicine* 307(24): 1476–1480 (Dec. 1982).

Prasad Kedar, et al. "Scientific rationale for using high-dose multiple micronutrients as an adjunct to standard and experimental cancer therapies." *Journal of the American College of Nutrition.* 20 (5 Suppl: 450S–463S; discussion 473S–475S. (Oct: 2001).

Renshaw, Domeena. "How Cancer Patients and Their Families Cope with Cancer." *Medical Opinion* 73: 843–848 (August 1975).

Scott, Diane W., et al. "The Antiemetic Effect of Clinical Relaxation: Report of an Exploratory Pilot Study." *Journal of Psychosocial Oncology* 1(1): 71–84 (Spring 1983).

Silverfarb, Peter, et al. "Chemotherapy and Cognitive Defects in Cancer Patients." (review article). *Annual Review of Medicine* 34: 35–46 (1983).

Smith I. E., et al. "Low-Dose Oral Fluorouracil With Eniluracil as First-Line Chemotherapy Against Advanced Breast Cancer: A Phase II Study." *J. Clin. Oncology,* vol. 18: 2378–2384 (June 2000).

Speigel, David. "Health Caring: Psychosocial Support for Patients with Cancer." *Cancer* 74(4, Supplement): 1453–1457 (1994).

Spiegel, David. "Facilitating Emotional Coping During Treatment." *Cancer* 66(6, Supplement):1422–1426 (1990).

Speigel, David, et al. "Effect of Psychosocial Treatment on Survival of Patients with Metastatic Breast Cancer." *The Lancet* ii: 888–891 (1989).

Stoll, B. A., and Santilal Parbhoo. "Treatment of Menopausal Symptoms in Breast Cancer Patients" (letter). *The Lancet:* (June 4, 1988).

Trounce, J. R. "Antiemetics and Cytotoxic, Drugs." *British Medical Journal* 286(6362): 327–329 (Jan. 1983).

Welch, Deborah, and Keith Lewis. "Alopecia and Chemotherapy." *American Journal of Nursing* 80(5): 903–905 (May 1990).

Welch-McCaffrey, D. W., et al. "Surviving Adult Cancers (part II): Psychosocial implications." *Annals of Internal Medicine* III(6): 517–524 (1989).

Wieneke, Mary H. (1996). "Neuropsychological sequelae of cancer chemotherapy in adult breast cancer patients." Doctoral dissertation, California School of Professional Psychology, Berkeley/Alameda.

Winningham, M. L. "Walking Program for People with Cancer: Getting Started." *Cancer Nursing* 14(5):270–276 (1991).

Winningham, M. L., et al. "Effect of Aerobic Exercise on Body Weight and Composition in Women with Breast Cancer on Adjuvant Chemotherapy." *Oncology Nursing Forum* 16(5): 683–689 (1989).

Index

About the Author

Nancy Bruning is a twenty-year breast cancer survivor and author or co-author of more than twenty books. She has counseled cancer patients informally, has volunteered at the Memorial Sloan-Kettering Cancer Center, and is a former board member of Breast Cancer Action, an education and advocacy group. A writer with a particular interest in health and medicine, her other books include *The Real Vitamin & Mineral Book* and *Dare to Lose: 4 Simple Steps to a Better Body.*